THE HEARTBEAT OF INNOVATION

The Heartbeat of Innovation

A History of Cardiac Surgery at
the Toronto General Hospital

EDWARD SHORTER, HUGH E. SCULLY,
AND BERNARD S. GOLDMAN

UNIVERSITY OF TORONTO PRESS
Toronto Buffalo London

ISBN 978-1-4875-2681-8 (cloth)
ISBN 978-1-4875-2683-2 (EPUB)
ISBN 978-1-4875-2682-5 (PDF)

Library and Archives Canada Cataloguing in Publication

Title: The heartbeat of innovation : a history of cardiac surgery at the Toronto
General Hospital / Edward Shorter, Hugh E. Scully, and Bernard S. Goldman.
Names: Shorter, Edward, author. | Scully, Hugh E., author. |
Goldman, Bernard S., 1936–, author.
Description: Includes bibliographical references and index.
Identifiers: Canadiana (print) 20210324015 | Canadiana (ebook)
20210324112 | ISBN 9781487526818 (cloth) | ISBN 9781487526832 (EPUB) |
ISBN 9781487526825 (PDF)
Subjects: LCSH: Toronto General Hospital – History. | LCSH:
Heart – Surgery – Ontario – Toronto – History.
Classification: LCC RD598 .S56 2022 | DDC 362.1/9741209713541 – dc23

We wish to acknowledge the land on which the University of Toronto Press
operates. This land is the traditional territory of the Wendat, the Anishnaabeg,
the Haudenosaunee, the Métis, and the Mississaugas of the Credit First Nation.

University of Toronto Press acknowledges the financial support of the
Government of Canada, the Canada Council for the Arts, and the Ontario Arts
Council, an agency of the Government of Ontario, for its publishing activities.

Canada Council
for the Arts

Conseil des Arts
du Canada

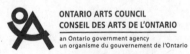

ONTARIO ARTS COUNCIL
CONSEIL DES ARTS DE L'ONTARIO

an Ontario government agency
un organisme du gouvernement de l'Ontario

Funded by the
Government
of Canada

Financé par le
gouvernement
du Canada

Canadä

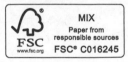

MIX
Paper from
responsible sources
FSC® C016245

Contents

Part Three: The Team

Part Four: Today

Colour plates follow page 272

Plates

Preface

Looking at Cardiac Surgery

In 1977, Dr Wilfred (Bill) Bigelow, the father of cardiac surgery in Canada, noted, "There is not a hospital or centre in the world that has contributed as much to the development of the whole field of cardiovascular surgery than the Toronto General Hospital."[1]

There are two ways to look at the early days of cardiac surgery. One, as envisioned by cardiac surgeon Dwight McGoon at the Mayo Clinic, is lyrical. "Cardiac surgery represents a challenge in surgical technic [sic] comparable to that of the music of Liszt to the pianist, the Olympics to the athlete or Mount Everest to the climber. The reward of the surgeon is not only the thrill of accomplishment, as it might be to the musician or athlete or climber, but is also the health and happiness of many of his patients."[2]

The other is realistic. Cardiac surgery is a difficult, demanding profession. It demands technical expertise and an ability to lead an integrated team through often complex, high-risk operations and unexpected emergencies in the operating room, the intensive care unit, and the ward. Of the surgeon, it requires personal qualities of determination, physical durability, courage, curiosity, optimism, flexibility, patience, humility, resilience, and compassionate support of patients' families and other team members when patients die. When a patient does die in the face of best efforts, a cardiac surgeon must not take this personally but must learn from the experience and move on.

Today it is recognized that the frequency of "burnout," depression, substance abuse, and suicide within the medical profession is significantly higher than in society generally. It is estimated that for every one hundred promising young medical students and resident doctors who aspire to be cardiac surgeons, *one* succeeds.

The additional years and hours of demanding, intense training (eight to nine years – greater than all other specialties in medicine with the exception of neurosurgery), together with the physical and psychological pressures, exact a high price in personal identity and development. These young professional "superstars" often fail to "grow up" as balanced adults until later in life. The incidence of failed relationships and marriages is high. Unhappily, we have lost cardiovascular surgery colleagues to substance abuse and suicide along the way.

Notwithstanding this reality, the majority of the surgeons portrayed in the story that follows feel very satisfied and fulfilled with the great success of their careers as cardiovascular surgeons, having contributed to major advances in cardiovascular care and science and to the health and happiness of their patients and their families.

Hugh Scully and Bernie Goldman together worked under Bill Bigelow in 1966 and subsequently remember the "early days." Scully, a junior intern on the cardiovascular service at Toronto General Hospital (TGH) in 1966, recalls, "Surgeons like Bill Bigelow, Jim Key, Ray Heimbecker, Al Trimble, Bernie Goldman, and Dave McGregor had great courage and a determination to 'make a difference' in the fact of challenging odds. Bill Bigelow often talked with humility about their great opportunity. I was so impressed that I applied for entry and was accepted into the cardiovascular thoracic training program, changing from the neurosurgery program."[3]

Goldman, a young cardiovascular staff surgeon at TGH in 1966, remembers, "Until the coronary bypass came along, heart surgery was a little bit rough and tumble in that you had to move fast because we didn't have good protection for the heart (nourishing the heart muscle). Instead of carefully placing twelve to sixteen sutures around the annulus to secure an aortic valve implant as is done today, you had to go Bang! Bang! Bang! Bang! and get the hell out. If you did not have the speed and accuracy of Al Trimble, but only speed and sloppiness, you can see why you'd have heart block, bleeding, and strokes."[4]

There is a dramatic story to be told about the development of cardiovascular surgery at the Toronto General Hospital. The story is very much alive in the minds and hearts of those who have worked there and been patients there. It was at TGH that cardiac surgery became a jewel in the crown of Canadian medicine.

More than a Local Story

In 1967 Bill Bigelow, one of the founders of cardiac surgery in Canada, paused for a moment to look back: "There was very little surgical treatment for arteries and hearts 15 years ago. This large mass of patients (hearts), representing 25% of all medical admissions, has suddenly become amenable to surgical treatment. There has never been a special area in medicine that advanced as rapidly."[5] This is indeed an extraordinary story: an entire field of medicine that would make a major difference in the human condition created within a decade!

Hugh Scully had been considering this project for some time. Encouraged by Viv Rao, the current chief of cardiovascular surgery at TGH, he consulted with former chief Ron Baird and invited Bernie Goldman to collaborate.

Edward Shorter adds, "Speaking for myself for a moment, I was very pleased when they invited me, in the History of Medicine Program at the University of Toronto, to take the lead in writing the history of cardiac surgery at the TGH.

"Initially, I thought that this might be a rather narrow topic. However, when I told friends about the project, their eyes would light up. A neighbour excitedly proclaimed, 'I had cardiac surgery at the TGH two years ago. If it hadn't been for that, I wouldn't be here.' Hugh and Bernie also heard great enthusiasm for the project.

"We arranged for detailed searches through historical records at the university and hospital archives. Fern Baird, Ron's widow, gave Hugh access to her late husband's extensive records and personal memoirs. Hugh arranged for fifty-two interviews with surgeons, cardiologists, anesthetists, administrators, nurses, perfusionists, and others in or knowledgeable about the division and the hospital.

"But as I started to get into this story, it became apparent how little of it is known abroad, and it is especially unknown in the United States, where the basic assumption is that all important medical events are American in origin. And thus, a light went on in my mind: This story is unknown! The Toronto newspapers published news about some of the new successes (and challenges) in cardiovascular surgery from the 1950s on, but there was no cohesive history of these developments available. So this book, supported by two very able fellow scholars, is a journey into terra incognita. Nobody outside a narrow circle has ever heard of the heroes of the story – and they are real heroes – such as Gordon Murray and Bill Bigelow. This book fixes that. Canadian hearts may beat with pride at the knowledge that one of the major stories in modern medicine took place here – and continues here. Last year, TGH was rated the seventh-best hospital in the world, attributed in significant part to its record in transplantation and the Peter Munk Cardiac Centre. This book tells the story of the great men and women who made that happen."

Cardiac surgery is a surgical subspecialty with a vocabulary of its own that presupposes an intimate knowledge of cardiac anatomy and physiology. Most readers will not have this. We have therefore been at pains to make this material accessible to the general reader, without making it less authoritative, so that readers may catch the great drama inherent in cardiac surgery. The surgeons endeavour to maintain their cool – so as not to demoralize the rest of the operating-room team – when the new heart valve won't fit or the artery is too kinked to accept the balloon pump. There is drama in every area of medicine. This is what makes medical history such an exciting subject. But in cardiac surgery many readers will be on the verge of tears as these awful struggles are waged in the operating room and sometimes lost – but increasingly won.

These struggles were fought in the bosom of one of North America's great academic hospitals, the Toronto General Hospital. Bill Bigelow knew that he was teaching in a special institution. In 1971 he wrote a hospital administrator, "We have the exciting and challenging possibility of being the greatest hospital in North America ... The tradition and background, presence of a first-class medical school, adequate density of population, and the geographical location, which lends itself to being a 'national hospital,' are all factors in its favour."[6]

This story is thus a "local" one, but it is a local story situated within the larger panoply of the history of Canadian medicine. And on that broader sweep, one recalls that Canada was once a very British colony, and that Canadian medicine reflected the British interest in bedside teaching and clinical acumen. Clinicians in the United Kingdom rarely evidenced a fundamental commitment to research, and in the common rooms of Oxford and Cambridge overt enthusiasm for research was taken more as evidence of being a "striver" or a "thruster" rather than as a badge of merit. These mannerisms were copied to some extent in medical Canada, where research was often viewed as a matter of indifference.

This began to change as Canadian medicine swung on its great axis from England to the United States, and from an amused tolerance of research to making it the very centre of the medical enterprise. Johns Hopkins University in Baltimore played a key role in this pivot. At the Johns Hopkins Hospital around the turn of the last century, William Halsted organized the first training program in the United States for surgeons, and William Osler did so for physicians. These events were followed with great interest in Canada, and in the 1920s and 1930s William Gallie mounted the first Canadian program for training surgeons, Duncan Graham for physicians. Gallie's trainees were called "Gallie Slaves." The name Johns Hopkins has always had reverential status at the Toronto General Hospital, and, as we shall see, the cardiac surgeons at the General were no exception to this.

Even though this is a local story, it gets at questions that are national and international in nature. The Americans now ask urgently, are we doing too much coronary bypass surgery, too much angioplasty (dilating clogged arteries with catheters and stents)?[7] These questions seem rather less urgent in Canada, which has a low angioplasty rate.[8] The surgeons at TGH felt themselves under siege by the many heart-attack patients clamouring for a life-saving operation. The idea of preaching unnecessary procedures would have struck them as delusional. And TGH was the governor that set the engine speed for much of the rest of Canada.

So in recasting the history of cardiac surgery at the General we get at the remarkable recency of this branch of medicine. Even before Gallie, surgery on the heart had been attempted and stories abound of what were essentially medical curiosities. It turned out that in 1912 a patient at the General had been operated on for an unnamed cardiac problem. One Toronto surgeon, who wished to remain anonymous, commented in 1914 that "there were a good many cases known of in Italy." But as for operating on the valves of the heart, "the doctor thought that was past surgery [impossible]."[9]

Then surgery on the heart started to become reasonable. After the Second World War, specialist training became the watchword in both medicine and surgery at the General. The emergence of these specialties is a huge story, one that has been told elsewhere.[10] The growth of the specialist program in cardiac surgery has been deftly charted by Vivek Rao and several colleagues in the Division of Cardiovascular Surgery, who conclude, "TGH has always been proud of its contributions in medicine as a center long devoted to superb patient outcomes, research productivity, and the education of the next generation of academic surgeons."[11] As Bigelow said in 1962, "The Toronto General Hospital is at an important crossroads and it faces a challenge. It is a challenge to meet the need for some place in Canada to supply advanced training in the specialties, which is not available in many instances anywhere in Canada."[12] In the past, specialists had gone to the United States for gastrointestinal work; to Bristol, England, for chest surgery.

Within surgery, cardiac surgery was among the later specialties to emerge, not because of the listlessness of the practitioners but because surgery on the heart is very difficult. The training program in cardiac surgery was the work of Wilfred G. Bigelow, whom everyone called "Bill," or – but not to his face – "Uncle Bill." McGill had an important cardiac training program too, but the program that made the greatest impact on Canadian surgery and on the world was Bill Bigelow's at the Toronto General Hospital.

Striding Down the Hall

And he and his residents were proud of it. Bernard Goldman, a younger surgeon, said, "There is the drama end of it. Bigelow sat atop the world like a colossus, and there was nothing like striding down the hall as a cardiac surgeon. Nobody can take that away from us, the drama." But then Goldman added a caution: "Bigelow always reminded us that if you want to be a movie star, you got to learn to take bad press, so that is where his humility came in, and you had to be very careful with the colossus syndrome, because the very next day you could really screw up."[13]

Bigelow and his students launched several important innovations in heart surgery. The first part of this book is about the work of these clinicians and scientists. The second part is about other members of the cardiac team, without whose collaboration these advances would have been impossible.

We admittedly shave the story closely by concentrating on the General. Some of the major achievements in the history of Canadian cardiac surgery came from the Hospital for Sick Children and from the hospitals of Montreal. But the work of William Mustard and the first Canadian bypass operations are told in an excellent study, *SickKids*, by David Wright[14] and it is unnecessary to comment further upon them here (except to note that the term "Sick Kids" was a later press agent's creation; never did physicians and surgeons of Bigelow's generation refer to the hospital as anything but "the Children's Hospital" or "HSC").

Often drowned out by the noisy prancing to the south, Canadian medical accomplishments have not received the attention they deserve. In his account of hypothermia and the pacemaker in 1984, Bigelow wrote, "Perhaps the most compelling reason for writing the book is that this is a uniquely Canadian story and there is some unawareness of this on the part of many Canadians and, of course, non-Canadians … It is reasonable to review the Canadian origin of these advances for the new generation and to share the adventures. This may serve to bolster what some consider our inadequate Canadian self-image."[15] True, that.

Acknowledgments

When Hugh Scully agreed to undertake this "Book Project" after discussion with Vivek (Viv) Rao, current chief of the Cardiovascular Surgery Division of the Toronto General Hospital, it was an easy decision to invite his friend and colleague Bernard (Bernie) Goldman to share his memories and stories about the exciting evolution of cardiac surgery at TGH. We then invited Edward (Ned) Shorter, Hannah Professor in the History of Medicine at the University of Toronto, to take the lead in writing this book, aided by his resourceful and accomplished assistant, Susan Bélanger. There followed many discussions, research in archival files and records, and fifty-two interviews with surgeons and others associated with the division, arranged by Hugh.

Hugh has funded this project from donations from his grateful patients and their families to the University Health Network (UHN) Foundation, previously known as the Toronto General and Toronto Western Hospital TGH/TWH Foundation.

THE HEARTBEAT OF INNOVATION

Introduction

Surgery goes back to the Ancients, but because of the twin problems of preventing infection and relieving the pain of surgery, the great body cavities were inaccessible to the knife. Because of the lack of asepsis and anesthesia, in other words, only such "peripheral" procedures as amputations were possible. This then changed in the nineteenth century with the advent of ether and chloroform anesthesia and the discovery that germs caused infections. The abdomen, the thorax, and the brain all became accessible to the surgeon's incision.

The Problem of Heart Surgery

Of the great surgical terrains, only the heart lagged behind, in large part because the heart – a moving organ – was so difficult to operate on. And circulation could only briefly be suspended without causing irreparable damage or death. Some reluctance due to the symbolic and cultural significance of this unique organ may have played a role as well.[1]

This was the situation that surgeons confronted to a greater or lesser degree until after the Second World War. Apart from suturing wounds to the heart (itself considered impossible until Ludwig Rehn of Frankfurt, Germany, proved otherwise in 1894[2]), few procedures were attempted. And the need for safe interventions was great.

Before antibiotics were widely available, rheumatic fever resulted in stenosis (obstruction) of the mitral or aortic valve, claiming countless young lives. Yet only a handful of attempts at repairing or replacing valves were made before the late 1930s.

A few "closed heart" operations were developed during the 1930s and '40s to treat or alleviate congenital cardiac defects, yet without direct access to the heart's chambers and the great vessels, these efforts were limited.

A growing epidemic of smoking and obesity claimed countless adults as coronary artery disease became one of the leading causes of death in Western countries. A couple of procedures had been developed to revascularize the heart muscle, with modest success, but there was no question of operating directly on the coronary arteries.

Of all areas of medicine where the lot of humankind could be improved, it was cardiac surgery that cried out most for innovation. And it was primarily in American centres – Baltimore, Boston, Philadelphia, and Minnesota – that the first tentative efforts to make heart surgery a possibility began. In Canada, these early efforts began in Montreal and Toronto. These developments were all more or less simultaneous. But up to now, it is mainly the American (and occasionally the British) version of the story that has been told.[3]

The Toronto (General Hospital) Story

This book tells not the Canadian but the Toronto version, indeed focusing on a single key institution. Why such a narrow focus? We have an important point to make: great innovations take place within great institutions. And the Toronto General Hospital (TGH) provided a nurturing environment for early Canadian innovations in heart surgery, innovations that followed on the heels of pioneering work in Montreal. So this is not just the story of a handful of brilliant surgeons. It is also the story of the hospital environment that became an incubator to these men and women – skilled perfusionists, dedicated nurses, and pioneering cardiologists, to name only a few of the specialties that participated in the revolution in heart surgery that took place along Toronto's University Avenue, or "Hospital Row," as it is also called.

Toronto General is one of Canada's oldest hospitals, founded in 1819 and opened a decade later in what was then the town of York. The original two-storey brick building, located near the garrison,[4] was supplanted in 1854 by a much larger facility located on Gerrard Street in the growing city's east end, "far away from the original site," as historian James Connor put it, to "help ensure that the past would be forgotten."[5]

The hospital provided bedside training for medical students as early as the 1830s, before Toronto or Upper Canada had a medical school. Until the University of King's College, an Anglican institution, established a medical department in 1843, prospective physicians had to enrol in the Montreal Medical Institution (founded in 1824), forerunner of McGill University's Medical Faculty, or study abroad, preferably in Scotland.[6] A succession of private medical schools followed between the 1850s and 1880s, until the University of Toronto's present Faculty of

Medicine (recently renamed the Temerty Faculty of Medicine in honour of a historic $250 million donation),[7] was launched in 1887. By this time, the General was already firmly established as Toronto's teaching hospital, providing instruction in anatomy and the clinical subjects.[8]

As additional hospitals were founded, a growing network of teaching institutions quickly evolved in parallel with the rising number of medical students. St. Michael's Hospital (established in 1892) became a teaching facility almost immediately; the Toronto Western Hospital (founded in 1896) brought an additional 250 teaching beds to the undergraduate medical program when it joined in 1912.[9] And the Hospital for Sick Children, begun in 1875 as a six-bed charitable institution founded by a group of philanthropic women, had several of the faculty's professors among its consultants as of 1887, and by 1894 was providing instruction in the new field of pediatrics.[10] Today, twelve Toronto hospitals, including the four comprising the University Health Network (TGH, Toronto Western, the Princess Margaret Cancer Centre, and the Toronto Rehabilitation Institute) are fully associated with the University of Toronto, while a further twelve centres in southern Ontario are community affiliates.[11]

In 1913 the aging east-end hospital was replaced by a magnificent new building at the southeast corner of College Street and University Avenue in midtown Toronto, adjacent to the university. The present General would later expand from this auspicious beginning to encompass an entire city block. Among its numerous world "firsts" in the years that followed were the clinical introduction of insulin (1922)[12] and of the blood thinner heparin – essential to cardiovascular surgery and in which surgeon Gordon Murray played a capital role (1930s).[13] In 1949 came the world-famous experiment demonstrating that open-heart surgery was possible using hypothermia, followed in 1950 by the invention of the pacemaker.[14] The central figure in both these advances was Wilfred G. "Bill" Bigelow, who would go on to create the first Division of Cardiovascular Surgery in Canada; along with his friend and colleague William T. "Bill" Mustard at the Hospital for Sick Children, Bigelow would organize Canada's first postgraduate training program for cardiovascular surgeons. More recently, TGH's Division of Thoracic Surgery has become the world leader in lung transplantation, with Joel Cooper's team performing the first single (1983) and double (1986) lung transplants, a tradition built on by the hospital's current surgeon-in-chief Shaf Keshavjee, who is working on making more donor lungs available for transplantation.[15]

In October 1986 TGH and the Toronto Western Hospital were merged into a single entity, the Toronto Hospital, with the General and the

Western becoming its two "divisions."[16] (The hospitals' original names were reinstated in 1999 as both, along with the Princess Margaret Hospital, became members of the University Health Network.[17])

Following the original merger in the 1980s, areas of specialization were consolidated at one site or the other: the cardiovascular, thoracic, and transplantation programs were based at TGH, while neurosurgery, ophthalmology, and orthopedics went to the Western. Merging the two cardiac surgery programs into one was a lengthy and difficult process for all concerned: according to Ron Baird, a former division chief at both sites, it was not completed until 1992. In the long run, however, the results have been spectacular. The Peter Munk Cardiac Centre, established in 1997 through the philanthropy of Barrick Gold founder Peter Munk and his wife Melanie, is mentioned prominently in a 2019 *Newsweek* profile of the world's top ten hospitals in which TGH ranked seventh and was the only Canadian hospital on the list. (In 2020 TGH rose three positions, ranking fourth, and it maintained that position in 2021.)[18]

PART ONE

Getting Going

Chapter One

Gordon Murray

Motto: "It ticketh and ticketh forever, until it ticketh no more."

Murray Becomes a Surgeon

Many of the great figures at the University of Toronto grew up on farms in small-town Ontario, and Murray was no exception. He was born in 1894 in a farmhouse near Paris, Ontario, and went to high school in Stratford. Gordon's father, John Murray, a Scotsman, arrived in Canada in 1873. Of Gordon Murray's home environment, Bigelow said, "His mother was probably the profound influence in Gordon Murray's life. She must have been a remarkable woman, with unusual imagination and knowledge and a never-ceasing interest in nature. She always had time to demonstrate its wonders first-hand to her children."[1]

She was also a resourceful woman. When two-year-old Gordon fell and lacerated his scalp, "In spite of swooning remonstrances from onlookers, she produced the sewing basket, selected a fine stout needle with a good-sized eye, put in a number 20 cotton thread, and placed both in a pan of boiling water." Holding the screaming young Gordon between her knees, "she proceeded to repair the damaged epidermis ... with a neat running mattress suture."[2] The family doctor, who inspected things the next day, gave her a thumbs up – and for the rest of his life Gordon rather proudly bore the scar.

And the curiosity about the wonders stuck. As Murray was growing up on the farm, he had a neighbour whose horse kept falling over, always on the same side. As neurosurgeon Bill Keith (who knew Murray when Keith was an intern and Murray a resident) tells the story, "One day Gord heard that the horse was dead and had been buried. He went and dug up the head and examined the brain and found that there was a brain tumour in an appropriate position to produce the fits that always threw him onto one side ... I guess we'd call it a meningioma in a human."[3] So Murray was scientifically curious, for sure.

Murray enlisted in the army in 1915 as a first-year medical student. He was not in the medical service but in the ranks. Bigelow later said of Murray's military experience, "He ... joined the army in 1915 as a gunner, in the 26 Battery Canadian Field Artillery. All four Murray brothers joined up – three were old enough for overseas duty, one was killed, and Gordon, who experienced Ypres, Somme, and Vimy Ridge, was blown up and buried with major wounds. It is said that the site in which he was buried was taken by the Germans, then recaptured before he was disinterred and discovered to be alive. He advanced from being the rider of the lead horse in a gun carriage to the rank of sergeant major."[4]

The First World War was, as for so many, a formative experience for Murray. Bill Keith said, "He had a very bitter core of thinking about World War I because he had been in a class where they called for volunteers and he volunteered and went overseas and classmates who didn't, came over two or three years later as fully fledged doctors. Gordon Murray got trench fever [a louse-born rickettsial disease]. He recalled that he was very sick and he recalled that his liver was impinging on the ileum on the right side. It was so big from trench fever, I guess. This remained as feelings of bitterness long after the war, between himself and those who had chosen that other course, I guess he was paranoid as well."[5]

After gaining his medical degree in Toronto in 1921, Murray spent six months as a house physician and six months as a house surgeon in the Toronto General Hospital, then another six months as house surgeon in the Stratford General Hospital. He concluded his North American training with a final six months as junior assistant pathologist at the Mayo Clinic. In September 1923 he sailed for Britain, where he practised as assistant to a general surgeon in Edinburgh for eighteen months, during which time, he said, in applying for a scholarship in 1926, "I performed over two hundred major operations and had charge of the accident surgery of a plant employing 1200 men." Once in London, he held the post of resident medical officer to the West End Hospital and house surgeon to the Hampstead General Hospital. At the time of the application, for three years he had been a demonstrator of anatomy at St. Mary's Hospital and clinical assistant to All Saints Hospital.[6] In 1926 he became a fellow of the Royal College of Surgeons of England (he passed both of the English exams on the first go). He ended his stay in London by heading the Naval Surgical Post-graduate course at the London Hospital, where he also lectured in surgical anatomy and demonstrated anatomy at the "primary" Royal College of Surgeons class.[7]

Murray returned from London, to fellow briefly in New York, with a certain set of airs. He later reported, "While I made no effort to acquire an English accent, I learned an improved method of speaking from an educated fraternity."[8] Murray, new method of speaking and all, returned to Toronto in 1926 (and quickly acquired the Fellowship of the Royal College of Surgeons in Canada too). In June 1928 he was appointed to the surgical staff at Toronto General Hospital as chief resident to Professor Clarence Starr and in 1929 became a staff surgeon at age thirty-five.[9]

During this long apprenticeship Murray acquired the reputation of being a gifted instructor. As Elsinore Macpherson Haultain retold the story some years later, "In London he taught a class of nineteen medical students who were trying for their fellowship in anatomy. Usually only seventeen percent passed this examination. Under Murray's tuition, eighteen of the nineteen passed."[10]

Brilliance

Murray's technical brilliance was soon appreciated. Clarence Starr, the professor of surgery, was heard to say, "This resident is the handiest man I ever had around the department."[11] (This is an almost eerie foreshadowing of the praise for technical brilliance that Tirone David would garner half a century later.)

Murray's contemporaries admired his superb knowledge of anatomy. Said Bill Mustard, who founded cardiac surgery at the Hospital for Sick Children, "He could have easily put his finger through mitral valves [between left atrium and left ventricle] because his anatomy was so perfect ... He was the best surgeon I've ever seen. But he was cynical and that didn't go down too well with his colleagues. They were always a little jealous of him too, you know."[12]

But it wasn't just anatomy. Murray had a special economy of movement that would again be celebrated in the work of his much later successor, Tirone David. Bryce Taylor, surgeon-in-chief at the University Health Network from 1999 to 2010, writes that with Murray, "There were no wasted moves, as every action and every minute served a purpose. Some surgeons of the day had what was referred to as 'a flair,' as the upper body would move as though they were being filmed for a documentary with Fred Astaire – like exaggerated movements that appeared to emphasize that this was basic carpentry complemented by a distinct flavor of artistic virtuosity. Not so with

Dr. Murray – he was a consummate practitioner who got the job done masterfully and quickly."[13]

When Hugh Scully informed D.L.C. Bingham, chairman of surgery at Queen's, himself a master surgeon trained in Edinburgh, that he wanted to remain in Canada for training in surgery rather than going to Edinburgh, Bingham said, "Then you must go to Toronto to work with a true master surgeon, Gordon Murray."[14]

Murray was a general surgeon, not specifically a cardiovascular surgeon, and he was a master of all the procedures in general surgery. Around 1932, John D. Hamilton, later dean of the faculty, was a second-year medical student and developed an acute appendicitis. Hamilton's father was a distinguished figure, and so young Hamilton figured that he had enough leverage to demand that Professor Gallie, head of surgery, perform the appendectomy. "So Dr. Gallie came," said Hamilton later, "and he was very good and very helpful and he said he thought I had appendicitis alright, but I don't do that very well, and that was true, because he was an orthopaedic surgeon not an abdominal surgeon, but he said I have a young man that is just the slickest young man I have ever had, and he called Gordon Murray and Gordon Murray took out my appendix and Dr. Gallie stayed with me right through the night."[15]

In 1963, Murray explained to a Venezuelan colleague how he had found his way in the 1930s from general surgery to cardiac surgery. "Early in my career I became interested in experimental work. This involved my early investigation of thrombosis and embolism and heparin and its effect in preventing these conditions. From that naturally it led to experiments in vascular surgery in which heparin was an adjunct in preventing thrombosis. From there on it was another step to some experimental work and then a great deal of clinical work in cardiac surgery."[16] (On Murray's clinical work, see "Heart Operations," later in this chapter.)

It wasn't that Murray went over to heart operations and left the rest of general surgery behind. About half of his cases were not cardiovascular, and he continued to do routine procedures. One of the surgical services would supply him with residents to help out. In January and February 1965, in the Pavilion Operating Room (POR), we find him ligating a varicose vein, doing a hemorrhoidectomy, a thyroidectomy, and a sigmoidoscopy, among other procedures.[17] He may have done these bread-and-butter operations to maintain his income, but the fact is that even as a world-famous surgeon, he continued to do them.

Jacob Markowitz

Murray's world in the 1930s was alive with interest in experimental (animal) transplanting. At the centre of it was Jacob Markowitz, born in Romania in 1901 and brought to Canada as a baby. He earned a medical degree in 1923 from the University of Toronto and thereafter worked in the Department of Physiology with J.J.R. Macleod on insulin (PhD in physiology 1926). After an excursion to Glasgow, Markowitz progressed in 1927 to the Mayo Clinic as an assistant of Frank Mann, where he spent "3 busy and happy years," as he later put it. "I was known as their physiologist." At Mayo, "I was struck with the ease with which a heart could be kept pulsating vigorously with saline solution, so suggested to Dr. Mann that we sew a little dog's heart to the carotid [neck artery] of a large dog." This is a classic contribution to science (1929), "the homotransplantation of the canine heart." This apparently unpublished work, Markowitz noted, was later erroneously cited as being "Russian" in origin.

In 1930 Markowitz went to Georgetown University, a Jesuit institution, as professor of physiology and head of the department. There, he did no further dog-heart work but published the Mayo research. He mentioned that they had used heparin as an anticoagulant. The article, co-written with Mann among other authors, appeared in 1933. The longest survival was eight days.[18] At this point the Georgetown Jesuits apparently discovered he was Jewish and did not reappoint him, causing "half the senior faculty" to resign. Unable to find a job now during the Depression, Markowitz returned to Toronto to practise medicine. After his arrival in Toronto, in 1933 Charles Best invited Markowitz to become a "research associate" in physiology. At this point he wrote his classic text *Experimental Surgery* (1937). He himself paid $3,500 for the first printing, although it later sold thousands of copies. At this point Markowitz had now launched cardiac transplantation.[19]

In his 1937 book, written in Toronto, Markowitz devoted a whole chapter to "the experimental [dogs] surgery of the heart." Displaying some of the tongue-in-cheek humour that would stand him in good stead in the coming years of imprisonment in a Japanese prisoner-of-war camp, he wrote, apropos heart-lung preparations, "It is a surgical operation demanding a high degree of skill even though what results is not a 'dog' but a 'preparation.'" Apropos achieving "heart-lung-kidney perfusion," he wrote, "This exercise requires nimble fingers and nimble wits. It teaches the surgeon how to go about building up a dog out of its constituent parts. Using the heart (with attached lungs) as a pump, a pair of kidneys, a liver, and a hind leg can be added."[20]

So transplantation started to become prevalent. Transplantation articles appeared in several Toronto newspapers in these years.[21] But to what extent Murray – and later Bigelow and the team in the Banting basement – were influenced by Markowitz is unknown.

Heparin

Following the lead of Charles Best, who had reactivated interest in heparin in Toronto in 1929, Murray began his experimental work with heparin, studying its effect on thrombosis in the laboratories of the Experimental Research Committee.[22] It was then in May 1935 that Murray administered heparin at TGH. Murray, Best, and their two assistants published a brief article on heparin in the *Canadian Medical Association Journal* in December 1936,[23] "obviously designed to establish precedence in the clinical use of heparin," said surgeon Ronald Baird, chief of the University Division and chief of cardiac surgery at the merged Toronto Hospital from 1988 to 1998. "For the five years from 1935 to 1940, Gordon Murray had a virtual international monopoly on the clinical use of heparin. Only Clarence Crafoord in Sweden had a similar supply."[24]

Yet introducing heparin to the clinic in Toronto was not so easy. Throughout this experimental and early clinical work with heparin, Murray felt himself opposed by "the Toronto School." He later said in his autobiography, "The theory having been developed and tested, the school was in a position to expand and lead the whole world in this new departure of anticoagulants, blood vessel surgery and everything related thereto. Because of human weaknesses, the opportunity was sacrificed and the fame that undoubtedly could have been gained for the University was allowed to go in large measure to other centres." Meanwhile, Murray received "a steady stream of visitors from many countries," all curious about heparin in conditions such as pulmonary embolus.[25]

An obdurate Duncan Graham, the crotchety professor of medicine, in particular established a long tradition of Medicine resisting Surgery's innovations. In 1938, William Gallie, as professor of surgery, wanted to enlist Graham's cooperation in heparinizing patients with various clots, including pulmonary emboli. Graham was completely resistant, and his exchanges with Gallie make harrowing reading as an example of the consequences of benighted medical vision. On 4 March 1938 Gallie said that he had called Graham again. "He replied that the Medical

Staff had decided that heparin could not be of any value in coronary thrombosis and could therefore not be used." As for the use of heparin in cases of pulmonary embolism resulting from coronary thrombosis, Graham said the number was quite small. "He stated that such treatments might even be injurious as they often showed heart failure and this would be accentuated by the quantity of fluid administered with the heparin." For these reasons the staff was unwilling to use heparin. As for arterial embolism, Graham said the "suction boot" was "satisfactory."

Gallie said, "I told him I was disappointed in the answer of the Department of Medicine as I felt that heparin was a preventive of thrombosis and might be of value in treating diseases in which thrombosis was a feature."[26] Indeed.

Relations between Murray and Gallie were cool. Gallie was a figure of great distinction, and just as Bill Bigelow's students would later come together and found a "Bigelow Club," W.E. Gallie's students organized a "Gallie Club," which held rotating meetings at various academic centres – and Murray was not along when, in May 1948, the Gallie Club met at the Mayo Clinic in Rochester, Minnesota. (There turned out to be a problem. There was to be a staff meeting and dinner at the Mayo Clinic at eight o'clock that evening. "When it was pointed out that the Chief [Gallie] and many others had reservations for the train leaving at 8 p.m., Dr. Balfour quietly turned to Dr. Clagett and said, 'We'll arrange to have that train held over for an hour or so, Jim.' Which they did."[27]) This anecdote shows the power that Gallie had, and indicates the enthusiasm of the Gallie Club. Murray found this kind of slavishness offensive.

Murray didn't really require Gallie's imprimatur. He forged ahead on his own, and the *President's Report* of 1938 was positively agog with Murray's doings regarding Murray's work with heparin: "It is now definitely established that it is of great value in all operations on blood vessels and the heart, in preventing thrombosis, and the results in spontaneous venous thrombosis suggest that it is of value in preventing the extension of thrombus ... Dr. Murray has enlarged the field of blood vessel suture to include free transplants of veins to replace gaps in arteries. This can be done with a high percentage of success in animals and its possibilities in wounds of great vessels and in tumours and aneurysms are highly interesting. He has also made some progress in an attempt to replace damaged heart valves."[28]

It was 1939, and the shadow of war lay over Europe. In October, six weeks after the outbreak of hostilities with the German invasion of Poland, George Grey Turner, the professor of surgery at the British

Post-Graduate School of the University of London, came to Toronto to lecture. He was an old friend of Murray's. Casualties are certain, he said, when the German air raids come. Note that he did not say "if," and the prediction was totally prescient. But he said that the London hospitals were ready for them, and, referring to heparin, he said that Murray's discovery "would be of immense value to the surgeon in wartime. Many limbs will undoubtedly be saved by the use of heparin."[29] Murray's discovery of the clinical uses of heparin had an international importance second only to the discovery of insulin at the University of Toronto two decades previously.

Bigelow dates the beginning of vascular surgery – at TGH and in general – with Murray's clinical introduction of heparin in 1935. "At a time when pulmonary embolism or phlebitis occurred in about 15% of general surgical patients post-operatively, he ran a series of cases in which Heparin was used post-operatively as a prophylactic measure and from his report it prevented pulmonary embolism in all cases." Bigelow noted this as a classic finding, and it established heparin's value surgically, "although the medical department of the hospital [under Duncan Graham] did not accept it."[30]

In 1940, Murray proposed using heparin in blood-vessel surgery and embolisms of various kinds. He also suggested the use of venous grafts in arterial surgery together with heparin, evidently the first time that this procedure was reported as a success in the literature: the vessels stay patent.[31] (This was the first major advance in vascular surgery since Alexis Carrel pioneered vascular suturing around the turn of the century.) Later scholars have attributed the use of venous grafting in vascular surgery to a variety of sources – but this is apparently the real first. In this 1940 paper, Murray said they had heparinized 22 patients with pulmonary embolism, some of whom were near death. All survived. By 1946, Murray had used heparin on 149 patients with pulmonary embolism, "all of whom were saved," as Murray told the American College of Surgeons.[32]

With anticoagulation in place, the stage was now set to take on surgery on the heart. An interest in the heart specifically seems to have begun for Murray at the Banting Institute in 1933, when he asked Professor Gallie "for permission to conduct experiments on the heart."[33] In 1936, he initiated surgery on the mitral valve of the dog, replacing it with venous tissue. Of the eight dogs, two survived and were "perfectly well, now 6 months following the operation." In January 1938, he gave a talk at the surgical staff meeting on "experimental surgery on the heart," evidently reporting these results. In April 1938 he reported the dog research in the *Canadian Medical Association Journal*.[34]

What he did not report, however, was that in 1938 he had already replaced several incompetent mitral valves in humans. This would have been the beginning of mitral valve surgery. All this came out in his autobiography, the first volume of which was published in 1960. Colleagues at a meeting who looked on in "supercilious amusement" as he described his dog research sat shocked as he talked about his human operations. "The physicians on the hospital staff made quite certain that none of their patients would be so unorthodoxly treated."[35]

Murray's first public excursion into surgery on the heart and the aorta occurred around 1943. This is the story: A female patient, who had been suffering from rheumatic heart disease but was otherwise able to move about, "noticed a scatter rug slightly out of place on the living room floor. Instead of bending down to reposition it, in a moment of exhilaration she placed both feet on the rug and, making a small skip, skillfully slid the rug into position. Immediately, without warning, something dreadful happened. The quick, sudden movement must have displaced a pre-existing clot in the heart and started it on its way into the general circulation." The patient soon went into shock, and her very survival appeared in question.

She had the symptoms of an aortic embolism: Her feet and legs were cold and she had a blotchy blueness in the upper thighs. What to do? Until that point, surgery on the aorta had been a no-go area. But Murray decided to remove the clots from her lower aorta and the branching (iliac) arteries. "The aorta above was pulsating violently ... struggling against the obstruction produced by these massive clots which plugged into the lower two inches, along with two inches on the left side and three inches on the right side of the adjacent common iliac (pelvic) arteries." What Murray did was simple: he made an incision of about an inch in one of the iliac vessels "and through this all the clots were expressed [squeezed out]. The involved vessels were next irrigated thoroughly with heparin solution to make sure there were no remaining fragments." He neatly stitched up the incision, and the blood rushed back into her lower limbs, "which immediately changed from their deadish, whitish appearance to a nice rosy pink."[36] Murray described this and six further cases in an article in 1943.

Murray's secrecy, quarrelsomeness, and paranoia began to emerge early in the game. Don Wilson was a resident in Ward C just after the war, and he recalls that Murray "was not the easiest person to get along with. I often wondered if he didn't enjoy fighting with everybody, as a bit of a challenge. He would go out of his way sometimes to make it difficult for somebody." Wilson helped Murray in his dog lab on the top floor of the Banting Building, where Murray would try out new experimental ideas. "The interesting thing is you would sort of be sworn to secrecy, after you had finished something he would say, now don't talk about this, we'll just see how it gets along."[37]

Heart Operations

In the 1940s, Murray undertook a number of cardiac operations. By 1950 he had operated on six patients, evidently adolescents and young adults, for the narrowing of the aorta called "coarctation." "It is very satisfactory, immediately after operation, to feel the first pulsation in the lower extremities and to find blood pressure in the legs equal to that in the arm," he wrote in 1950.[38]

Blue Babies

It was after the war that Murray began operating systematically on "blue babies," infants whose cardiac output was somehow compromised. Murray's first blue-baby operation occurred on 16 February 1946, at the Wellesley Hospital on a twelve-year-old girl for the correction of tetralogy of Fallot. As Stephen Evelyn, who administered the cyclopropane anesthetic, said, this operation "opened the gate to the new field of cardiac surgery in Toronto … This first operation required five hours to perform. But at the end of this time the child's color was much improved." Evelyn said the operation was "a success."[39] It was apparently accomplished without onlookers.

The procedure for the tetralogy of Fallot had been pioneered by Alfred Blalock, who published about it in 1945. Tetralogy of Fallot involved several developmental problems: the pulmonary valve is stenosed, causing pulmonary hypertension (pulmonary damage from the stuck valve because of the left to right flow through the ventricular septal defect [VSD]); the VSD itself – a hole in the wall separating the left from the right ventricles – is present; and the aorta arises partly from the right ventricle, causing the problem of unoxygenated blood. It was a not uncommon developmental defect and was often fatal. At some point Murray went down to Hopkins to watch Blalock operate, then returned to Toronto to perfect his own version of the operation.[40]

The second operation by Murray took place in March 1946; his patient was thirteen-year-old Isabel Douglas of Toronto. Murray believed that several members of the Department of Surgery at the General were "undercover reporters for several of the newspapers" [!], and it was for that reason that he chose once again to perform the operation at the outlying Wellesley Hospital on a Saturday morning rather than at the General.[41] This attempt at secrecy failed, however, and many surgeons and physicians cancelled their weekend plans to be present. (Murray later presented this operation as the first blue-baby procedure, but his memory must have failed him.)

In the Blalock-Taussig operation, after a long dissection of the places where the lung had become attached to the chest wall, Murray proceeded to divide the right subclavian artery and to bring a portion of it down to hook up with the right pulmonary artery (thus increasing the amount of blood available for the lungs to oxygenate). But "there was a gap of probably an inch between these two vessels, and the ohs! and ahs! in the audience made it quite obvious that it seemed improbable to those who could see in the restricted field that these two delicate friable structures could ever be brought together and sewn so that they would not leak." Yet Murray mastered this work of great complexity; heparin was instilled, and the anastomosis (the joining of two vessels) was completed.

But would the anastomosis hold once the clips were removed and the arterial blood started gushing into the lungs at high pressure? "A nurse on the other side of the table and a medical student at the back promptly fainted and were lugged out of the operating room."

Shortly, "the area was as completely dry as the young bride's quivering finger receiving the wedding ring." Further clips were removed: "the artery became distended to its full size, delivering a torrential flow of blood into the lung field, with no deleterious effect on the anastomosis.

"The final act of the great drama was unfolded as the anaesthetist shone a light on the young patient's face. Before, it was blue, almost as ink; now, within two minutes after the circulation from the aorta passed into the lung fields, the colour of the child's face was changing to a blueish-pink and in the next few minutes it was a great satisfaction to everyone to see both the face and the finger tips turn a lively, reddish pink. To the onlookers the miracle had reached such an emotional crisis that many left the operating room dabbing their eyes with the corners of their operating room gowns.[42] This is surely one of the most dramatic descriptions in the history of modern surgery, even if it was the second successful heart surgery and not the first.

"Isabel left the operating room early Saturday afternoon," reported the *Globe and Mail*, "with her lips pink for the first time." Yet she developed a cerebral embolism and died almost at once. Her father nonetheless accorded to Murray credit due: "If medical science has benefited, then the sacrifice will not have been in vain," he said.[43]

In June 1946 Murray operated on a third "blue" child, Viola Ireland of Burks Falls, age five and a half. The operation on Isabel had been a failure, but this effort was crowned with success. Viola's father had died of a heart condition a week before the operation, and her mother said, "It was a hard decision she had to make, for she felt there was little hope that her daughter would recover."[44] Viola lived to adulthood and went on to have children of her own. Viola, said a journalist not quite accurately, "became the first Canadian blue baby to turn a healthy pink."[45]

What the press trumpeted as the first successful "blue baby" operation in Toronto received huge media play, despite Murray's precautions. Murray's name became synonymous with miracle worker. By September 1946 he had done six more.[46] Baird said, "When I entered medical school in 1948, 'Gordon Murray, the blue-baby doctor,' was a household phrase, not only in Toronto, but across Canada."[47] "There was so much excitement and interest not only in the profession but in the public that it was useless any longer to try to keep it under cover." Murray moved the operation to Ward C of the General.[48]

In August 1946 Murray went down to Hopkins to demonstrate his own technique, and Blalock later thanked him effusively.[49] A number of beds in Ward C were reserved as "blue baby" beds, and their occupants were continually replenished. By April 1947, Murray, as the *Toronto Star* stated, "was on 'Blue Baby Nr. 46.'"[50]

Billy Lopen, on whom Murray operated in 1948 for a septal defect, said afterwards, "I had the best doctor in the world."[51] By January 1949, Murray was said to have performed 190 such operations, and as he told the *Globe and Mail* newspaper, "at least 90 per cent were successful."[52] (Of the 342 operations that Murray had done for tetralogy of Fallot by October 1953, 6 per cent were fatal; of 260 operations for mitral valve disease, 6 per cent fatal.[53])

Murray himself reported on his series of sixty-two congenital heart operations (in children) at a meeting of the Canadian Medical Association in Winnipeg in June 1947. Conducted at the General, the operations included forty-one "tetralogies," twelve patent ductus arteriosus cases and nine others. (The ductus arteriosus is a shunt that exists between the aorta and the pulmonary artery in utero, when lung oxygenation is not required. If it fails to close, unoxygenated blood is pumped into the circulation.) The overall mortality was 11.3 per cent; in the tetralogies 7.3 per cent. The "PDAs" (patent ductus arteriosus) were fairly straightforward, involving often just a simple ligature. The tetralogies were much more complex, involving, as we have seen, bringing down the subclavian artery (which originates on the arch of the aorta) and anastomosing it to the pulmonary artery (increasing the amount of blood that the lungs are able to oxygenate). This was the original "blue baby" operation that Blalock and Helen Taussig had originated at Johns Hopkins in 1944. Murray noted in his 1947 paper, "The patient turns from blue to a satisfactory pink colour immediately."[54]

These operations had a transformative impact on the lives of the little patients. One mother wrote Murray in September 1947, "I wish you could see her [the patient] now. She is quite sun-tanned. She can swim a little – just loves the water. If it hadn't been for having to stop taking her to beaches because of the polio epidemic here, she'd likely be swimming *very* well now." The mother concluded, "You really are a very good and wonderful man, Dr. Murray. May God bless and continue to assist you in your life-giving work."[55] In August 1948 a grateful father wrote, "When I see my little son playing with an energy he never knew before, a layman like myself feels that the medical profession is a godly one and that men like yourself are the glories of it."[56]

And the parents! Murray recalled "a great Swedish six-foot-three father [from Northern Ontario] who had brought his tiny two-and-a-half-year-old flaxen-haired daughter to the hospital in a pitiable state of shortness of breath, very great cyanosis and complete disability, so that she had not stood on her feet even in her crib." The operation went well, and the father was advised to come and pick her up. "As he entered the door of the ward, the child was at the far end of the corridor. He saw the pretty nurse in her starched uniform and her trim nursing cap leading by the hand a tiny little tot, who was jabbering gaily and walking quite freely and joyfully toward the door. With her screams of 'Daddy!' she ran to his enfolding arms, while the great tears rolled down his twitching weather-beaten face."[57]

Valves

Since 1932, Murray had been doing experimental operations on the valves of dogs' hearts, some of which were successful, the animals surviving with their new mitral valves. As noted above, in 1938 he initiated surgery on mitral valves in humans for regurgitation (leaking).

In 1945 Murray began, or resumed, operating on humans with mitral stenosis. He described the operation: "The approach is made through a small incision in the left ventricle through which is passed a cannula guarded by a valve, much as is used in a cystoscope. The punch or knife is guided through the opening in the valve by palpation with a finger which has invaginated the left auricle into the funnel shaped orifice.

Either a cut is made or a portion is taken out, as desired." Eight out of ten survived.[58] He replaced the mitral valve with a ball cage valve and did not use commissurotomy (cutting the leaflets apart).[59] This work clearly antedates the 1948 commissurotomies of both Charles Bailey in Philadelphia and Dwight Harken in Boston, who conventionally are credited with introducing operations for mitral valve stenosis.[60] Indeed, in his autobiography, Murray says that Bailey and Harken were following his, Murray's, lead. Murray is maddening about dates, except to say that his operations were the first.[61]

No one else in the world had Murray's record with intracardiac operations; no one else could repair or replace the mitral valve. Surgeons would come up from Buffalo to watch Murray operate. According to one (who was apparently unaware of Edouard Gagnon's work in Montreal), "Dr. Murray is performing operations inside the heart which make him 'completely unique' and doing it so often it is becoming 'routine.'" Murray's Buffalo medical admirer continued, "I don't think many surgeons in the United States know how far advanced Dr. Murray is in heart surgery. I'd say he is 10 years ahead of us. He is the only man I know of who is doing actual cardiac surgery."[62]

In May 1948, at a meeting of the American Surgical Association in Quebec City, Murray reported on his operations on atrial and ventricular septal defects in children (ASDs and VSDs). This was closed heart surgery, not opening the heart. Using a very refined knowledge of anatomy, Murray guessed where the septa might lie and inserted sutures. In the VSDs he used "a living suture removed from the fascia lata of the thigh." For the ASDs he used conventional fabric sutures. Blalock, who was at the meeting, said, "You all remember the amazing paper on coronary occlusion presented by Dr. Gordon Murray at the last meeting of the Association, and now he comes forward with an even more amazing presentation. Certainly it never would have occurred to me to place sutures blindly in this manner."[63]

Murray was well aware of the historic importance of this first closure of an interventricular septal defect. "The patient made a rapid recovery and was out of bed in a few days. On investigation before leaving hospital, it was found that all evidence of an opening in the septum had disappeared. The murmur had gone. The patient was in much better physical condition, had much more energy and his condition seemed ideal in all respects." X-rays showed a great reduction in the size of the heart and "striking changes in the shape of the heart. On the left border there had been a bulge. Following the operation this had completely disappeared, and the heart had returned to a normal shape." Fifteen years later [in 1963], "He was now a strong and vigorous man with a regular labouring job, driving a truck, loading it himself and carrying on as well as any other person with a normal heart."[64]

The valve operations were almost as celebrated as the tetralogies. In January 1950, the *Toronto Star* – which ran endless enthusiastic stories about Murray's operations – said that doctors had virtually given up on thirty-nine-year-old Audrey Dufton, advising her to go home and "rest" – until she referred herself to a doctor who referred her to Murray, who repaired her mitral valve. She was said to have had a heart "the largest Dr. Murray had ever seen."[65]

The acme of this valve work was transplanting a cadaveric (homograft) aortic valve in 1953,[66] with publication in 1956. This was a historic first. While working in his private laboratory near the Wellesley Hospital, Murray successfully transplanted an aortic valve in a dog. He was doubtless inspired by Charles Hufnagel's report in 1954 on placing an artificial valve in the descending aorta. Hufnagel's work began in September 1952. Of twenty-three of Hufnagel's patients with severe aortic insufficiency, seventeen survived and improved.[67] (These pioneering operations could be harrowing: in the spring of 1955 Baird, as a junior intern on Ward C, watched a patient bleed to death within a minute or two as one of these mechanical valves dehisced.)

Murray said, "We first applied this principle [of transplanting valves] in 1953 on patients who were deteriorating rapidly from the lack of proper valve function in their own hearts. They would have died but these patients are alive, well and working at the time of this writing. [1963]" But he didn't write it up, so his work wasn't publicized. Murray's first publicized aortic valve transplant in humans took place in 1955, using the valve of a postmortem patient, age thirty-two, thirty-six hours after death. They then did two more. Where these operations took place is unclear, but they were possibly not at the General, because of Murray's paranoid fear that colleagues (such as, presumably, Bigelow) were about to steal his ideas. "The valves functioned well," he wrote in an obscure Italian cardiology journal in 1956, "and one could, on the surface, feel the valves closing ... Following the [first] operation, the patient's heart diminished in size considerably. His energy was much improved and he has continued to go on perfectly to date, now eight months postoperative." The other two patients had similar results. (Murray did one mitral valve as well.)[68]

Ray Heimbecker, who alone had good relations with Murray, assisted Murray in one of these operations in 1955. This was done at the General. Heimbecker recalled, "Murray and I had discussed many times the flood of patients who had become cardiac invalids because of the ravages of rheumatic fever and heart valve damage." Heimbecker and

Murray often met for lunch in the cafeteria of the General and "discussed the concept of transplanting a healthy heart valve into a patient whose own valve had been destroyed by rheumatic fever."

The patient, "JP," from northern Ontario, had a history of a leaking aortic valve. "Gradually, his heart was enlarging so that finally, at the age of 25, his life had become a bed-to-bathroom existence." Heimbecker recalled, "Excitement was at a high pitch in 'C' operating room that day. I had harvested the heart valve under sterile technique from the hospital morgue 24 h before. After taking routine cultures, I placed it in a sterile-capped bottle along with some gauze moistened with the new wonder drug, penicillin."

Then Heimbecker tried to pretty-face Murray's paranoia. "Because we wanted no publicity, the operation was booked simply as a left-lateral thoracotomy. In spite of the secrecy, we had more than enough visitors looking over our shoulders."

They clamped off the aorta, split it, and put the new valve in place. "Forty minutes later, the clamps were gradually released. The transplanted leaflets began to open and close with each heart beat. Our excited fingers could feel the vigorous throb as the fragile leaflets closed and opened with each contraction. As I placed my hand on the heart muscle, it too had dramatically changed to a much quieter and more peaceful contraction ... In a few days, JP was back with his jubilant family. The world's first heart valve transplant had been a thrilling success."[69]

Baird said, "In October 1955, while I was still working in Bill Bigelow's lab, he performed the first clinical operation [in Ward C]. The operation was kept secret and the cardiac surgeons in Toronto first heard about it when they received copies of Murray's report in the October 1956 issue of *Angiology*, a rather obscure journal printed in Italy." Baird said, "The valve was still functioning well 19 years later."[70]

Nobody read that particular obscure Italian journal and nobody had heard of it. It was only in 1962 when, in an article in the *New England Journal of Medicine*, Don Wilson and collaborators reported on the first patient's condition, that the actual date of the first operation was given.[71] Murray did not leave it here but did a series of aortic valve transplants, all of which were apparently "functioning well" by August 1957.[72]

Bigelow inscribed on the title page of his copy of a later article he had written with Murray, "Gordon Murray's successful use of a homograft valve in the descending aorta in 1955 in humans initiated the whole subsequent era of biological valves."[73] This operation did begin a new era, but it is maddeningly unclear how many early operations there were and exactly when they happened.

As a result of all this innovation, Murray became world famous. Invitations to lecture in Europe, Latin America, and Australia were breathlessly followed in the press,[74] and Murray was unquestionably Canada's most distinguished surgeon, which makes his downfall all the more painful. One could see it coming. He had a pathological suspiciousness of his colleagues and, as cardiac surgeon Don Wilson remembers, "When he got into the blue baby business, he would book the case as a hernia, he wouldn't book it as a blue baby. Then, you know the little window you have looking into the OR, there would be a towel over it so you couldn't see what was going on."[75] Once, as related by Scully, when Bigelow appeared at the door of Murray's OR, "Murray draped the patient first with a sheet before saying, 'Yes, Bill, can I help you?'"[76] Because Murray was so secretive and had irritated so many colleagues, he really was without a following.

Murray proposed other cardiac procedures that transfixed the field. That verb is not too strong. At a meeting of the American Surgical Association in Hot Springs, Virginia, in March 1947, Murray described increasing the survival of dogs, after inducing in them massive heart attacks, by excising a portion of the damaged cardiac muscle. He speculated that humans would benefit from the same procedure. Murray tied off the left coronary artery in cats to see exactly what happened to the myocardium. "The infarcted area is easily visible." But then, Murray excised the infarcted area with a scalpel. "Following removal of the infarct, the area is again oversewn and a satisfactory repair can be obtained ... The results of removing this infarct produce an astonishing effect in the animal. The cardiac output increases considerably and the blood pressure rises moderately." Instead of dying, "the animal survives quite satisfactorily and most of them have made quite a good recovery."[77]

Alfred Blalock, who was in the audience, said, "I was sitting next to Dr. Rudolph Matas while Dr. Gordon Murray was presenting his paper and he stated to me that this work may be epoch-making. [There was little discussion.] This lack of prolonged discussion is probably due to the fact that others are as amazed by these brilliant experimental observations as I am ... The fact that Doctor Murray was able to prevent the death of animals following coronary occlusion by excision of the infarcted area is a magnificent accomplishment."[78] Although this publication was based on experimental (dog) research, in fact Murray performed the aneurysm-resection operation three times successfully on humans before meeting so much resistance that he found it "discreet to discontinue."[79] Murray's student Ray Heimbecker was later to resurrect it. (See chapter 3, section titled "Raymond O. Heimbecker.")

There was more to come. The key to later aortocoronary bypass was taking a saphenous vein from the leg, reversing it, and using it to work around the obstruction in the coronary artery. The historical record is a bit unclear here, but it was apparently Murray who pioneered reversing the saphenous vein in vascular surgery as early as 1937.[80] First to describe it in the literature was Jean Kunlin in 1949, in a femoral bypass.[81] But according to Ray Heimbecker – as Baird reports – "Kunlin had visited Gordon Murray in 1947 or 1948 and had picked up the idea from him." Baird said, "[This] further embittered and twisted Murray's thoughts on priority."[82]

In 1953, Murray, piqued at the refusal of Robert Janes, the professor of surgery, to cut him a special deal, resigned his university appointment – although he did accept a university appointment in June 1959 as graduate lecturer in the Department of Surgery.[83] So he didn't actually leave the University Department. He merely pretended to do so to make a point and continued to operate in the Private Patients Pavilion and perhaps elsewhere – and was sufficiently involved in clinical care to send to a colleague in 1960 the horrendous statistics on cases of pulmonary embolism treated with anticoagulant (heparin): 1955: seventy-six cases, forty-six deaths; 1956: eighty-one cases, thirty-eight deaths.[84]

Hostile Murray

In 1948 Murray was promoted to head surgeon on Ward C on the third floor of the College Wing, replacing the retiring Norman Shenstone. Shenstone and Murray apparently cordially disliked each other, although this would have been true of the rest of the surgical leadership as well. As Goldman tells the story, "[Bigelow] was mentored by Gallie although at that time [1948] Gordon Murray was doing incredible lab and clinical work, including infarctectomy, subclavian-coronary anastomoses, 'blue-baby' operations, blind closure of atrial and ventricular septal defects, mitral splits, closed mitral slings for regurgitation, etc. He probably did the first Blalock operation in Canada and is credited with starting heart surgery in Brazil and Australia after invited visits in 1953. But he was secretive, competitive, arrogant, and deceitful albeit a truly gifted surgeon and he was shunted aside politically for Bigelow."[85]

So here was the problem with Murray. He was difficult to work with, and this in a department that prized collegiality. In such a department, Bigelow fit perfectly. Murray didn't fit at all. Early on, Murray had established a reputation as a surgeon's surgeon, but he alienated many in the department. Cardiologist Robert MacMillan remembered,

"He was always a stormy player. But they couldn't let him go, I guess, because he was just too good ... Gallie, I am sure, would have removed Murray had he been able to get away with it. But I think Gallie recognized that if he did this, some of his other senior staff would be upset."[86]

Contemporaries' comments were filled with collegial unease. On the basis of Murray's trip to New Zealand, Auckland surgeon Douglas Robb commented, rather unusually in what was intended to be a laudatory "biography," that "his relations with others were sometimes strained." While Murray inspired his juniors, "he seemed to the outsider not as capable at working with his contemporaries."[87]

Murray wasn't close to anyone except perhaps his very junior students such as Heimbecker. Bigelow later wrote, "Murray was a loner, and suspicious, and medical science was the loser. He had a fear of plagiarism and a strong desire to be sure he received the recognition he felt he deserved ... During early heart and blood-vessel operations he hung a towel over the window in the operating room to prevent prying, and excluded everyone, including myself."[88] Murray never used an anesthetist from the department (Anaesthesia Associates) and brought along his own, Stephen Evelyn.[89]

Murray bristled at the idea of even mentioning in print the names of the members of the Division of Cardiac Surgery who, he felt, had scorned and obstructed him. In 1959 Lorne Pierce, Murray's editor at the Ryerson Press, asked for a bit more detail on personalities in the draft of Murray's forthcoming autobiography *Medicine in the Making* (1960). Murray replied, "I will submit [some names] only when we pulled together and worked well as a team in the routine work. However, as they did not assist, but rather opposed my investigative work, it is not easy to include them."[90] That apparently applied above all to the hated Bigelow.

In the mid-1960s Murray launched his ill-conceived "serum" for breast cancer. His admirers beseeched the Canadian Cancer Society: Why was support for Murray's work not forthcoming? R.M. Taylor, executive vice-president of the society, replied to the director of the society, "We have had certain problems in our relationships with Dr. Murray for a number of years." Murray had rejected the society's advice to consult about the cancer serum with colleagues in immunology – a subject of which Murray understood little. Of course, Taylor continued, Murray was free to apply to the society for a grant at any time. "Between you and me, the problem is that Dr. Murray would be required to give full details of his proposed experiments, and he has felt in years past that to do so is to reveal plans which he would prefer remained known only to himself."[91] Thus, the paranoia gathered.

The early 1950s found Murray at the height of his fame. The introduction of heparin, the first dialysis machine, kidney transplant, and
the blue babies had resulted in him being ranked him among the chief
medical personalities of Toronto. When New Zealand surgeon Rowan
Nicks visited Toronto in May 1952 – in the course of a large trip of
inquiry across several continents – he was literally awestricken at Murray's presence. Murray had already got cardiac surgery going in New
Zealand in the course of a trip Down Under. But here was Murray at
home: "the most outstanding personality in this city." Nicks gushed,
"He is generally conceded one of the world's most delicate and expert
craftsmen; as well as this, he is a deep philosopher on world issues as
well as in medicine." Nicks met Bigelow as well and mentioned hypothermia in passing; ditto for Bill Mustard and his oxygenation of the
blood with monkeys' lungs.[92] (It evidently did not strike Nicks that
these two figures were initiating intracardiac surgery.)

But clouds were gathering for Murray. Perhaps overly impressed
with his own fame, he overplayed his hand. His resentments accumu-
lating, and in May 1947 Murray wrote Eric Phillips, chair of the board
of governors of TGH, complaining about under-recognition and the
Department of Surgery's general failure to give him the resources he
deserved. The letter struck a grandiose note: "I am enclosing the letters
received in one mail, as well as others, and these are arriving daily, to
illustrate my point. Also enclosed is a list of my publications, for which,
requests for reprints from all corners of the earth, reaching into many
thousands."[93] His note to Phillips proved unavailing.

In August 1947 Murray petitioned Bob Janes, professor of surgery, to
cut him a special detail, asking that chemists be assigned to him, that
a considerable amount of money be assigned to a special budget for
him, and that his special program be independent from control by the
Department of Surgery. Janes straight-armed him: none of the requests
could be met. Moreover, "I see no reason why your service should be
[more] autonomous than that of any other division of surgery and I
could not consent to an independent chair in surgery over which I had
no control." Janes also deplored Murray's refusal of a personal meeting. "I am sorry that you have not found it possible to find time to have
lunch with me some day so that we could discuss the problem you
raised in your letter."[94]

Deeply offended, Murray withdrew increasingly from the department. We shall later see how Bigelow ended up running Ward C at
TGH even though Murray was the nominal chief. In 1949 Murray transferred his lab work to the quarters of the W.P. Caven Memorial Research
Foundation on Homewood Avenue, becoming their "medical director."

The Caven Foundation had been created through a five-year donation from J.S. McLean, president of Canada Packers, and wound up its
work in August 1954, as the McLean Charitable Foundation apparently
declined to renew the grant.[95] (Murray continued to operate at TGH.)

From around 1954 to 1974 Murray's research was supported by the
Gardiner Medical Research Foundation, and it was here that he studied
the tissue samples for his cancer research and dissected the rats for his
spinal cord research, both of which projects ended haplessly (see "Dis-
grace," later in this chapter).[96]

It is often said that Murray "withdrew" from the Department of Surgery. Yet to some extent he was pushed, and that would have started
in 1947 when Robert M. Janes became professor of surgery. Shelley
McKellar underlines the growing friction between Janes and Murray.[97] The last reference to Murray's activities in the annual *President's
Reports* comes in 1948, as Murray's promotion to assistant professor
was noted.[98] Thereafter, silence descended on his activities in Surgery;
in these reports, submitted of course by Janes, Bigelow figured as the
chief of cardiac surgery. It is not difficult to understand why Murray
evidently hated Bigelow.

Murray in Person

In personal terms, Murray was, as Goldman recalls, "a slim, vigorous, and quick-witted man, popular with students and nurses."[99]
As an intern, Ernest McCulloch, the later co-discoverer of stem cells,
remembered Murray around 1948 from the Wellesley Hospital (then
part of the General), where Murray was a staff surgeon: "He was a
slight grey undistinguished looking man. You wouldn't think anything
of him to meet him." At the Wellesley in those days surgery was conducted by general practitioners who, McCulloch said, had little idea
what they were doing and would hack out great pieces of flesh. Then,
however, McCulloch scrubbed in with Murray, whom he did not previously know. "I thought, my god, this is another retractor job." Instead,
Murray proved amazingly dextrous. "I just stood there. Well in about
seven minutes, he fixed this hernia. I don't think he lost three drops of
blood in the whole operation ... I was superfluous. He was technically
magnificent and intellectually magnificent."[100]

George Trusler, later a pediatric heart surgeon, was a resident under
Murray. Trusler and his fellow residents perceived no hint of the com-
bativeness that alienated the staff. "To the residents, he was a fine
man, and very skilled. One of the most skilled surgeons that I came
across, and he had a lovely feeling for the tissues and getting in and out

without disturbing the tissues, didn't clamp off a lot of vessels, so that patients by and large did well."[101]

Ron Baird echoed this praise: "As a medical student in the early 1950s, I regarded Gordon Murray with awe. He was a charismatic teacher, a brilliant innovator, and a magnificent surgical technician. He was the most famous surgeon in Canada ..."[102] Regarding Murray's operating skills: "These procedures required exceptional surgical skill, could not be performed by the average surgeon, and have been superseded by methods that became possible with open-heart surgery ... For several years he added a footnote to his articles stating that the work has been supported by private funds only and without assistance from the hospital or university. (Although probably true, this did not ease his way in the academic community.)"[103]

Murray seems greatly beloved by his patients (in contrast to his colleagues). His files are thick with notes of gratitude, and many comment on his low fees. Indeed, for many patients he dispensed entirely with a fee.

Murray was a difficult man to get hold of. He was not out for money. He had fame aplenty. But his constant complaints about his colleagues' scheming against him suggests some kind of thirsting for acceptance by the establishment. He arrived in Edinburgh and London basically as a farm boy and returned three years later as something of a swell. He prided himself on all the famous people he knew, and of particular importance were the Christmas gifts: who had given what. In 1960, for example, two days after Christmas he had his secretary, Ethel Kerr, type up a list of the gifts received: From William F. McLean, president of Canada Packers, there was a holiday hamper of meats; from F.R. Gardiner on Old Forest Hill Road, "dinner for assistants"; from neighbours on Sandringham Drive in suburban Downsview, a "Christmas Dinner, silk tie, and Old English cup and saucer."[104]

And then, there is this: the possibility that this thirst for acceptance, amid real triumphs, may have led to some invented ones. Bernie Goldman writes, "I recently performed coronary bypass on a patient with a sternotomy incision for apparent 'blue baby' surgery performed by Murray in the 1950s with newspaper accounts of the successful procedure. Strangely, there is no evidence the pericardium had ever been opened or the heart sutured in any way."[105]

A particularly painful episode occurred in 1957 when he made it appear as though it was his secretary, Ethel Kerr, who was soliciting friends and colleagues for contributions to a "biography" that she was supposedly ginning up without Murray's knowledge. (It wouldn't do to appear to be seeking recognition.)[106] In his handwriting appears a considerable list of individuals who were to be circularized: colleagues such as surgeon Don Wilson, Governor General Roland Michener, Lord Webb-Johnston, and so forth. Tellingly, most did not respond to the invitation. Internist John Oille did, however: "I am sorry but I do not feel able to contribute anything that would be of value in preparing such a biography as you mentioned."[107]

Disgrace

Emboldened by pride, fame, and a complete lack of good judgment, Murray pressed into areas of medicine where he had neither training nor knowledge. The first was cancer chemotherapy. Murray asserted in 1955 that he had developed a serum for the cure of breast cancer and, perhaps, all cancers in general. This was quickly exposed as nonsense, yet the episode did not seriously tarnish his prestige.[108]

A graver assault on Murray's prestige began in 1965 when he claimed to have a cure for spinal paralysis and paraplegia. He wrote, "The problem of cord injury in human beings with fracture of the spine or other injury is that it has never been possible to bring the divided ends of the cord into apposition as we had accomplished in these [rabbit] experiments ... Under proper conditions (good apposition), the cord does regenerate."[109] This was the gist of a lecture Murray gave in November 1965 at the Toronto Memorial Society, where he revealed that he was thinking about undertaking the operation in humans, then clammed up when he learned that a reporter was present.[110]

These claims, too, quickly dissipated but not without drama. In 1972, Murray completely divided the spinal cord in three paraplegic patients. In one, a twenty-one year-old whom historian Shelley McKellar identifies as Purvis Damms, there seemed to be some slight restitution of movement in the left toes and ankle, and of "vague sensations" in the feet, before the patient is lost to follow-up.[111] Another patient, quadriplegic Bernard Proulx, was introduced as much improved at a fundraising dinner; but then, it turned out he hadn't received a spinal resection after all, and Murray's claims began to dissolve in a puff of smoke.[112]

There was great skepticism from colleagues and from the field, as McKellar documents.[113] (A public slanging match between Bill Drucker, the head of surgery, and Murray rocked the press from about November 1967 to February 1968.[114]) This is the research that left Gordon Murray a virtual non-person in the Faculty of Medicine. Murray had done the procedures covertly in the Private Patients Pavilion, and the hospital publicly disavowed the research. Said Drucker at a press conference, "I don't believe him in this particular instance because I can't get the data that says this patient really improved."[115] This whole episode caused Drucker – and the Department of Surgery – much distress. When Bryce Taylor, as an intern, went to see Drucker about his application to be a resident, Drucker asked him what he thought about Murray's presentation of Proulx the day before at the Toronto East General. Taylor hemmed and hawed. Drucker "stood out of his chair and said, 'The man's a goddamn liar!'"[116]

Probably the most distinguished surgeon in Canada at one point, and unquestionably a pioneer of cardiac surgery and dialysis, Murray passed from the scene in silence: aside from an annual Gordon Murray Lecture on Gallie Day in the Department of Surgery, established in 1981, nothing was named after him; there were no memorial funds, no plaques, no nothing. There was silence, so deeply was the Department of Surgery and the Faculty of Medicine embarrassed by what was perceived as his ill-judged recklessness at the end of his career. Nobody else, to our knowledge, has ever attempted again this experiment of cutting the spinal cord, stripping away the dead nervous tissue, then firmly reapproximating the ends. When a snide obituary in the *Globe and Mail* in 1976 dwelt on the spinal issues and glossed over virtually everything else,[117] James Fallis, director of emergency medicine at HSC, protested: heparin, the blue baby operations, the artificial kidney. To be sure, "controversy ... attended some of Dr. Murray's claims to fame. However, these situations are far overshadowed by his real and diverse accomplishments."[118]

Despite everything, Bigelow did indeed hold a high opinion of Murray and later wrote, "In general Dr. Murray contributed a superb example of surgical technique. He is one of the best surgeons that I have ever observed. As a teacher he used the Socratic method and stimulated thought." Bigelow then listed Murray's contributions, which, aside from heparin, include first use of vein grafts in humans ("thanks to the use of Heparin") and the transplantation of an aortic valve from one human into another. He might have added, but didn't, the first clinical use of the artificial kidney.[119]

Murray resigned his hospital appointment in 1967 amid the furor over his spinal cord resections. It was, in a sense, just in time. A new era was about to dawn in cardiac surgery. Murray never used the pump.

Chapter Two

Uncle Bill

Motto: On the occasion of a gathering for his wife Ruth's eighty-fifth birthday, which she was too ill to attend, he signed a very affecting note to her, "God bless you dear Stuffy, all my love, Uncle Bill."[1]

"From Brandon to Bigtime"

The Bigelow family came from England to New England in the seventeenth century; then in 1761 their descendants migrated from Connecticut to Cornwallis, Nova Scotia. Bigelow's father, Wilfred Abram Bigelow, was born in Cornwallis, in 1879. As a young man he started teaching school, then in 1898 he was lured by his sister to Winnipeg to stay in their home and work as an apprentice to a surgeon. A year later, in 1899 he enrolled as a student at Manitoba Medical College and graduated in 1903.

From the get-go, the father, Wilfred Bigelow, practised scientifically – which was not at all the rule in those days. He took postgraduate training in surgery at the Mayo Clinic and at several hospitals in New York City. After moving about small-town Manitoba as a general practitioner, he migrated to the town of Brandon in 1906, to take over a busy practice where he specialized in surgery. He bought his first X-ray machine the following year. Bigelow decided that medical teamwork was much better than solo practice, and in 1913 organized in Brandon an outpatient group practice that he called a "clinic." This was, apparently, the first group practice in Canada. The same year, Wilfred Bigelow became a founding member of the American College of Surgeons.

Bigelow's father, said a journalist, had "fierce bushy brows and one of the brightest and steadiest pairs of eyes I've ever seen ... [He] was, to my mind, the very personification of the country doctor. He was full of bounce and spirit and often sang lustily as he moved about the cottage."[2] Bill Bigelow, who doubtless wanted to romanticize his origins, called his father a "horse-and-buggy country doctor." But the image is rather patronizing, even though Wilfred Bigelow senior did deliver his share of babies in farmhouses and perform emergency operations on the kitchen table.[3] The father wrote in his memoir, "The concept of a clinic where a complete examination and treatment could be provided by specialists working together and submitting one common account proved to be successful."[4] These are not the lines of a simple rustic practitioner.

It was into this household that Wilfred Gordon ("Bill") Bigelow was born in 1913. Bill was a nickname that stuck, and all his life he was known as Bill Bigelow (some medical colleagues, striving to be formal, might address correspondence to him as "Dr. William Bigelow.") Bill's mother, Grace Ann Carnegie Gordon, was a nurse of Scottish origin. One of thirteen children, she had grown up on a farm and studied nursing at Sunderland Infirmary School of Nursing. Wilfred Abram Bigelow noted of his wife, "The church was her chief hobby."[5] Of his mother, Bill wrote, "She ran the household with adequate help and the finances with Scottish skill. Her spare time was spent in intellectual pursuits, preparing weekly lessons for a large young women's Bible Class."[6]

Bill Bigelow later told an interviewer, "I had a fairly happy childhood. I guess our family was athletic and sort of nature oriented. We played hockey practically every day from November to March in the Prairies, and I continued to play hockey when I went down to university of course."[7]

Evidently, to polish off a few rough edges, Bigelow's family sent him to Brentwood College in Victoria, BC, for a year, then to Brandon College in 1931, and the University of Toronto, where he harvested a BA in 1935 and an MD in 1938. (A University of Toronto medical graduate worked for Bigelow *père*, and it was for that reason that Toronto was chosen for *fils*.)

During the war, Bigelow served from 1941 to 1942 as a captain in the Royal Canadian Army Medical Corps with the Field Transfusion Unit, and then as a battle surgeon with the Sixth Canadian Casualty Clearing Station in Normandy and Belgium, which counted as "a front-line facility."[8] Both Bigelow and surgeon Harry Botterell were stationed in England: "Harry asked me about my plans for training. I told him I was applying to the Mayo Clinic for surgical training. He said, 'Why don't you apply here?' He knew they only appointed 3 each year and I explained that I had no personal contacts on the TGH staff (coming from Brandon) and did not think I had much chance. 'Hell,' he said, 'apply here and tell them, you plan to go out West and work with your Dad in his clinic. That will probably get you in, because you will not represent any future competition!' What wisdom and perception."[9]

In 1945 Bigelow returned from the war to work under Murray for a six-month residency at TGH on arterial sutures. The concept was apparently that Bigelow, outfitted with these new skills in anastomosing arteries with venous grafts, would return to the army.[10] But in the meantime the war ended.

From 1946 to 1947, at Gallie's suggestion, Bigelow went down to Hopkins to study with the Blalock group. Bigelow wrote Fred Kergin, professor of surgery: "[We] both worked in Richard Bing's laboratory at Johns Hopkins without having actually performed the catheterizations, although we always assisted and learned a great deal."[11] But Bigelow did watch Blalock in action too. He later wrote, "There evolved the astonishing spectacle of a heart operation every morning. This was the key to the 'birth' of heart surgery ... Here for the first time was an established, routine heart operation."[12] ("We both" refers to Ray Heimbecker, who went down at a different time.)

These were epochal events. There had been other, earlier heart stories, but the modern history of cardiac surgery really began in 1944 in Baltimore, Maryland, as Alfred Blalock, a staff surgeon at Johns Hopkins Hospital, did his first "blue baby" operation, publishing the following year.[13] Ron Baird later said, "A blue-baby became a pink baby. What a fantastic occurrence! Surgeons flocked to Baltimore" – including, from Toronto, Murray, Bigelow, Mustard, and Heimbecker. "Blalock remains one of the most revered surgeons in history."[14] In June 1945, Dudley Ross in Montreal was first to conduct the operation in Canada.

Bigelow returned later in 1947 to Ward B at the General, then migrated to Ward C, alongside Murray. In that same year Janes was appointed professor.[15] Ward C was for "public" patients, in contrast to the tonier Private Patients Pavilion.

It was now 1949. "The vascular pot was beginning to boil," said Bigelow later. "There has never been more excitement than at that time."[16] The previous year, 1948, Dwight Harken in Boston and Charles Bailey in Philadelphia had both done surgery on the heart "with the crude but successful 'closed heart' dilations of stenosed mitral valves," as Baird put it.[17]

Relations between Bigelow and Murray were said to be cool; Bigelow had been a student of Gallie, not of Murray. But what is interesting is how Bigelow seemed to take over control of the ward even while Murray was the nominal chief. In February 1951, for example, it was

Bigelow, not Murray, who represented Ward C at a meeting with Professor Janes on space requirements.[18] In January 1953, months before Murray's resignation in November, Bigelow was proposing to Professor Janes that TGH set up a children's service. (On the third floor of the College Wing, Ward C had six child beds for blue-baby operations.) Bigelow's note had a kind of sovereign tone, as though he were the ward chief.[19] It is unclear whether this was because Murray, his paranoia growing, was already absenting himself from routine hospital procedures, or because the energetic Bigelow was just taking command.

It was with Murray's resignation later in 1953 that under Bigelow the golden age of cardiac surgery as a team effort began, Bigelow's team undertaking, with the use of hypothermia, operation after operation on patients who previously would have been unsalvageable.

But Ward C was full of sharp elbows. The ward was really for general surgery and orthopedics, and it was as a general surgeon that Bigelow began his career. In 1953, forty-two orthopedic patients per month were admitted, thirty-five general surgery, and eleven cardiovascular.[20] Orthopedics was very aggressive about taking beds originally assigned to cardiovascular surgery. On one occasion in 1959, Bigelow complained, "[In the current situation], where we have five or six of our beds occupied by another service, or bed spacers [patients "boarding" from another service], I find that I cannot obtain a routine admission in under three weeks and urgent admissions, in spite of our potential bed space, are very difficult."[21] Heimbecker joined in, "Last Monday I had two urgent admissions for Ward C, one of which was an expanding aortic aneurysm. The waiting list was a month long."[22]

Bigelow maintained a private office until 1967 in the Medical Arts Building at the corner of St. George and Bloor Street West, where he saw private patients "a little more than one half day every two weeks." Thereafter he moved his office to the eighth floor of the University Wing of the General.[23]

"We Have Sad, Sad News Regarding Our Hibernation"[24]

Bigelow's first scientific adventure was in fact a misadventure. As early as 1951, he was already exploring the idea of hypothermia in surgery, as a way of slowing the metabolism of the body – reducing oxygen uptake from the blood – so that the heart could be stopped and operated on without damaging tissues. Hibernation was well known. Groundhogs (woodchucks) were true hibernators, their bodily temperature dropping with the ambient temperature and their heart rates slowing. "The study of this animal," Bigelow later wrote, "might yield the clue to safe, deep hypothermia!"[25] Humans could not be cooled to temperatures less than 20°C without killing them. What was the secret of the groundhog that let it reach much lower temperatures and emerge from the winter sleep unharmed?

In 1951 Bigelow asked John McBirnie, a recent fellow in the cardiovascular lab at the Banting Institute, to collect some groundhogs. The effort failed because burrowing groundhogs are devilishly difficult to find and retrieve. The Bigelow team finally asked Earl Terreberry, a professional trapper, to organize a "groundhog farm" near Port Colborne on the Niagara Peninsula, where ultimately up to seven hundred groundhogs were kept in hibernation, nestled in their individual burrows and available for shipment to the Banting Laboratory in Toronto. (Goldman recalls returning the animals to a "farm" in Collingwood in 1961.)

For the next decade, the Bigelow team tried to isolate the "hibernation factor" – they called the chemical formula "hibernin" – from the groundhogs' brown fat. Early efforts seemed promising. In 1953 the Bigelow people reported on their hypothermia work at the annual meeting of the American College of Surgeons in Chicago. "The hottest subject at the opening session," breathed a big story in the *Chicago Daily News*, "was cold."[26]

And then, by 1961, apparent success! On the ultraviolet and infrared spectrophotometer graph, a new substance appeared in the extract! They identified it chemically, and their chemist synthesized it in the laboratory. The university set out to obtain a patent. The Bigelow team worked into the night, and Bigelow himself stopped his surgical practice. "Some NASA scientists made enquiries. A university photographer took a picture of the team, in view of our impending important announcement to the scientific world." Two hypothermia patients received extracts of the new hibernin. "The nurses in the recovery room said the patients acted as if they were drunk."

Four articles were drafted, ready for scientific release. Meanwhile, the US patent office were heard from, "stating that hibernin had been patented 20 years before as a plasticizer, a chemical that maintains the pliability of plastic tubes." Alarm bells started to ring. A controlled experiment was run: in one, hibernin was extracted using the normal plastic tubes of the lab; in the other, no plastic tubes were used. In the former, plenty of hibernin, in the latter none. The hibernin was nothing less than a chemical used in plastic tubing, and "you could buy our precious hormone by the barrel!" Bigelow later said.[27] They had used the same tubing over and over to save money. The draft papers never, of course, went out, and a horrible scientific embarrassment was averted. "Mother nature does not release her secrets without a struggle, and thus far we have been unable to open this door," Bigelow said.[28]

There was much bitterness in the lab. Almost ten years of research was down the drain. The groundhog farm was dismantled. Al Trimble, who had driven the research forward from the early days, was, as Goldman later said, "livid about the failure of Hibernin and the realization that it actually came from his overused IV tubing; he would come to the lab after the OR and verbally assault and abuse the lab-techs – and especially Goldman, the 'kike,' who destroyed his reputation."[29] (For more on the anti-Semitism of the era, see chapter 9.)

What of value came of the hibernin fiasco? Bigelow had required the nine or ten residents and fellows who trained with him to do a stint in the lab in the basement of the Banting Building in this fruitless search for "the secret of hibernation," as Goldman said. "It was a futile attempt in the long-term but it taught us all the basics of research."[30]

Bigelow as a Person

Bigelow had a distinctive gait, as Scully put it, "a way of ambling along that was different. Sort of sideways." His residents called it "the Brandon Shuffle." Goldman said, "There was a certain … It was not forward totally. It was kind of sideways."[31]

Bigelow was frank. Saying it outright may have been a characteristic of Canadians of his generation, who liked to think of themselves as plainspoken, but Bigelow was capable of an almost brutal frankness, whether assessing colleagues, residents, or former secretaries. (In his letter in 1950 on behalf of a former secretary, there is a hint of his mother's Scottish Presbyterian moralism as he commented on her personal life.) Was he ambitious? Not really. Or at least not ambitious to rise within medicine. In 1966 a search committee asked him if he was interested in being considered a candidate for dean. Not at all, he said. "Actually, I possess neither the ability nor the desire to do that type of work."[32] But he *was* ambitious for the Toronto General Hospital and its Cardiovascular Division, and wanted the General to become one of the world's great hospitals and his own service to rank in the senior class. (It was therefore, for Bigelow, a continual exasperation that American scribes consistently omitted Canadian contributions from their chronicles – see chapter 7.)

Bigelow was not a "titan" but a modest man. He was not puffed up about himself, though others in his shoes might have been. On 17 February 1967, at the first meeting of "the Bigelow Club" of alumni at a surgery meeting in New York, Bigelow put an end to this "Bigelow Club" nonsense. He later told Dick Weisel, "I felt uncomfortable with the name because of the major role of Bill Mustard, Don Wilson etc in training so I wrote the president George Trusler and asked that the name be changed to the Toronto Club."[33] Trusler was Bigelow's former student and an important cardiac surgeon at the Children's Hospital. Bigelow did not want the kind of idolatry that the previous professor of surgery, William Gallie, had received with the "Gallie Club."

Even though Bigelow talked often of his "boys," and of surgeon colleagues as "men," he was not one of those "half gods in white coats" who treated non-MDs as inferior creatures. Scully said of those days, "When we had Friday morning rounds, he would invite input from the nurses, from the residents, from the senior orderly in terms of what the traffic flow was like and whether it could be better. It was an open process, and though the buck stopped with him at the end of the day, he invited opinion openly."[34]

If there were one word that was key to unlocking Bigelow's personality, it would be humility. He said, "After years of the study of creativity I believe the single most important factor is 'intellectual humility.' It is a sissy word with a religious connotation but it carries a powerful message." He defined it as "an open-mindedness which is acquired by an understanding of the meager state of our knowledge in relation to the vastness and elusiveness of the ultimate truth. [Such humility requires] a special breed of scientist. This special breed of scientist, including the present company, usually 'hangs loose' and 'laughs and chuckles a lot.'" His 1969 paper, "Intellectual Humility in Medical Practice and Research," became an almost instant classic.[35]

Many were struck by Bigelow's modesty and absence of posturing. At his death in 2005 one correspondent wrote, "I met Wilfred Bigelow as a third-year medical student. I could not believe that this kind, soft-spoken, intelligent gentleman would not only have the time for undergraduates but also treat them with respect and courtesy – it did not seem possible that this was the man who had made open-heart surgery possible."[36] Bryce Taylor, later chief of surgery, remembered interning in a rotation with Bigelow: "I was helping Bill Bigelow stick his index finger through toasty mitral valves [stenosis]. The coolest guy I have ever worked with. I never saw him raise his voice, never saw him phased. He was the kind of character that could build something just by the force of his character."[37]

Scully, who was present at this interview with Taylor, said, "Just to reinforce that, never getting phased. I was getting upset on a case, and he put his instruments down, reached out, and tapped me on the glove and said, 'Scully, settle down, we'll be fine.' [laughter]."

In resident Bernie Goldman's judgment, "Bigelow cautioned me to approach the wonders of our field and the accompanying respect and adulation it created with a degree of humility."[38] Wayne Johnston, who did a rotation with Bigelow in cardiovascular surgery in the context of the general surgery program, said that Bigelow taught him how to "talk to a patient. 'Remember, you know, it's a huge day for the patient.' Either doing the consent or giving them some bad news, whatever you're going to give them, 'always be sure that you go and sit down.'"[39]

Goldman recalled, "We used to operate on a lot of patients from way up north or Newfoundland. Bigelow always reminded us of the anxious family back home awaiting news. We were instructed always to call the local GP and ask him to relay info to the outlying family."[40]

Said Bigelow on the need for humanity in dealing with patients, "I may be out of date, but I feel that in modern medical practice there are too many doctors who appear to pay insufficient attention to the patient as a psycho-social entity. There is insufficient caring, compassion, and inadequate communication."[41]

Bigelow put these principles into practice. Wilbert Keon, later a distinguished Ottawa heart surgeon, had trained with Bigelow and recalled him on the wards: "To him, a heart operation was not just a technical undertaking – it was an interface with patients of enormous consequences to them ... When preparing for new procedures, his preparation was meticulous. He emphasized [to us residents] that these undertakings would have enormous potential for progress and good, but must be tempered with the awesome responsibility to avoid harm to a patient."[42] The cardiac surgeons were highly mindful of the need to avoid harm, as their patients – especially in the early days – regularly died under their eyes on the table. Some coped by pacing the corridor, smoking, and taking Valium. Some took to alcohol, and there are whispered stories of the surgeons who drank at night. Bigelow did none of these things.

For a scientist, Bigelow was surprisingly open-minded about what might be called paranormal experiences. This anecdote begins with Hugh Scully in the operating room. "The patient is not doing well, and I was aware of that, the anesthetist was losing interest, and the resident was – when is this going to be over. And the perfusionist wasn't paying a lot of attention." But Scully wasn't about to give up, he tried a few things, and "we turned it around, all of a sudden the patient started to get much better. Just like a switch." Scully talked to the patient subsequently.

"I want to tell you something," said the patient. "I was watching what you were doing."

Scully asked, "What do you mean?"

The patient said, "Well, you have a gallery in your operating room. And I was up there watching what you were doing." The patient identified exactly who was there.

Scully went on: "The patient said that, 'where people seemed to give up, you didn't give up. I decided that I had a decision. You hear about the blue light? Off in the edge of the gallery there was this very soft music and a blue light. Very attractive, but you didn't give up, so I decided to come back.'"

Scully continued, "So that was the switch in the operation, I took that to Bigelow. He said, 'Hugh, I've seen that a number of times.'"[43]

Chapter Three

"Bigelow's Boys"

Motto: "They were not all giants, nor heroes nor great researchers. Many were simply dedicated, talented, innovative, and resourceful clinicians who worked long hours as they perfected their craft in a rapidly evolving field ... Most had the courage and tenacity to create a rapidly expanding new discipline, despite the challenges of ... disappointing early results and often reluctant support."[1]

– Bernie Goldman, 2005

Bigelow's students were invariably referred to as "Bigelow's boys." This is in contrast to colleagues elsewhere, who were always called "men." There were at the time no female heart surgeons, and the usage, though grating, is understandable.

For the young men grouped around Bigelow in these founding years of cardiac surgery, so intense was the excitement that the division out-published the entire Department of Surgery. In the years from 1956 to 1965, of the 197 publications of surgeons at the General, 36 per cent (61 articles) came from the Cardiovascular Division. (The next runner-up was General Surgery, with 50 articles.)[2] Entering the 1960s, a series of technical innovations took place that made cardiac surgery swifter and safer. The baton had now started to pass to Bigelow's students, such as Hugh Scully and Al Trimble.

Al Trimble

Born in 1932, Alan Trimble grew up in the Toronto suburb of Scarborough; he earned an MD degree from the University of Toronto in 1956, interned at the General, and worked as a research fellow in the Department of Surgery from 1959 to 1961. By 1963 he completed his residency in surgery, was a R.S. McLaughlin Travelling Fellow, then in

1964 joined the Division of Cardiovascular Surgery as an assistant surgeon, filling the slot that Baird had just vacated with his departure for the Western; Trimble was also a research associate of the Ontario Heart Foundation, with a salary of $9,500 paid for by the foundation, making him "full time."[3]

As he joined the staff at the General, Trimble was given charge of the cardiovascular laboratory in the basement of the Banting Building. In 1964, while still a senior resident, Trimble was lead author of a paper co-written with Bigelow and Heimbecker on the experiences in Toronto with the implantable cardiac pacemaker.[4] At this time, plans for transplant were being bruited, and Trimble was tasked with "bringing the Toronto centre up to date." He went down to Mississippi to study with James Hardy, who had, unsuccessfully, attempted an early transplant. Trimble then went on to Palo Alto, California, where Norman Shumway was founding cardiac transplantation in North America.[5] In July 1968 Bigelow made Trimble director of "the laboratory."[6]

Hugh Scully's recollection of Trimble was that "as a young resident and staff surgeon, I learned more about anticipating and staying out of trouble in the operating room from Alan Trimble than from anyone else."[7]

Goldman's recollections of Trimble are generous: "[He] was a superb resident: tireless, intelligent, creative, technically gifted and devoted not only to his patients but also to his mentor, Dr. Bill Bigelow ... I was in Bigelow's Bungalow [the Cardiovascular Investigation Unit] on a cardiology rotation and saw first-hand Trimble's remarkable productivity. After long days in the OR he would return to his office, working with pencil on large clinical spreadsheets, with smoke curling up from endless cigarettes and inevitable nips of scotch and vodka." Goldman said, "Those were heady days for the division and entirely sparked by Trimble's innovations and dedication." Goldman saw a "father-to-son air" in Bigelow's relationship to Trimble and says that Trimble, "dominated cardiovascular surgery in the city ... He was the Tirone David of the TGH in the latter 1960s and 1970s."[8]

Trimble's further contributions will be noted in due course.

Bernard Goldman

Bernard S. Goldman, universally known as "Bernie," was born in Toronto in 1936 and took most of his training there. He graduated MD in 1960 as the silver medalist of his class and finished his postgraduate training in cardiovascular surgery in June 1967. Goldman had "star" written all over him. In 1960 Bigelow told Fred Kergin, "I have seen Doctor B.S. Goldman who is currently interning at Mount Sinai. He is an A.O.A. [Alpha Omega Alpha, the medical honour society], and expresses an interest in cardiovascular surgery. I would be glad to take him on in our laboratory in research although interestingly enough he is allergic to animals, particularly dogs. He is going to investigate his allergy in the next few months. Perhaps the hibernation research would be better than doing pump work."[9] Out of his experience with hibernation research in the basement of the Banting Building, Goldman got in 1962 a bachelor of science, writing a thesis, "Studies in Hypothermia with Special Reference to Natural Hibernation."

The "hibernin" research, as we know, was a bust. Yet it launched Goldman's research career, and by 1972 his bibliography had grown to thirty entries.

As a resident, Goldman lodged at the General and was given a room there as well (and his unhappiness is a reminder of what it meant to be a trainee then): In January 1966 he wrote the assistant medical director of the hospital that he could live with the intense heat of the uncontrolled radiators, the dust, and the "peeling paint and filthy walls. What I am getting a little peeved about is the fact that I can barely see in my room, because it is so dark and dingy. The light in the bathroom works intermittently and continually blows out the bulbs. The light over the dresser also does not work, making it somewhat difficult to shave in the morning." All told, "these are my living quarters, inadequate that they may be, and unhappy as I am to live in them ... All I am asking is that I have some light."[10] This is a reminder that there is a hierarchy of prestige in cardiac surgery: at the bottom are trainees such as Goldman; at the top the grand barons who are so powerful that a mere word from them can hold the trains at the station for an hour or so.

Goldman trained briefly abroad, at Bristol in lung surgery with Ronald Belsey and at the Massachusetts General Hospital with Gerald Austen, after which he returned for what normally would have been a layover until receiving a provincial posting. In 1967 Bigelow told John Hamilton, vice-president of Health Sciences, that Goldman would be returning from Bristol, "and is about to take up a 'temporary staff appointment of one to three years [here], which is a maturing period and will fit him for a senior cv surgical post in some other university.' We need to finance this."[11]

But Goldman was never shipped out. The story is this: Bigelow had wanted Goldman to go to Queen's, a prospect in which Goldman had zero interest. What prompted Bigelow to think of placing Goldman at Queen's is unclear, because Bigelow had quite a high opinion of Goldman. After Goldman had worked for Bigelow a bit at the lab in the Banting, in July 1962 Bigelow wrote to Ian Macdonald, who was the surgeon-in-chief at the Wellesley Hospital: "Of the eighteen or twenty bright young men that have gone through my hands in the research laboratory, he is one of the brightest and most gifted I have encountered." Bigelow noted a "beautifully organized mind," and said that Goldman would do well in his general surgery rotation at the Wellesley.[12] (The backstory is that Bigelow felt the need to extract Goldman from his first clinical rotation in cardiovascular surgery, under Al Trimble, where Trimble, furious that Goldman had identified the real composition of "hibernin," was berating him with anti-Semitic tirades.[13])

Yet there was a catch. "Bigelow said I had to follow the Bell Canada Concept of going away," said Goldman, "making my name away, and then coming back to the Big House, which was an interesting concept. I didn't really know what to do. Herb Basian and I talked about [Doctors' Hospital], about the last place I wanted to go [a community hospital on College Street with enormous business]. So I spoke to Bruce Tovee [university chair of general surgery], who, like everyone, I thought of as a personal mentor. Then he asked me about my research, teaching, my results, etc., and he was satisfied. He told me he was going to go speak to R.A. Mustard [head of surgery at the General] because Bigelow had a meeting scheduled with Mustard. He said, 'I'm going to tell him [Mustard] that if Bigelow doesn't want you then I'd like you to come and start vascular surgery on Ward A.'"

Q: And did that force Bigelow's hand then?

GOLDMAN: Sure, because if you lose portal cavals [shunts around the liver], it was just a fraction of what we did; but to lose vascular surgery – I mean, we were doing amputations that orthopods should have done. We were a full and busy vascular service at that time, and general surgery wanted to pare or hive vascular from cardiovascular.

Q: So setting you up in Ward A as a vascular surgeon would have meant the loss of all that business for the division. So that's why Bigelow collapsed. That's very interesting.

BERNIE LANGER: That's the first time I've heard that story.[14]

In 1972 Goldman became assistant professor of surgery at the University of Toronto and staff surgeon, Division of Cardiovascular Surgery at the General (he had an appointment at the Mount Sinai Hospital as well). All academic hospital staff had dual appointments at the University and at the Hospital.

In the late 1980s a waiting-list crisis was brewing. Community cardiologists, said Goldman, "had every expectation that their patients would have timely and appropriate access to revascularization surgery [bypass]." But the funding wasn't there. With the death of a waiting-list patient at St. Michael's Hospital whose surgery had been postponed numerous times, the province finally acted and established in 1988 the Metropolitan Toronto Triage and Registry Program (later the Cardiac Care Network of Ontario), of which Goldman and Ron Baigrie were co-chairs. Goldman said that it gave physicians, for the first time, a single number to call to get cardiac care for their patients.[15]

In 1989 Goldman moved to Sunnybrook Hospital. Baird said, in 1980, "Jim Key resigned his longstanding role as cardiac surgery consultant at Sunnybrook and [Key] asked Goldman to assume that position." There had been talk in the 1970s about opening a heart surgery centre at Sunnybrook, but Bigelow had opposed it, Baird said, "for the obvious reason that it would significantly impinge on the TGH referrals and volumes." But Bigelow retired in 1977. Thus, Goldman worked as a cardiovascular consultant at Sunnybrook during the 1980s. He said, "I came [to Sunnybrook] weekly to review cases presented by their active cardiology and catheter lab and brought them back to TGH to distribute among the CV staff." Goldman then headed the cardiovascular surgery unit that officially opened at Sunnybrook on 27 November 1989. "Goldman took with him 2 exceptional residents from TGH ... Stephen Fremes and George Christakis." Baird was very supportive.[16]

Thus, Goldman was in charge when in June 1994 a journalist was given several weeks of access to the service. He wrote, "No one in the [operating] room is more conscious of medicine's tacit assumption of divine function than the chief surgeon. Dr. Goldman is an unlikely gift to his staff, an eminent man who enjoys his underlying earthiness, sometimes reveling in blunt talk (he is unafraid of profanity) and a theatrical sense of humour." The staff said that Goldman definitely did not have the characteristic "God-complex" of a cardiac surgeon.[17]

Wilbert Keon

Willie Keon, who became a distinguished cardiac surgeon in Ottawa, trained in Toronto under Bigelow and died in April 2019, just as this text was being completed. Bernie Goldman contributed the following:

There has always been a sense of rivalry between the Departments of Surgery at McGill and the University of Toronto. So there was heightened anticipation among those of us training with pioneer heart surgeon Dr. Wilfred (Bill) Bigelow at Toronto General Hospital, concerning the impending arrival of a storied McGill surgical resident named Willie Keon. Was he really as good a surgeon as his cousin Dave Keon was at hockey?

The story that preceded Willie's arrival 1 July 1966 was that as a senior general surgery resident in Montreal, he had expeditiously taken a critically ill trauma victim to the OR without a supervising staff man present, and expertly repaired his torn liver, thereby saving his life. In appreciation the grateful patient had given young Willie a Ford Thunderbird automobile. Thus there was a certain sense of awe, perhaps even a degree of tension, as we awaited this surgical superstar, as Bigelow's next resident. I had just completed my time with "Uncle Bill" and had moved up to the next training level at the Hospital for Sick Children across the road. However, as often happens, fate intervened: a week or so into Willie's first clinical experiences with Bigelow, a postoperative patient needed a tracheotomy, a rather standard procedure. Willie was all set when Bigelow hesitated – and then told him to get me to come back over, perform the tracheotomy, and demonstrate "the Toronto method." Needless to say, Willie was taken aback, and the both of us were feeling a trifle embarrassed. But residents did not argue with their chiefs, and I must admit a frisson of glee did pass through me as I dutifully showed Willie "our way."

The rest is history. Willie Keon was a superb resident, energetic, a skilful surgeon, and a delight to know and work with. We later both went to Boston on overlapping rotations at different Harvard hospitals. I returned to Toronto General to work my way up the academic ladder, and Willie went and founded the University of Ottawa Heart Institute early in his career.

We were colleagues and friends throughout our respective careers. His contributions to Canada as a heart surgeon, teacher, researcher, mentor, administrator, and later as a senator were immense, and his legacy is outstanding.

Hugh Scully

Hugh Scully, born in Windsor, Ontario, in 1940, and grew up in Ottawa and Europe. His father (having been denied support to train as a physician by *his* father) was with the federal Department of Trade and Commerce after serving in the Royal Canadian Navy for five years during the Second World War. His mother worked for many years in the Department of Nutrition at the Ottawa Civic Hospital.

At around the age of fourteen, Scully decided that he wanted to become a doctor. Dr. Howard Hamlin, the father of a good friend, was an inspiring role model. "I liked to work with my hands, so I decided to become a surgeon."[18] He went to Queen's University rather than Toronto because he would have had to live with his grandparents in Toronto (and his grandfather was as disapproving of his grandson's career choice as he had been with his own son). Scully graduated from Queen's with a BA (1961), MD (Silver Medalist – 1965), and MSc (1967).

At one point, Scully and his brothers attended a French community school (La Celle St. Cloud) not far from Versailles. He passed the high school qualifying exams with honours. "The Entrée à Lycée written, oral, and physical education exams were more comprehensive than any I took for the rest of my education." He then attended the exceptional private American Community School in the Bois de Boulogne in Paris, and spent a term at the International School of Geneva (50/50 English and French), where, like former Premier Bob Rae, he was president of the International High School; his education was completed at Fisher Park High School in Ottawa.

Lest anyone think that Scully was just a bit too "fine" for medicine in Toronto, in addition to Cancer Society summer fellowships, he did work for three summers as a labourer in heavy construction in Labrador, "driving a cab after finishing shift work." About half the workers were French Canadian and half Newfoundlanders. The local First Nations people spoke French. Scully later said, "Because I spoke both English and French, I got along well with everybody. Between my regular and overtime salary working construction and cab fares with generous tips I was able to cover almost all of my expenses at Queen's. I must say that having grown up internationally, that experience living in crowded bunkhouses and working from ten to fourteen hours every day with men and local people, most of whom had, at best, grade school education, familiarized me with a whole sector of society that I had never known. It was simply invaluable in terms of my practice. I could talk and empathize with anybody at any level of society."[19]

Scully interned at TGH from 1965 to 1966. Having initially been accepted into the neurosurgery program at University of Toronto, at the recommendation of Tom Morley, professor of neurosurgery, he returned to Queen's from 1966 to 1967 to complete an MSc in neuroanatomy and neurophysiology under John Basmajian. However, during a later rotation on cardiovascular surgery as an intern at TGH in 1966, he was captivated by the dynamism of the specialty and switched to general surgery, to be followed by cardiovascular-thoracic surgery. "Bernie Goldman is significantly responsible for my change of heart, along with Bill Bigelow, Jim Key, Ray Heimbecker, and Al Trimble."

At that time, with the Royal College of Surgeons of Canada and the Department of Surgery at the university, one had to complete training in general surgery before going on to train in cardiovascular and thoracic (CVT) surgery. Scully completed his general surgery training in 1970, became a fellow of the Royal College (FRCSC, General Surgery), and entered the CVT program.

Bigelow wanted Scully to get additional training in cardiovascular physiology. Arrangements were made for him to spend two years at Harvard and the Massachusetts General Hospital (MGH) under the direction of Gerald Austen, professor and university chair of surgery at Harvard, surgeon-in-chief at the MGH, and research supervision of Bill Daggett.

Scully was awarded a Canadian Centennial Fellowship and received additional support from the Cardiovascular Division at TGH. With the signed agreement of Bill Drucker (University chair of surgery), Robert Mustard (surgeon-in-chief at TGH), and Bigelow, it was agreed that Scully would return to Toronto to complete the final senior residencies in CVT surgery from 1972 to 1973 at HSC with Bill Mustard and George Trusler in pediatric cardiac surgery and at TGH with Griff Pearson in thoracic surgery. His final year as senior resident was planned for the adult cardiovascular unit at TGH from 1973 to 1974.

Thereafter, performance proving satisfactory, he was to be appointed to the staff of TGH as a CVT surgeon and to the University Department of Surgery.

In October of 1973, Scully made an appointment with Dr. Bigelow to confirm the earlier arrangements for his joining the staff of the division in July of 1974.

Bigelow said, "Hugh, I don't have a position for you in July. Those arrangements before were really to secure your Centennial fellowship. Maybe I can secure a position for you in a year or two in Saskatchewan ..." (The awarding of a Centennial fellowship was dependent on written confirmation of a staff appointment at the hospital and university.)

Scully remembers, "I was devastated ... especially as I had turned down an offer from Dr. Austen to become chief resident in cardiac surgery at the MGH the year following my time there, and then to join his staff and Harvard.

"The next day, I called Gerry Austen and related my dilemma. He immediately invited me to come to Boston, have dinner with him on a Friday night in the fine hotel that had been booked and paid for by his executive assistant, Connie Martino, and meet with him privately in his office at the hospital on Saturday afternoon.

"During our conversation in his office, he again offered me a position at the MGH (but now delayed by two years with an interim position at a MGH referral hospital). He also presented what he was confident would be assured positions at universities and hospitals in Chicago, San Francisco, San Diego, and New York.

"Dr. Austen said, 'Hugh, there would be no problem securing these positions, but my sense is that you are a committed Canadian.' (We would meet frequently to discuss our respective healthcare systems and physician human resources ... more than my lab research!)

"He continued, saying, 'My suggestion is that you go back to Dr. Bigelow and seek his advice and support as you consider any of these opportunities in the United States.'"

So Scully returned to Toronto and made another appointment with Dr. Bigelow:

BIGELOW: Hugh, we met two weeks ago ... what's new?

SCULLY: Yes, sir ... and you said that you do not have a position for me in July.

BIGELOW: I still do not ...

SCULLY: Sir, I went to Boston last weekend and had a good meeting with Dr. Austen.

BIGELOW: You did *what*?

SCULLY (OPENING A FILE FOLDER WITH INFORMATION ABOUT AMERICAN OPPORTUNITIES): Sir, these are positions in the US that he is confident that he could secure for me in July. I would appreciate your advice and assistance in making a good choice ...

BIGELOW (VERY AGITATED): Scully, you are NOT going to the States or anywhere else!

Dr. Bigelow called an urgent staff meeting that evening. He called me at 7:00 the next morning: "Okay Scully ... Hugh ... We would like you to join our staff in July, on condition that you pass your CVT Fellowship written and oral exams in the fall."

Scully joined the staff of the Division of Cardiovascular Surgery at TGH and the Department of Surgery at the university on 1 July 1974.

He passed the fellowship exams in CVT surgery (FRCSC, CVT, 1974).

At the MGH, while doing research on atrio-ventricular synchrony and teaching Harvard medical students, Scully got involved with Bob Leinbach and Chip Gold with the cardiac assist intra-aortic balloon pump program that they were initiating. Bernie Goldman, when he had spent some time earlier at the MGH, had also been exposed to this promising new program to support ischemic or failing hearts.

Scully and Goldman were lifelong friends, comparable to the friendship between Bigelow and Jim Key. Scully said, "The two of us had a reputation for being more calm than agitated during a crisis. Both of us sort of stopped talking and asked everyone to focus.

"The other thing that's important as I was starting out was that if I got into a situation I didn't recognize, I never hesitated to ask for help. I'd ask Bernie to come in or call Al Trimble for advice."[20]

It was a modest comment, born of a long friendship. But at the level of Canadian medicine as a whole, it was Scully who would be called in, and one writer suggested that Scully might be deemed "the Dr. Fix-it of Canadian medical care."[21]

On the friendship between Hugh and Bernie, Dr. Goldman contributes the following. The two surgeons have been colleagues and friends since training in the mid- 1960s: indeed Bernie, as senior cardiac surgical resident in 1965, suggested that Hugh, the junior intern, switch from neurosurgery to cardiovascular. Each became well known for their respective skills and contributions. Hugh married Vanessa Harwood, principal ballerina of the National Ballet of Canada, and Bernie married the lovely Fran, daughter of the Loblaws president, while his own father became president of Shoppers Drug Mart. Fran and Bernie went to New York to see Vanessa dance with Nureyev. Thus they each enjoyed a degree of social prominence combined with recognition in their careers.

Hugh became known "for his excellence in redo valve surgery" as Tirone David put it. He became expert in the saga of failing Björk-Shiley tilting disc mechanical valves. (The story about the failing Shiley valves and the model of the bileaflet St. Jude mechanical valve with the toxic silver-impregnated sewing ring is told in chapter 13.)

Bernie was a particularly skilled coronary surgeon and world leader in pacemaker surgery. Early in their careers, Bernie and Hugh had worked together to bring the intra-aortic balloon pump assist to Toronto for patients with unstable angina or post-op left ventricular failure. They were both recognized as superb, compassionate clinicians, teachers, and mentors, particularly in the OR.

Bernie was very successful academically. His leadership potential was recognized as he left TGH to establish a highly successful new cardiac surgical division in the Department of Surgery at Sunnybrook Health Sciences Centre. He served as chair of the Medical Advisory Committee, and was then selected as surgeon-in-chief at this important teaching hospital. He was the second president (and first Canadian one) of the North American Society of Cardiac Pacing and Electrophysiology during the late 1970s and early '80s.

From 2001 to 2011, Bernie was chair of Save a Child's Heart Canada, a UN-sponsored Israeli NGO that has sponsored heart surgery for more that five thousand needy children from sixty-two countries in the developing world, more than 50 per cent of these Muslims from various Arab countries. He has received numerous teaching awards from the University Department of Surgery, the Division of Cardiovascular Surgery, and the Canadian Society of Cardiac Surgeons. In recognition of his many contributions to cardiovascular health in Canada and internationally, Bernie was awarded the Order of Canada in 2010.

Hugh pursued his interests in leadership and professional activism in medicine at local, provincial, national, and international levels (along with his passion for motorsport; see the section "The Story Continues" in chapter 24). While training in general surgery in 1968 and 1969 he was founding president of the Professional Association of Interns and Residents of Ontario. Representing all doctors in postgraduate training in Ontario in negotiations with the Ontario Hospital Services Commission, he and his team secured the template contract model used to this day to determine reasonable work and on-call duty hours, protected personal time, and adequate salary support. This contract model was quickly adopted by all the other provinces.

At the time, it was certainly true that some academic-physician leaders (and the Ontario Medical Association [OMA]) expressed the opinion that "this radical young resident" should be fired. However, with the support of the dean and chair of surgery at the university, the surgeons-in-chief and heads of general surgery at both TGH and TWH, Bill Bigelow and Ron Baird, he was able to persevere. It must be said that this venture could not have succeeded without the many extra hours of work carried out on his behalf by his extraordinarily talented – and tolerant – assistant resident, Bryce Taylor. Equally important was the generous understanding of his then-wife, Anne Johnston, during these time-consuming additions to his already busy duty schedule away from home.

In 1982, in negotiations on behalf of the OMA (representing all physicians in the province), Scully again militated successfully against the provincial government for a pay increase. In July 1987 he was elected president of the OMA amid a fierce battle over "extra billing" and withdrawal of elective services. Not generally known is that he effectively terminated the strike when some physicians began to advocate for limiting hospital emergency services, including teaching hospitals such as TGH.

Scully was chair of the TGH Medical Advisory Committee (Chief of Staff) as well as deputy surgeon-in-chief and deputy head of cardiovascular surgery during the stressful merger of the Toronto General and Toronto Western hospitals in the late 1980s. While there had been agreement by the boards and leaders of both institutions, there had *not* been adequate information shared at the level of leadership that would have to make it work.

This experience was followed by numerous elected positions in national and international bodies including the Canadian Medical Association (president from 1999 to 2000), the Canadian Cardiovascular Society (president from 1998 to 2000), and the Royal College of Physicians and Surgeons of Canada (RCPSC) (council member from 1994 to 2002). As a board member of the World Medical Association (2001 to 2003) he chaired the committee that created the Ethical Recruitment of International Medical Graduates guidelines, later adopted by the World Health Organization. Between 1998 and 2008 he co-chaired the national multidisciplinary task forces that made recommendations to reverse the net loss migration of Canadian physicians to the United States and developed guidelines for physician human resources that remain relevant today.

Scully was governor of the American College of Surgeons (ACS) (2008 to 2013), representing the RCPSC. Between 2009 and 2015 he was the only non-American ever appointed to the ACS's elite Health Policy Advisory Group in Washington during the intense debates about "Obamacare."

It must be said that Scully's political activism was not typical for an academic surgeon. Much of what he did has never been carried out by any other physician, let alone a surgeon, from UHN-TGH. John Wedge, when university chair of surgery (and grandson of Emmett Hall of Hall Report fame) was supportive, and later said "Hugh, I think it's fair to say that you were not exactly encouraged." Very true about some colleagues, but many others have been very helpful.

Both Hugh and Bernie suffered significant personal crises at different times in their careers. Having completed a successful double heart valve "redo" on a Thursday afternoon in 2001, Hugh awoke the next morning virtually unable to use his hands, a terrifying nightmare for any surgeon. Guillain-Barré syndrome was the diagnosis, unusually concentrated bilaterally, affecting C-5, 6, and 7 of the brachial plexus. Motor-nerve conduction velocity was diminished to 12 per cent of normal on the left and only 8 per cent on the right – and Scully is right-handed!

Functional recovery was very doubtful. Leading neurologist Vera Brill said, "We have rarely seen complete recovery from such severe ulnar and median nerve compromise."

Scully replied, "Don't tell someone who works with their hands that they cannot make it back."

Brill later said, "You were so stubborn and determined that you would not give up!"

Over twenty-eight months, with the dedicated help and support of his wife, Vanessa, and family, various colleagues at UHN and the university, and expert professional advice from colleagues in the world of motorsport, he regained 98 per cent function and returned to full complicated cardiac surgical practice. Lynn Koven, the administrative director of the Cardiovascular Division at TGH at the time, was of great assistance in sorting out the frustrating maze of arrangements for disability insurance.[22]

Bernie's father suffered a cardiac arrest in the cardiovascular investigation unit (Bigelow's Bungalow) after cardiac catheterization / angiography in 1980. Heroic attempts at resuscitation, including emergency coronary bypass surgery by Tirone David, were not successful. He had suffered major brain damage and languished in the intensive care unit for weeks, ultimately dying at age sixty-nine. An inquiry revealed serious errors in his clinical management. Bernie and his family suffered greatly from the tragedy of his father's untimely death. This may have been partly responsible for his move to Sunnybrook Hospital a few years later.

Thus, these two surgeons, colleagues and friends, who had clinical and personal lives that contributed to their social and professional standings, were the obvious choices for the collaboration on the history of cardiac surgery at the Toronto General Hospital, a project suggested and funded by Scully.

Not Students but Early Colleagues

Two other surgeons were not really students of Bigelow's yet worked alongside him in the early days: Ray Heimbecker and Jim Key.

Raymond O. Heimbecker

Ray Heimbecker was Murray's student, virtually his only one. Heimbecker served as an intern to Murray during 1952 and 1953, then continued under Bigelow. In March 1953 Heimbecker wrote Murray, "I want to thank you again for the wonderful year I spent with you. It was certainly the most stimulating and instructive year I have had – or could ever hope to have."[23]

In 1952 or 1953 at their annual banquet, the interns composed a song in honour of Murray – who was present – to the tune of "Waltzing Matilda":

> Dissecting with Murray, dissecting with Murray
> You'll come dissecting with Murray and me.

And we'll laugh and we'll cheer with unadulterated glee
As he does another commissurotomy.

Heimbecker recalled that Murray "enjoyed it very much."[24]

Then Heimbecker segued smoothly to the Bigelow regime and became Bigelow's most important early collaborator. After Heimbecker left Toronto for the University of Western Ontario in 1974, he achieved fame independently by performing Canada's first successful heart transplant with the immunosuppressant drug cyclosporine.

Born in Calgary in 1922, Heimbecker earned a bachelor's degree from the University of Saskatchewan in 1944 and an MD from the University of Toronto in 1947, just as Bigelow was returning from Johns Hopkins. After training in cardiac and vascular surgery in Toronto – and after a stint with Blalock at Johns Hopkins – in 1955 Heimbecker joined the Department of Surgery as its first "full-time member"; his salary was paid by the Ontario Heart Foundation. Simultaneously he attained the rank of clinical teacher in the Department of Surgery (university post) and assistant surgeon in the General (hospital post). In the Cardiovascular Division he worked mainly with cardiologist Ramsay Gunton in the investigation unit, and participated in all the big innovations on the surgical side. From 1950 on, he and Bigelow collaborated on the clumping together of red blood cells (sludging, intravascular agglutination) in traumatic shock, and "sludging" became an important Toronto research achievement.[25]

In 1959 Heimbecker introduced a "heat exchanger" to the heart-lung bypass circuit (extracorporeal support for open-heart surgery) that would rapidly cool the patient's body, and by cooling the blood pumped into the heart, stop the beating of the heart so that open-heart surgery could begin on a stilled organ. The heat exchanger then rewarmed the patient at the end of the operation. (He is said to have begun this research around 1955 by drilling holes into his wife's pressure cooker.) Previously, ice packs had required hours to cool the patient's body, rather than minutes with the heat exchanger.[26]

But Heimbecker's heart belonged to Murray. When in 1947 Murray published an article on exactly what went wrong in the heart in coronary thrombosis, he thanked Heimbecker for the photography.[27] Surprisingly, the article made no impact on the field. Nobody tried excising the area of myocardium damaged in an infarct, despite the availability of hypothermia.

Nobody except Heimbecker, now a mature and highly innovative surgeon, twenty years later. Heimbecker followed Murray in other ways as well. In 1960, seven years after Murray's retirement, Murray and Heimbecker described an instrument for removing emboli (embo-lectomy).[28] Murray had already done twenty of them.[29] The extent to which Heimbecker was Murray's "best student" has probably been overlooked, so keen have people been to see Murray as a lone wolf.

(Heimbecker's further contributions will be reviewed as we encoun-ter them chronologically.)

Heimbecker could be exasperating. Goldman said, "Ray was so dif-ferent from the rest – he mumbled, was reticent, somewhat secretive, committed to his external life – sailing gliders, farm in Collingwood, Georgian Bay, cottage, raised Cornish hens, etc."[30] Bigelow was very circumspect and he put in writing little direct criticism of Heimbecker. Yet his irritation shone through. Furious at a lack of progress in build-ing new space for experimental (animal) work in cardiovascular sur-gery, Bigelow composed in October 1961 an irate note to Fred Kergin, the aggressive chest surgeon known as "Fearless Fred" who was now the professor of surgery.[31] Some pokey committee had been appointed to draw up plans for an addition to the Banting Building. "I do not know who appointed the committee, but I understand you and Doctor Heimbecker are members." Really? He "understood" that Heimbecker was a member, rather than consulting closely with him? Bigelow then added that the committee had to be completely "revised": "Replace Doctor Heimbecker with Doctor Baird on this committee."[32] (Ron Baird was head of cardiac surgery at the General from 1977 to 1987.) This is not a ringing vote of confidence in Heimbecker. In July 1961, Bigelow asked that his name be removed from an article that Heimbecker had submitted to a journal. "If the journal asks why, say I didn't have that much to do with the writing." But the real reason is otherwise. "Ray, I do not agree with your premise that aortic valve surgery has a higher mortality rate simply because the patients are a poorer risk. There is another factor, and that is that it is a more difficult and complicated operative procedure and reflects to a degree the skill of the surgeon. [Thus it] reflects rather badly when I am writing an article with 2 deaths out of 11 for aortic insufficiency."[33]

It turned out there was another burr under the saddle in the Heim-becker relationship. Bigelow told Kergin he was furious that Heim-becker was making so much money, given that he was receiving a full-time salary from the Ontario Heart Foundation. In 1963 Bigelow had gone to the trouble of checking on Heimbecker's operations on private patients (where the patients paid the surgeon directly) and, as Kergin mentioned in a memo, "It is apparent that he [Heimbecker] is earning, in addition to his salary of $12,000, up to two or three times this amount. Dr. Bigelow thinks this is not proper."[34] The Heimbecker salary issue threatened to become a *cause célèbre*: Bigelow wanted Greenwood's Cardiovascular Committee to recommend a salary cut for Heimbecker. In a conversation with Heimbecker, Bigelow had asked him if he would accept a salary cut, and Heimbecker said no. In September 1963 Kergin minuted, "Dr. Bigelow states that even the St. Michael's people are beginning to complain about the amount of practice that Dr. Heimbecker is doing on a theoretically full-time support."[35]

There were other grumbles. One colleague said of Heimbecker, "He was the only man I ever knew in heart surgery that would finish a case and go off sailing down at the lake. Well, god bless him for sailing. But you know most of us lived in super anxiety in the first hours after any case." Under the circumstances, it is clear that there might have been several dry eyes in the house when Heimbecker left for the University of Western Ontario in 1974.

Yet Heimbecker was much beloved by patients, and at his passing in 2014, he was fondly remembered by some. Honor Nivin, a Toronto woman, recalled having had an atrial septal defect repaired, and a second surgery the next day for hemorrhage. "I vaguely remember Dr. Heimbecker coming to see me at my bedside and asking me if I had nail polish on my toes and finger nails. I was guilty of wearing a pearly white colour, which must have frustrated him, as he was doing a manual check to see how the blood was circulating in my hands and feet by checking the colour of my nails.

"I was very lucky to have had such wonderful pioneering cardio doctors helping me at the young age of 22."[36]

James A. Key

James Key was born in Dundee, Scotland in 1915, the youngest of three siblings (he had an older brother and sister). He attended George Watson School and graduated from medical school in Edinburgh, where he completed his postgraduate training in surgery. It was there that he met his wife, Mora Smeaton, who graduated in medicine. He joined the medical corps of the British Army from 1939 to 1945 and was stationed in North Africa, Italy and the Far East. On a hospital ship, he provided medical care to POWs in Singapore.

Key joined the Department of Surgery in Newcastle, England, in 1946. In 1949 he won a one-year Rockefeller fellowship to study medicine and surgery at Johns Hopkins in Baltimore, and in Canada in Montreal and Toronto, thereafter returning to Newcastle for two years.

In 1952 he was invited to return to Toronto to join the Department of Surgery at the university and the Toronto General Hospital. He thus emigrated to Toronto with his family, and the following year joined the new cardiovascular surgery group. Jim Key was Bigelow's first close collaborator and joined Ward C in 1953. The two men became fast personal friends. Like others, he got involved in research on hibernating groundhogs at the Banting Institute.

Jim Key was a wonderful and supportive teacher on the cardiovascular service until his retirement in 1980. Quite apart from his skill as a surgeon – or perhaps related to it – he was an accomplished concert pianist and possessed a mellow baritone singing voice.

He retired near Collingwood, serving as medical officer of health for Simcoe County for a number of years. He passed away in 1996.

While in Toronto he became known as a specialist in abdominal aortic aneurysms (AAAs)[37] and reported a series of 146, "all removed without a death," as Bigelow later said. In Key's follow-up study of these patients

- ten had celebrated a golden wedding anniversary;
- ten had celebrated a silver anniversary; and
- they would live to see the birth of fifty-nine grandchildren and thirteen great-grandchildren.

But Key also did open-heart procedures, exactly as all the other cardiac surgeons. For a Toronto *Telegram* reporter in 1968, the high point of watching a mitral-valve replacement came at 10:29: "Dr. Key turns his head towards the gallery. He looks directly at me. 'We're ready to slide the valve into the heart.' It disappears and I turn my eyes wet at the marvel of it." (The reporter had just had a valve replacement himself six months previously.)[38]

Key was not very productive as an academic but was loved by colleagues and the residents. Scully said, "Jim Key, Gentleman Jim. I think I only heard him swear once in the operating room in ten years. He was a wonderful teacher, a very, very competent technical surgeon, vascular surgeon, and cardiac surgeon, the important cardiac stuff. Fantastic with us. Showed us what to do. Helped us do it. Always there if we had a problem; he'd step away and say, 'Wait a minute. What are you going to do next?'"[39] Goldman added, "Jim was a slightly built, elegantly dressed man with the most beautiful long fingers. He was invariably polite, soft spoken, and *always* available to bail us out when in technical trouble in the OR."[40]

Key was a gifted pianist, a "concert-level pianist," as Scully said. He also sang beautifully. "He would invite us to his apartment on Prince Arthur Avenue, and we could go on for hours."

Key and Bigelow fished together, and their families holidayed together. "There was a perennial New Year's Eve party at our cabin on the Collingwood mountainside," said Bigelow, "where together with the Ted Dewars and Donald McKays [Toronto surgeons] we had a bonfire, skating, square dancing, fireworks, and much singing."[41]

Key will have been among the few Toronto surgeons who publicly celebrated the drinking of Scotch, telling the Canadian Health Forum in 1963, that four "S's" were essential to the preservation of cardiac health. One was no smoking. The other three were "plenty of salad, Scotch and sex."[42]

Chapter Four

Hypothermia Discovered

Kindling Interest in Hypothermia

The therapeutic induction of hypothermia was not unknown in medicine. At McLean Hospital, a psychiatric facility in a suburb of Boston, ten schizophrenia patients had been experimentally deep cooled (made "hypothermic") in the early 1940s. The patients were numbed with a barbiturate, then cooled with special refrigerator blankets. Four of the ten showed some improvement.[1] There is also a long history in Europe of treating "nervous" patients with "Priessnitz treatments" in cold-water spas.[2]

It is doubtful that Bigelow knew about any of this. His own interest in hypothermia arose when, around 1940 as a resident in surgery, he presented at rounds a case of frostbite that he had treated by amputating the fingers of "a young man from the Canadian Northwoods." He had read the literature and discovered how little attention frostbite had received. Bigelow said later, "I was very disturbed that we Canadians should know so little about frostbite."

Later, over coffee after rounds, Gallie said to Bigelow, "Why don't you pursue this?" Bigelow read more and learned that cold reduced metabolism.[3]

With this knowledge of cold, Bigelow went off to Europe as a staff surgeon with the Canadian Army Medical Corps. William Mustard, later a distinguished pediatric cardiac surgeon, was said to be his anesthetist. "Muss" and "Buss" they called each other.[4]

In London, Bigelow's thoughts turned again to hypothermia. "Whiling away the hours in Britain before the second front opened, I made some connection with a British refrigeration engineer and we designed the cabinet which was supposed to be mobile and could presumably be used to cool the lower extremity or the upper extremity of a wounded soldier and keep the tissue viable until they could have a revascularization procedure."[5] The War Office gave the contract to a British firm, and the machine was completed on V-J Day. "I think it weighed something like, well, the better part of a ton I would think. It certainly didn't look very mobile to me."

As well, while in France, he undertook to save some limbs from amputation and "was concerned about the fact that amputations were still being carried out for poor circulation or disruption of the femoral artery." So he made a few attempts to reconstruct damaged arteries, which were largely unsuccessful. At that point "these trials ... were interrupted by my recall to Toronto to act as Dr. Gallie's resident."

When Bigelow met Gallie in Britain, Gallie advised him to go into vascular surgery. Once back in Toronto, Gallie sent Bigelow down to Johns Hopkins Hospital, "[where I] became exposed to blind closed heart surgery; it was obvious that someone had to find a method of getting inside the heart to properly correct the lesions." At Hopkins, Bigelow ended up studying with the great cardiac surgeon Blalock but more, as we have seen, with Richard Bing, who was just introducing cardiac catheterization in humans. Bigelow said, "It was a fascinating six months that I spent with him. [Leroy D.] Vandam, who later has become very famous in anesthesia, and I watched the blue baby operations and we talked heart surgery and the frustrations of not being able to fix the blue baby and correct the ventricular septal defect. During the six months that I spent, I heard about [John H.] Gibbon with the heart-lung pump. And this may sound very dramatic, but in my little old rooming house near the hospital I woke up one night and the whole picture of hypothermia was very clear to me. You cool a body; you interrupt the circulation; and you get inside the heart."[6]

Bigelow said later, "The idea of cooling the body to reduce the oxygen requirements as a means of doing heart surgery occurred to me while engaged in some postgraduate cardiovascular training at Johns Hopkins after the war, and I could hardly wait to get back to the Banting Institute to put the theory to the test. It is interesting that, at this time, most of the scientific articles suggested that cooling the body actually increased the oxygen requirements."[7]

Operating on Dogs

Once back in Toronto, Bigelow went to work. "We used the cold room at the air force base on Avenue Road which could be manipulated down to 40°C below zero and our early experiments were carried out with the experimenters in flying suits and flying boots." R. Cameron Harrison from the University of Alberta, in Toronto for a year's surgical training, evidently led this work.[8] The investigators then moved to the Banting Institute, and, together with colleagues from the departments of pathological chemistry and anesthesia – and with W.F. (Bill) Greenwood in cardiology (who would become a long-time collaborator) – the Bigelow team established that, contrary to conventional wisdom, metabolism fell as body temperature declined. By 1949 a paper describing this work was ready. The key finding was that lowering the dogs' temperature reduced their demand for oxygen rather than, as previously thought, increasing it. "Hypothermia to 18°C was induced in dogs by exposure to cold air ... Oxygen consumption fell consistently with reduction in body temperature down to 18°C, and rose in proportion during rewarming in a way that was parallel." This relationship had eluded previous investigators, who found that metabolism increased as temperature dropped. Yet the Bigelow group determined that once shivering was reduced, metabolism was reduced.[9] The scientific basis of hypothermia had been established.

In August 1949, Bigelow gave L.W. Billingsley at the Defense Research Board a progress report on hypothermia. The Defense Research Board had financed the work in response to Bigelow's request for a grant. But what is of interest is how willing the National Research Council (NRC) was to help out in the absence of any formal grant application. Bigelow told Billingsley that the NRC had loaned them Jack Hopps quite readily, and had "not only given us the services of Mr. Hopps but supplied us with a great deal of technical equipment without charge. [B.G. Ballard, the NRC director] understands that this is essentially a Defense Research Board project, and we have received this aid from the National Research Council without ever having made any formal application."[10]

Indeed, the NRC "loaned" Hopps full-time to TGH and the University of Toronto, paying his salary. (In 1956 Hopps acquired the academic rank of research associate in the Department of Surgery.) Those familiar with the convoluted, highly compartmentalized, and totally bureaucratic process of obtaining research funding today will read these lines with stupefaction. In those days, one could simply pick up the phone. And, as we shall see, out of this easy, spontaneous communication came the pacemaker!

In November 1949 Bigelow did the world-famous experiment establishing that open-heart surgery was possible under hypothermia. He cooled the dog, clamping off the circulation of its heart, opening the heart as though to do surgery on it, closing the heart, and rewarming the dog. The media began to pick up on the work in the basement of the Banting Building. "While a dog will die at most three to five minutes in normal temperatures once the heart is cut out of circulation, he can be kept alive much longer when his body is 'living more slowly.'" This operation had never been performed before, and opened the prospect of surgery on the human heart. Continued the journalist, "Dr. Bigelow's operation is a new approach to the age-old problem of how to keep the heart motionless long enough and sufficiently clear of blood, to make surgery possible."[11] In April 1950 the Bigelow team presented these results at a meeting in Colorado Springs of the American Surgical Association.[12]

In 1953 and 1954 the cooling technique was used in humans, first by F. John Lewis at the time in Minneapolis, then, following several others, by Bigelow. Bigelow said, "[We found] the safe body temperature to be 83F to 88F [28°C to 31°C] and at this temperature the circulation could be interrupted and the heart opened for periods up to ten minutes. This meant that only simple heart defects could be corrected in this period of time, and the two most commonly so treated were ASDs and pulmonary valvular stenosis." Then John Gibbon introduced the heart-lung pump technique, and "following that date both techniques [cooling and bypass] were used to an increasing amount and with rapid improvements each year."[13]

The next chapter discusses the application of these experimental procedures to surgery in humans. But this serves as a bridge: In the early 1950s, cardiac surgery was just getting going at the Hospital for Sick Children. Bill Mustard, then an orthopedic surgeon, refused to work with Murray and so set up a unit at HSC. And by 1954 Bigelow and Mustard had undertaken a series of intracardiac operations under hypothermia in children, including closing an atrial septal defect. The authors concluded, "Hypothermia would appear to be a physiologic approach to some of our problems in cardiac surgery."[14]

Hypothermia was the beginning of heart surgery. Goldman said in his obituary of Bigelow, "He is truly the father of heart surgery in Canada. His work in hypothermia is what allowed open-heart surgery to begin prior to the use of the heart-lung pump."[15]

Chapter Five

The First Operations

Hypothermia meant you had eight to ten minutes – maximum – to operate while the heart was stilled, before body tissues began to die from lack of oxygen. Bigelow said, "To violate this time frame might cause permanent brain damage or death. To keep the surgeon well informed of time, our anaesthetist would call out the minutes. He usually affected a mounting crescendo in announcing minutes eight, nine, and ten to stir up the surgeon. It was a rare outlet for the thespian that lurks in all anaesthetists and surgeons in the operating 'theatre.' There was no shortage of suspense and drama."[1]

Abdominal Aortic Aneurysm

Bulges in the abdominal portion of the aorta were not infrequent and were often fatal: "50% die of rupture 6 months after they are first diagnosed," was the wisdom. "Many of these are symptomless and diagnosed on routine examination."[2] They had always been the bane of surgery. But how about patching into the aneurysm a vein that has been reversed? As early as 1950 Don Wilson and Bill Bigelow were adopting Murray's technique of reversing the saphenous vein in operation, this time on the big artery in the pit of the knee (the popliteal artery). Yet aneurysms in the abdominal portion of the aorta were more challenging because they could instantly rupture, bleeding the patient out in minutes. And there had been no good means of repairing them. Instead, the bulging portion was simply removed. The first Canadian operation for abdominal aortic aneurysm (AAA) was undertaken in Toronto on 10 November 1953 by Don Wilson, then on 21 November by Bigelow. Both patients died. The first successful North American operation for AAA was done on 18 December 1953 by Frank Gerbode in San Francisco. (Worldwide, the first successful operation for AAA was performed by

Charles Dubost in Paris on 29 March 1951.[3]) Baird recalled that the "first successful operations for AAA in Canada were performed in 1954 in Toronto by Bigelow, Wilson, and Murray using the reversed saphenous vein of Murray." (The saphenous vein would be rather small to replace an aorta, yet that is what Baird said.) The surgeons used a vein until 1957, and then prostheses of Teflon or Dacron.

Yet in Toronto the surgeons never entirely abandoned the tradition of patching in the saphenous vein. Baird said, "Gordon Murray always insisted on using the reversed saphenous vein, and predicted the fabric grafts would not be in use in this area in 5 years." (Murray was wrong: Dacron is still used.) Mortality from the operation steadily improved. Baird did well at AAA operations; his last one was in the spring of 1992. (For more on Baird's work, see chapter 11.)[4]

Cardiac Surgery

Blalock and Taussig in 1944 were on the cusp of a revolution in cardiac surgery. Yet the war had played a role as well, and in 1946 Dwight Harken and Paul Zoll, still in the army, penned an important article on the removal of shrapnel from the chambers of the heart. To be sure, as they grasped for the shell fragments inside the chambers of the heart, the heartbeat became irregular. Yet "at the end of the procedure, upon the removal of the irritating forceps and missile from the ventricular chamber, the ventricular tachycardia ceased promptly and the P-R interval [of the electrocardiogram, or ECG] returned to normal in three beats. In our experience so far, these irregularities have been relatively benign."[5] This worked encouragingly. Donald Wilson, head of cardiac surgery at the Toronto Western Hospital, later said, "The war had proven that you could operate on the heart." (On Dwight Harken's classic 1946 paper about wartime surgery, see chapter 7, subsection titled "The Zoll Imbroglio.") "After the war the problem then was to develop a system so that you could operate on the heart and have it open and see what you were doing rather than sort of working blindly."[6]

The Vineberg Operation

Who was the real "father of Canadian heart surgery"? Chronologically, it would have been Murray, but he was such a difficult man that he left no school. Bigelow is often celebrated as "the father of heart surgery in Canada,"[7] and in a figurative sense that is true because the massive research engine that he assembled in Toronto overshadowed the man who actually did begin heart surgery in Canada, and that was Arthur Vineberg in Montreal, who discovered revascularization.

The problem was how to increase the blood supply of the heart muscle (the myocardium) – this is called "revascularization." Vineberg's ideas did not come out of nowhere. In the 1930s several centres experimented with this concept, and in 1935 Claude Beck, at the Lakeside Hospital and Western Reserve University School of Medicine in Cleveland, experimented with grafting a vascular structure to the wall of the left ventricle: Beck approximated the internal mammary artery to the roughened surface of the pericardium, holding it in place with pieces of the pectoral muscle and letting the blood supply of the little artery anastomose (connect) with the pericardium.[8] This did not work well because the scar tissue (granulation tissue) would choke off the circulation of the newly formed vessels.

But there was another possibility: inserting the far end (distal end) of the internal mammary artery directly into the myocardium: no roughening of the surface, no granulation tissue. This would be called "indirect revascularization." In 1946 Arthur M. Vineberg, affiliated with the Department of Physiology of McGill and a member of the Department of Surgery of the Royal Victoria Hospital, described transplanting in dogs the internal mammary artery into the wall of the left ventricle. Astonishingly, just pushing an artery like that into the heart muscle sufficed to form new connections (anastomoses) with the coronary circulation. In a heart attack, of course, the coronary arteries become blocked; the heart muscle, starved for blood, begins to die, and the left ventricle begins fibrillating, then stops pumping. (The left anterior descending artery – the "LAD," or "widowmaker" – which supplies the powerful left ventricle, branches off from the left main coronary artery, which supplies the left side of the heart.) Vineberg had essentially described a cure for heart attacks (in dogs): revascularizing the wall of the left side of the heart, especially the left ventricle, with the simple transplantation of a nearby vessel. (The internal mammary artery, often called the internal thoracic artery, arises from the subclavian artery; on the left side of the body, the subclavian artery arises directly from the arch of the aorta.) The article in the *Canadian Medical Association Journal* made no impact at all.[9]

When Vineberg presented his dog experiments at a meeting of the American Association for Thoracic Surgery at Quebec City in June 1948, he encountered considerable skepticism. Blalock said he had done some anastomosis research at Hopkins, and most of the dogs had died. "The point I wish to make," Blalock said, "is that this is a highly dangerous operation even in the experimental animal and that the incidence of thrombosis ... is quite high, ... Only yesterday [at the meeting] Dr. Churchill and I took a long walk with a surgical colleague who had had his first episode of coronary occlusion twenty years ago ... I think that both Dr. Churchill and I were more exhausted at the end of this walk than was our surgical colleague."

Vineberg listened to these comments with growing impatience. "The patients one would operate on are those who are no longer enjoying life; none of them would be able to take a long walk twenty years later. Many are totally incapacitated ... We are not ready to go ahead with human patients as yet, but this operation is extremely simple."[10]

In 1950, Vineberg transferred his dog research to humans. He reasoned that ligating the left anterior descending artery in dogs caused death or infarction. "It is reasonable to assume on the basis of our experimental work and the pathological facts of coronary artery sclerosis that an internal mammary artery implant may be of value in the treatment of human coronary artery insufficiency."

On 28 April 1950 Vineberg conducted the operation upon the first patient, a man of fifty-three with severe chest pain. The operation was an apparent success but the patient died two-and-a-half days later of a thrombosis of the left anterior descending artery. At autopsy, severe occlusion of the coronary arteries was found, but the implanted internal mammary artery was patent (open) along its entire length.

On 22 October 1950, a man aged fifty-four was admitted to the Royal Victoria Hospital with severe chest pain, unable to walk more than a city block. The operation this time was a success, and the patient was "discharged to his home five weeks after operation ... Recent communication from this patient states that he is completely free of pain and working." A third operation was an equal success.[11] This proof of concept, like Vineberg's initial paper in 1946, aroused little interest: it seemed just too unlikely that a major affliction of humankind, the "heart attack," could be relieved by simply poking an outside blood vessel into the wall of the heart. In 1955, Vineberg reported that of twenty-nine patients, "about 70 percent ... are markedly improved and have returned to work."[12] Few noticed.

Bigelow and Vineberg

Except, in Toronto, Bigelow noticed. In 1950 Bigelow visited Vineberg. "Arthur Vineberg's statistics were impressive. The operation was simple – that appealed to me. I went back to Toronto and did a series of dogs and confirmed everything that Arthur had said. The only thing unique about my experiments was that I did each operation myself, exercising care in the freeing of the internal mammary artery etc. On checking other negative reports that appeared in the literature … I found that they had all relegated the experimental surgery to a fresh-cheeked young research fellow – such was their reaction to this *improbable* operation." But Bigelow wanted to show support for another Canadian and pressed ahead. "I started my clinical [internal mammary artery] series in 1953 and with no preoperative angiograms available. I did most of the exercise tests myself, since the cardiologists were fearful of exercising these disabled patients. I had good luck. In the first series of nine, there was no mortality. The first fellow operated upon remained badly disabled for three months post-operatively. He would come to the clinic telling me that I had done my best. Then one day he arrived full of excitement, singing the praises of the operation with marked increase in exercise tolerance, demonstrating the frequently observed delay [sic] response. This fellow had been extremely disabled, and seven years later, while still living, an angiogram showed all his coronary arteries blocked, with the internal mammary artery apparently the sole source of his blood supply."[13]

Bigelow at the General was quite alone. The American Association for Thoracic Surgery, said Baird, "had accepted one publication from Vineberg in 1952, and had refused to accept any more."[14] Bigelow said, "Between 1953 and 1962 … Toronto was the only centre doing the internal mammary artery implant operations. Although patients were clinically improved, medical men did not accept this concept during this period."[15] By 1966, Toronto had done seventy Vineberg procedures.[16] (It was only in May 1962 that Donald Effler and colleagues at the Cleveland Clinic began doing Vineberg implants.[17])

Much later, Bigelow told cardiologist Bruce Fye, "I started my clinical series in 1953, with incredibly good results." But "clinical surgeons would not accept this operation because no one had proven that the blood actually passed down the implanted internal mammary artery into the heart." He told Fye, "Having heard of Mason Sones [at the Cleveland Clinic, cineangiography] I sent him a patient who was four years post-operative, who had come from almost total disability to full exercise tolerance. He did his expert coronary angiogram with insertion of the catheter into the internal mammary artery. This displayed a clear communication between the implant and the coronary artery system … He became quite excited about this and Vineberg sent him a patient with similar radiological findings."[18]

Bigelow said in 1968, "Actually it was sometimes a bit trying in those days when questioned about the rationale of implanting a bare artery into the heart muscle to observe a look of condescending kindly tolerance or frank disbelief in the eyes of one's associates."[19]

So, proof began to be provided of a Canadian first, but by an enraged Bigelow. "In 1961," Bigelow said (in a furious letter to the Ontario Health Services Plan, which had taken at face value a patient's statement that the Vineberg procedure was done poorly in Toronto), "I brought a group of patients back and with cardiac catheterization injecting dye directly into the internal mammary artery we proved for the *first time* that the internal mammary artery years later was patent and supplying blood to the heart." When Bigelow presented these findings in April 1962 to the American Association of Thoracic Surgeons in St. Louis,[20] "the Vineberg operation started to be accepted in surgical centres throughout the surgical world."[21]

In this paper, Bigelow thanks Mason Sones at the Cleveland Clinic for help with the cineangiography of one of the patients.[22] It was Sones who introduced cine coronary angiography in 1960.[23] Yet Bigelow saw his own paper on the angiography of the internal mammary artery as important. He later wrote on the title page of one of his copies, "This is the presentation together with an internal artery implant angiogram (by Mason Sones) that stimulated interest in the surgical treatment of cor. heart disease." And on another copy of the same paper, "This was the first angiogram (X-ray) proof that Vineberg's operation was effective."[24] Bigelow said of Sones, "The resulting X-Ray studies amazed the Cleveland Clinic physicians and surgeons." Sones's paper on the Vineberg procedure was published in October 1963.[25] "Dr. Vineberg, hearing of this work, sent one of his patients down who demonstrated equally remarkable function of the implanted artery." As for quality, Bigelow pointed out that in Toronto, between 1967 and 1969, the mortality rate of the Vineberg procedure was 3.4 per cent; at the Cleveland Clinic, 4.5 per cent. Bigelow concluded this missive, "Our centre in Toronto can perhaps be criticized for not advertising our skills as much as we should."[26]

The Vineberg operation was a clear success, and it is unclear why some authorities have persisted in dismissing it as a "failure." After Bigelow's paper, Cleveland took off, and the single or double Vineberg was the procedure used from 1961 to 1969. In 1994 Joseph Shrager, at the University of Pennsylvania School of Medicine, published in the *Annals of Thoracic Surgery* an assessment of Vineberg that appeared to vacillate about the effectiveness of the procedure.[27] In a later number of the journal, Shrager said, "Since publication of the article, I have heard from a large number of surgeons … The overall sense I get … is that many agree that the operation was of far greater benefit than generally has been credited."[28] (The finding of the article was hotly contested, and Shrager subsequently withdrew the aspersion.[29])

Vineberg, said Baird, became a "a rather sad figure as he repeatedly rose at medical meetings to defend 'his' operation," despite that bypass had overtaken it.[30]

Today, the internal mammary artery is frequently involved as a "conduit" of revascularization[31] – that is, a bypass, not an implant – although the eponym "Vineberg" seems to have been forgotten. In 1983 surgeon David Schechter deplored the lack of teaching of history to surgical residents: "This was reflected a few weeks ago on Rounds, when a Chief Resident in Surgery asked, 'What is the Vineberg operation?'[32]

Heart Valves

Earliest in the Toronto story were operations on the valves of the heart in the *closed* heart. Even though he was preceded by Murray, it was Bigelow who in 1949 began *the era* of operations on the heart valves. How this came about was that Bigelow and Bill Greenwood went down to Philadelphia in 1948 "to watch Charley Bailey at Hahnemann Hospital ... do, I think, his fifth or sixth mitral commissurotomy. When we came back, I am afraid we did not impress the cardiological staff of the General Hospital or the Department of Medicine. They felt that the technique was too new. I did personally receive support from Dr. Ian MacDonald of Sunnybrook and most of my first cases [in 1949] were Sunnybrook patients." Greenwood looked after the cardiological side, Bigelow said.[33] Greenwood then became head of cardiology at the General, which ended the obstructionism.

Years later, Goldman, in conversation, was telling fellow cardiac surgeon George Trusler about Bigelow and these early "mitral splits" at Sunnybrook:

GOLDMAN: The cardiologists wouldn't let him do it at the Toronto General but veterans were fair game for anybody, so ... [Laughter.]
TRUSLER: Unfortunately, that's true.[34]

Mitral Valve

The mitral valve is the guardian between the two chambers of the left side of the heart, the left atrium and the left ventricle; it is the left ventricle that pumps blood out into the body. Malfunction of the mitral valve can leave people disabled and lead to an early death. The earliest procedure on the mitral valve was called a commissurotomy, freeing up the leaves of the valves (commissures) that had become stuck together (stenosed) as a result of rheumatic fever.

Of all the problems in medicine, few were more vexing than that of the leaves of the mitral valve being stenosed, permitting only limited blood flow into the left ventricle. As early as 1902, London surgeon Lauder Brunton had lamented the problem of mitral stenosis. "Not only one of the most distressing forms of cardiac disease but in its severe forms it resists all treatment by medicine. On looking at the contracted mitral orifice ... one is impressed by the hopelessness of ever finding a remedy which will enable the auricle [atrium] to drive the blood in a sufficient stream through the small mitral orifice, and the wish unconsciously arises that one could divide the constriction as easily during life as one can after death."[35] London surgeon Henry Souttar famously undertook a successful mitral split in 1925 on a young woman.[36] (Souttar is also remembered for an enchanting little memoir *A Surgeon in Belgium*.[37]) Yet for the most part, nothing was done for the next four decades.

In November 1948 Dwight Harken of Boston and colleagues reported operating on five patients for mitral stenosis.[38] This was the beginning. As Charles P. Bailey, associate professor of thoracic surgery at Hahnemann Medical College in Philadelphia, pointed out in 1948 at a meeting (his paper on this topic was published in April 1949), "Stenosis of the mitral valve has long challenged the therapeutic ingenuity of the medical profession. It has seemed unreasonable that young persons in otherwise satisfactory health should be condemned to a life of invalidism and early death." He estimated that in the United States there were "at least one million cases of mitral stenosis, one-quarter of which are suitable for surgery." He presented three cases, one of whom survived. He added in the published version that since February 1949 he had operated on five more, two of whom "are doing very well."[39] Thus, mitral valve surgery was not to be undertaken lightly, yet it had the ability to restore the quality of life to patients otherwise invalided and doomed to early deaths.

Accordingly, the weight of decades of minatory remarks lay upon the shoulders of the Toronto surgeons as they contemplated the mitral valve.

Murray was said to have performed the first mitral valvotomy in Canada in 1950. "Bill Bigelow and Don Wilson soon followed," said Ron Baird, who, as a junior intern, started assisting at mitral valvotomies in 1954. As a graduate surgeon, he himself led the shift from closed to open valvotomy in the early 60s.[40]

Some of these earliest patients may have been lost in the mists of time. But we do know that in 1950 Bigelow performed a mitral commissurotomy (valvotomy) on patient William Brazier for "rheumatic heart disease." This may have been his first.[41] Brazier, thirty-three, the father of two girls, had been off work for a year. "My trouble must have started with rheumatic fever," he said, "although I never knew I had it." He went into the army in 1939 but was discharged for cardiac symptoms. He was admitted to Sunnybrook but remembered that Bigelow operated on him at the General. The *Telegram* said in September 1951, "Mr Brazier was the first man in this area to undergo this operation." Brazier said, "Dr. W.G. Bigelow operated on me a year and a half ago." He used a special knife extending his index finger.[42] This account would place Bigelow's mitral commissurotomy at around February 1950, giving him a tie with Montreal surgeon Edouard Gagnon, whose first commissurotomy – the first of two – was conducted on 27 February 1950.[43] This procedure on Brazier was the first of a series of five mitral valve operations done mainly at Sunnybrook Hospital.[44]

Why were so few children involved in the early procedures at the General (since children were operated on in those days at TGH)? Bigelow told Blalock he hadn't had much pediatric experience because, "in spite of prolonged overtures, I have not yet had access to the congenital heart group of cases in Toronto [in order to get intracardiac exposure with obstruction of the circulation]. I have cooled [hypothermia] one end stage mitral stenosis successfully." Bigelow then crossed this passage out in the draft letter, and it is unclear if it appeared in the final version.[45] (It is also true that in the developed world, rheumatic heart disease heavily affects people in midlife.)

Among the earliest patients in Toronto receiving a mitral "split," as valve commissurotomies are called, was Gordon M. Graham, later chairman of the board of the department store Simpson-Sears. Journalist Joan Hollobon said of him, "By 1951 his tightening mitral valve damned up the blood flow more and more until he was utterly exhausted. In his office he was often forced to work from a couch. When he got home, he fell into bed."

He said, "Life was no longer worth living for me or for my family."

In 1952 Bigelow took a chance on the fifty-two-year-old Graham and opened up his mitral valve. "Nothing could have saved me without it," Graham said later. After the operation, the cardiac team tried to get him out of bed. "The pain was dreadful," said Graham. "I said I wouldn't get up."

Then Graham said, "All right, you give me a Scotch and a cigaret and I'll get up." It was a bluff. He didn't really want either.

But they called his bluff. "Fastest thing I ever saw, there was a Scotch and a cigaret. So I had to get up."

He later said, "No one would have given two cents for me in 1951. We have some great doctors in this country. They deserve our support."[46] (Just as a footnote, the operation was evidently done through a long posterolateral thoracotomy, in which the ribs were fractured and spread wide; sternotomy is very tolerable.)

It is unclear if the operation on Mr. Graham was conducted under hypothermia. Bigelow puts the first hypothermia operation as "1954,"[47] yet the records for Mrs. Sleeman have survived, and she received a mitral valve "split" in June 1953. "Mrs. Doris Sleeman of Vancouver, 42, was admitted to the General in June 20, 1953 and operated on with a mitral commissurotomy on July 24. It was a closed-heart procedure. She had had an attack of rheumatic fever at age nine. Her operative note in July 1953 read, "This patient had chronic right heart failure with enlarged ascites [abdominal fluid] and peripheral oedema. as well as pulmonary congestion and cyanosis. She was considered a very serious operative risk."

She was cooled to 31°C using a Therm-o-Rite special cooling blanket.

"The left chest was opened through the fourth [intercostal] interspace, the lungs were found to be markedly congested, with a very large pulmonary artery." (The pulmonary artery pumps blood into the lungs.)

Bigelow prepared to insert a finger through a structure on the left atrium called the "auricular [atrial] appendage." "There was only a slight degree of regurgitation found on palpation, which was less than anticipated. There was a moderate degree of stenosis, and a long lateral commissure was found. This split readily at the periphery with finger pressure. This did not increase regurgitation and her valve worked much better, relieving the stenosis." (If you split the mitral valve too widely, blood starts to be regurgitated into the atrium from the ventricle.)

Bigelow noted, "This all took considerable time, during which time the blood pressure never fell below 90 mm. which was remarkable, considering the general condition of the patient before operation." She was rewarmed and returned to bed "in good condition, having been conscious since the termination of the operation."[48]

Present at the operation were, in addition to Bigelow himself, Don Wilson, Berton Grapes (a surgical trainee), John Evans (then a research fellow in Surgery, later president of the University of Toronto), two members of the NRC, and various anesthetists and nurses.[49] The operating room seemed crowded, Mrs. Sleeman later remarked. She asked if "admission had been charged."[50]

Mrs. Sleeman became therewith probably the most famous patient in the history of cardiac surgery at the General and the subject of countless news stories. The *Chicago Sunday Magazine*'s story prompted an inquiry from the *Encyclopedia Britannica* to the General, which hospital superintendent J.E. Sharpe fielded, explaining that "the circulation was not interrupted in order to permit direct vision surgery. The cold was used as an adjunct."[51] (This was not exactly Bigelow's view.)

When journalist Lotta Dempsey came to call at her home in Vancouver later in 1953, Mrs. Sleeman had just baked two pies, something that would have been inconceivable previously. "I'm sorry," she told Dempsey, "we've already eaten the peach pie; but I think you'd find the apple pretty good. They tell me I haven't lost my skill."[52]

Of the early operations under hypothermia, Bigelow wrote, "A new era had been launched ... Only congenital heart conditions that could be corrected in eight to ten minutes were amenable, but it was a breakthrough. Our background of fundamental research attracted a steady stream of surgeons and scientists from around the world to our Banting Institute laboratory."[53]

In the following years to 1957, thirteen more patients were operated under hypothermia for mitral stenosis, Of the series of fourteen, ten were women. Again and again, Bigelow pressed his finger through the stuck-together mitral valve to perform commissurotomy. Of the charts to have survived, one patient died. Heimbecker became the division's mitral valve specialist, and by 1959 he had conducted seventy-two successful mitral valvotomies, as a journalist put it, "without a single loss of life."[54] Of the first thirty-five patients followed up for six months to three years, sixteen "were able to carry on a normal life." For nineteen others, by contrast, the results were "less favourable," including four deaths. Some were "chronic invalids with cyanosis."[55]

It wasn't just the stenosed mitral valve. Many patients had disease in all heart valves, and Bigelow undertook "multi-valvular" surgery, always under hypothermia. Mrs. C.C., with mitral regurgitation and aortic regurgitation, was the first, on 28 April 1954. She was prepared with a "cocktail" of Phenergan (promethazine, a phenothiazine-class cousin of chlorpromazine), Largactil (chlorpromazine), and Demerol for an hour to reduce muscle tone and eliminate shivering, "then placed in cooling blankets and her temperature was brought down to 30°C." They examined her aortic valve, thought it was "not likely a serious disability," and freed up her mitral valve with the thrust of a deft finger. There was no increase in regurgitation (meaning they hadn't opened the valve too far), and she did well postoperatively.[56]

These are stories that seized the imagination of the public. In 1950, ten-year-old Helen Chevrette of Kitchener was picnicking in the park, then started to run home. "But she was caught in a rain storm," reported the *Toronto Star* later, "and was drenched. Within hours she was stricken with rheumatic fever." Her mitral and tricuspid valves were both affected, "narrowed so drastically that only a small amount of blood could be pumped."

"Three or four steps would leave the poor child breathless," said her father. "Her lips would turn blue and so would her limbs." She had to leave St. Theresa's school and stay at home. The family physician, Dr. N. Alister Morrison, said that an operation was conceivable, but that she had only a 15 per cent chance of surviving it.

"I hid nothing from the girl," continued her father. "And I told her she alone would decide. We gave her plenty of time to think it over. When she made up her mind I got in touch with Dr. Morrison and he consulted the surgeons. Next came a telegram asking when we could bring Helen to Toronto. Driving her to the city I found out what a brave daughter I had."

During the operation, Helen's heart stopped twice but was massaged back to life. The family waited tensely. "I noted the worried look during the operation, on the face of the hospital chaplain," said her father. "I knew something was up."

Yet the operation was a success. It was just before Christmas, 1955. Helen loved to sing, although she previously couldn't, and now on the public ward of this large hospital the patients sang, "Shepherds, why this jubilee. What the gladsome tidings be." A journalist asked her, "Now that you have been given a new life, what is your first wish. Some fine clothes? Jewelry? Plenty of money?"

"No," she replied. "I want to learn to sing well."

The journalist said that she loved the Christmas carols. "Angels we have heard on high." She hummed the words. "Why your joyous strains prolong, which inspire your heavenly song."[57]

The surgeons asked not to be named in the news story because it was "team work by the surgical staff." But the lead surgeon was Bigelow.

The self-confidence of the surgeons blossomed as they did long series of mitral splits. Bigelow said in 1954, "We analyzed our 150 operated cases of mitral stenosis over past 12–15 years; we could follow up 88 of them." (This would put the first operation around 1940, and Murray might have done it. But records have not survived.) Bigelow continued, "The patients operated upon have a much improved prognosis both as to survival and comfort in living ... Very advanced heart disease ... is not a contraindication to operation provided the disability is chiefly due to mitral stenosis."[58] (In mitral splits a mechanical dilator was often used to open the valve along the scarred commissural line. There being only one in Canada, Edouard Gagnon in Montreal and Bigelow would ship it back and forth via Canada Post as needed.)

Yet just as cardiac surgery triumphed over the stenosed mitral valve, rheumatic fever, the cause of all this terrible heart disease in the young, started to become a thing of the past. "Kager" (Keith John Roy – pronounced "Kaydger") Wightman, the professor of medicine, said in 1959, "Twenty years ago every cardiac ward had its little colony of boys and girls in their teens suffering from rheumatic heart disease, whose ultimate fate was often early death." Rheumatic fever, he continued, was now "a rare disease."[59] By 1960, there were only about three cases per 1,000 school children in Toronto, as opposed to twenty in 1941.[60] Penicillin had made the difference, and the emphasis in cardiac disease began to shift from bedridden adolescents to overweight adults, who would need repairs of their coronary arteries (and whose valves, later in life, would become affected too).

Aortic Valve

A tightening, or stenosis, of the aortic valve is among the most serious problems in the medical care of young men. The cardiac surgery staff at the General said that operations were urgent on these "usually husky, active males in otherwise good health. Most of them are dead 2 years after their first light headed spell, or precordial [chest] discomfort with exertion ... About 5 cases a year die before they reach the operating room and after the surgeon has seen them."[61] (This was from a brief for shortening waiting-list times.)

Then there was aortic regurgitation, blood being propelled back into the left ventricle from the aorta. In 1952 Charles Hufnagel designed a "floating ball-valve prosthesis" and inserted it into the descending thoracic aorta of a patient with aortic regurgitation ("aortic valve insufficiency"). This operation reduced regurgitant flow by as much as 75 per cent. In 1953 John Gibbon's development of the pump oxygenator at the Mayo Clinic (see chapter 4) made possible open-heart commissurotomies and valve reconstruction (because you could see what you were doing in the bloodless, stilled heart).[62] Then in 1965 C. Walton Lillehei at the University of Minnesota began the actual replacement of defective aortic valves with ball valves.[63] That's the big picture.

It was early in 1954 that Bigelow began the first of the operations under hypothermia for aortic regurgitation, replacing the leaky aortic value with a Hufnagel valve. (In December 1953 Bigelow had written to Hufnagel at the Gallinger Municipal Hospital in Washington DC, asking for some of the new aortic valves that Hufnagel had just originated.[64])

Bigelow was assisted by Ray Heimbecker and Don Wilson in operating on the first patient, Mrs. A.A., on 13 April 1954. (This was not
a pump bypass.) She was placed on her right side to gain adequate
exposure of her left chest. They opened her chest; the upper part of the
thoracic aorta seemed in good shape. They incised the pericardium (lining of the heart), ligated some of the vessels that originated in that portion of the aorta, then clamped the aorta above and below the stretch
they intended to work on. "The aorta was then carefully divided with
scissors midway between the clamps." They injected heparin and did
other necessary measures. "The appropriate [sized] Hufnagel valve,
filled with heparin, was then inserted into the distal [lower] end of the
clamped off aorta and pulled into place at the aortic valve." After a few
further manoeuvres, they took the lower clamp off. "There was surprisingly little retrograde flow. After another minute or two the upper
clamp was then slowly released at which moment the valve began to
function well." Mrs. A.A. was then stitched back up. "The patient left
the operating room in good condition, she had a normal blood pressure. The valve could be heard functioning adequately by means of a
stethoscope."[65] A success!

Of the fourteen patients on whom Bigelow operated for aortic regurgitation, there were four deaths: three on the operating table, one two
weeks later. But these were very sick patients, desperate for a shot at a
normal life and well informed of the risks of such a harrowing procedure. Mrs. B.B., for example, who died on the operating table, "has been
in some degree of chronic failure for a few years with regular diuresis,
salt restriction and digitalis. She is confined to the house, unable to
work and cannot walk up one flight of stairs."[66]

Confronted with a stenotic aortic valve, it was necessary to employ
some kind of dilator, and in 1950 Charles Bailey of the Hahnemann Medical College in Philadelphia introduced an instrument for this purpose,
the Bailey aortic dilator. But with what caution the Canadians approached
the purchase of this expensive instrument: early in December 1952 Bigelow asked whether this instrument, introduced as the Donaldson dilator but now the Bailey, could not be purchased. Yet on 15 December, H.S.
Doyle, the assistant superintendent of the hospital, was horrified to learn
that the price had jumped from $250 to $750. He asked Professor Janes
if the device was absolutely necessary. Janes got back to Bigelow: "Dear
Bill, What about this? It seems an awful lot of money unless it is established that this is *the* instrument." Bigelow ceded to this pressure from
the bean counters: maybe he could get one "on approval" to see if it was
suitable.[67] It was. And Bigelow had the reputation of introducing the

Bailey aortic [valve] dilator to Canada in 1953. Baird said, "Great caution and some luck was needed to avoid a torn leaflet and subsequent gross aortic leakage."[68] It is interesting that this exchange, and others implying Bigelow's chiefship of the unit, was conducted entirely without the inclusion of Gordon Murray, the nominal chief of Ward C.

In 1955, Gordon Murray performed several successful aortic valve transplants using a cadaveric valve in the descending thoracic aorta.

The following year, 1956, Bigelow at Ward C began duplicating these results in actual open-heart operations on pump, transplanting cadaveric human aortic valves into the heart. The first two patients died.[69] By 1964 they had done eight aortic valve homograft replacements; five of the patients survived. This was extraordinary for the day. A visiting surgeon from Auckland, New Zealand, Brian Barratt-Boyes who had pioneered the operation, conducted the first two, and Bigelow himself carried out the next six by 1964.[70] He did an additional four, so that twelve had been performed by the time the Ontario Heart Foundation held a celebratory program in June 1966. (On at least one of these deaths, there is a backstory. Goldman, an assistant resident at the time, recalls, "W.G.B. [Bigelow] had earlier invited Barratt-Boyes to come from New Zealand to demonstrate homograft surgery. Al Trimble assumed he was doing it with B.B. as teacher/first assistant. The operation was a mess as they got in each other's way, the patient died, everyone went out for dinner. I went home to sleep."[71])

By 1966, the General had organized a homograft laboratory that stocked cadaveric valves of all sizes. "The valves are sterilized on arrival," reported the press, "and put in a saline solution with penicillin and streptomycin. They are then placed in a refrigerator where they may be kept for two weeks." If not used by then, the valves were freeze dried and put into a nitrogen solution where they might be stored indefinitely. "A valve must fit a patient exactly," continued the account. "Too big or too small, just won't do. Surgeons allow less than one-sixteenth of an inch variation in size." The result was that the laboratory had to stock a wide range of valves.[72]

(For further developments in the valve story, see chapter 13.)

Open-Heart Operations

Many of the procedures described to this point were closed-heart operations, meaning that the walls of the chambers of the heart were not incised and their interiors not visualized. Closed heart meant the surgeon's finger entering via an appendage of the left atrium and exploring digitally the mitral valve, freeing up its leaflets.

Then came the first open-heart operations, actually opening up the heart and repairing its interior under the influence of hypothermia, the heart itself stilled. Bigelow permitted himself to be scooped on this. First to operate on an open heart under hypothermia was F. John Lewis in Minneapolis, who had heard Bigelow's 1950 lecture in Colorado Springs and, as Daniel Goor puts it, was among those who "rushed back to their laboratories and began their own experiments with hypo-thermia in man." In September 1952 Lewis repaired an atrial septal defect in a five-year-old girl, followed then in October 1952 by Charles Bailey, and in January 1953 by Henry Swan.[73]

Why wasn't it Bigelow who forged ahead? After all, by 1952 his lab had improved the open-heart technique with hypothermia that allowed them to cool monkeys to 20°C, and with twenty minutes' interruption of the circulation they had 100 per cent survival. They now sought a child with a simple atrial septal defect, thinking of an eight-minute interruption at 28°C temperature. They wanted a child because they had had greater safety in cooling *young* animals. But they couldn't get John Keith, the cardiologist at HSC, to cooperate. At some later point in 1952 or 1953 they did start getting referrals from HSC, and the TGH team performed an open-heart procedure under hypothermia on a three-month-old girl with tricuspid atresia. The child did not survive the operation, because after the clamps on the venous inflow had been removed, the surgeons discovered they had inadvertently created a hole in the posterior wall of the atrium. "But the two periods of occlu-sion were too much for the patient and she did not recover."[74]

So Mustard and Bigelow started operating simultaneously on the open heart under hypothermia at the General and at Sick Children's, both getting "very satisfactory results with low surgical risk, undoubt-edly a benefit from our years of research and experienced residents."[75]

Some valves were tougher because they required more time. In July 1954 Bigelow operated on Mrs. C.: "open heart relief of pulmonary ste-nosis." Mrs. C. suffered from a stenosed pulmonary valve (which is the valve between the right ventricle and the pulmonary artery, which leads to the lung). In this very early open-heart operation, they split the sternum, then pried it apart with retractors. There were various inci-sions. "It was obvious on inspection that there was a valvular type of pulmonary stenosis ... There was a very gross, harsh thrill palpable over the pulmonary artery but not over any other valve area. The right ventricle was moderately hypertrophied."

They then clamped the aorta "in readiness for the shut-off." The pul-monary artery was clamped. The venous input into the heart was shut off. The heart was let beat three or four times to clear its chambers of blood. "We now had a good view of the pulmonary valve." This is, of course, inside the heart. "Under excellent direct vision the commissures of the pulmonary valve were incised out to the valve ring." (One contrasts this with the blind groping of a closed-heart operation.) They removed the clamps and "the heart resumed the normal circulation without difficulty." They then closed everything up. Mrs. C. returned to the ward and "responded to questions." Bigelow's first open-heart operation was a success.[76]

Unfortunately, Bigelow's next adult open-heart operations, done for atrial septal defects were less successful. On 8 June 1954, he operated on Mr. D.D.: "This patient had been deteriorating progressively and had been in hospital the greater part of the last six months. Cardiac catheterization disclosed the presence of an auricular [atrial] septal defect. He had pulmonary emboli of source unknown. At the time he was operated upon his future was gloomy and he was keen to accept the risk with the hope of some improvement."

He was cooled in the usual way and given the standard cocktail of phenothiazine drugs. Once at 32°C, they anesthetized him. They first tried a closed-heart procedure: "With the finger invaginating the auricular appendage, the inter-auricular septal defect was palpated about two inches in diameter [huge!] with a small rim around all corners. For that reason, it was felt that a direct vision closure was most acceptable [open-heart]."

They clamped the venous inflow and the aorta. (They were evidently unaware at this point that clamping the aorta would create an air trap.) The heart emptied of blood after two or three beats. "The atrium was opened and a good view of the inside of the heart was obtained." They placed three sutures in the tear.

"The heart had stopped by the end of this procedure which was four and a half minutes." After a couple of compressions and cardiac massage, the heart started beating again. Blood pressure, respiration, temperature: everything looked good. Yet "as he warmed, he did not regain consciousness. As he approached the normal body temperature, about 94°F [34°C], his blood pressure fell, and he did not respond to methedrine. As his temperature approached normal, his pressure was unobtainable and he passed into cardiac arrest, no attempt was made to resuscitate his heart." (This raises the vexed question, When do you stop efforts at treatment and let the patient die? Bigelow's rule of thumb was, "The patient is biologically dead when the pupils are fully dilated and do not respond whatsoever to strong [cardiac] massage with good arterial pressure. In such cases it is usually difficult to maintain pressure because of the collapse of the peripheral vascular bed."[77])

What had been the cause of death? Said Bigelow, "I believe the most likely cause of death was cerebral embolus, very likely we did not remove all the air from the left atrium after the clamp … and allowed air to pass to his brain."[78] True!

It is unnecessary to rehearse further this chronicle of failed early operations. These surgeons clearly were feeling their way slowly into unexplored country. And here is a question: Do we need an electrocardiograph machine (an "EKG," using the German acronym, or "ECG") to track the heart's electrical activity? People today will be stunned that such a question could even have been asked, so fundamental is the EKG to determining the action of the heart. Yet in February 1954, we find Bigelow penning a rather uncertain note to Professor Janes. He thought that they might find an EKG useful for the future, but "at the present time it necessitates our transporting the electrocardiograph unit from the Banting to the General Hospital for such cases, which is detrimental to the instrument."[79] At the Banting Institute, of course, they used it on dogs, but for humans they occasionally had to push it through the tunnel to the hospital across the street.

By early 1954 these efforts had been sufficiently encouraging that in April Bigelow asked Professor Janes for permission to purchase a refrigeration unit. "We have now established an indication for hypothermia, and this would indicate that the number of patients which should be cooled in preparation for surgery will rapidly increase." There were already six patients in the queue, "and it would appear now that all patients with [cardiac] failure and all poor risk patients should have the benefit of hypothermia."[80] These were epochal lines and marked the beginning of the era of hypothermia.

Not Just Repairing Valves but Transplanting Them

In 1962 Heimbecker, assisted by Ron Baird and Bill Greenwood, turned to Murray's operation of transplanting a human (cadaveric) valve into a patient, but this time, on March 23, they transplanted the *aortic* valve from deceased human into the site of a patient's *mitral* valve. They first did animal experiments: transplanting the aortic valve (of a deceased dog) into the mitral valve of an experimental dog. They did this in fourteen dogs, four of whom survived more than twenty-four hours. Then they operated on a thirty-five-year-old salesman who had had two previous mitral commissurotomies. They grafted a human aortic valve into his mitral orifice under bypass. He died a month later of chest infection. "Autopsy showed the donor cusps to be completely normal, in good position and functioning well." This was "the first reported open-heart replacement of the diseased human mitral valve by an aortic valve homograft."[81]

Quite independently of Heimbecker at the General, Don Wilson at the Western, assisted by two cardiologists, Alf Kerwin and Susan Lenkei (who had studied medicine in Zurich), took up the torch Murray had ignited in 1955: replacing patients' defective *aortic* valves with cadaveric aortic valves. They had begun a series of nine patients in 1956 and reported them in 1962. Six of the nine were well at that point.[82] This was the operation that attracted international attention.[83]

Here is a sidebar: Lenkei, a Hungarian, had a fierce reputation and was said to be so disappointed by the general results of the cardiac surgeons at the Western under Don Wilson that she threatened to send all of her patients to Clare Baker at St. Michael's. This created a problem. Don Wilson asked Goldman to head the unit at the Western; Ron Baird would come to the General; Goldman went for a chat with the forbidding Lenkei and thought, "It was just crazy to go with this hostile negative cardiologist who refused to send any more patients for surgery." So he stayed at the General. Instead, Bigelow sent his resident Tirone David, whom Lenkei just loved – because David was, and is, a very charming man in addition to being a great surgeon. So Lenkei stopped cathing the patients post-operatively, which she had been doing to make sure the procedure had been done correctly! Surgeon Chris Feindel got on well with her and said, "She did put high-quality patient care as her number one priority."[84]

In the first days, the mortality of aortic valve transplants was about 50 per cent. This was in line with the generally horrendous mortality and morbidity (complications such as stroke) of valve surgery in the United States in the early days.[85] In 1968, one of the TGH cardiac surgeons explained to Bob Young, age forty-one and a father of two, that "of the first six patients, three had died. Would he like to become the seventh patient?" Young had been told that otherwise he had six months to live.

Young said yes. "I was willing to gamble death on the operating table in exchange for the possibility of even a few months of living a reasonably normal life." Young later said, "The gamble had paid off handsomely. The last two years have been a blessing and a gift beyond description. Rescue from certain death has given me new values, a new perspective on life." Young had started visiting prospective cardiac surgery patients and offering them comfort and counsel. "Life has never been more precious or beautiful," he said.[86]

The Success of Heart Surgery under Hypothermia

Hypothermia became celebrated. Dean John MacFarlane was not normally given to gushing. But this notice, in his *Annual Report* for 1954, was gush: "The most dramatic development in the work of the Department during the past year has without doubt been the progress in cardiac surgery. Operations upon the heart are now among the more common operative procedures ... All of this work has been under the direction of Dr. W.G. Bigelow who has achieved renown for himself and the Department in this field of surgery."[87]

Bigelow's celebrity began with a story in December 1949 in the Toronto *Globe and Mail* about him as the recipient of "a $100 silver tray" and $100 in cash for his "history-making operation involving use of an anesthetic to reduce body temperature. When the temperature is low," the piece explained, "the body lives at a slower rate, and needs less oxygen. It is then possible to cut off the heart's pumping for a longer period than usual." Bigelow had demonstrated this by cooling a dog, opening its heart, reclosing the wound, and reviving the dog. The importance of this was not lost: "the possibility of using the 'cold' anesthetic technique in other forms of surgery."[88] (Bigelow did not actually conceive of hypothermia as an anesthetic and used ether in clinical operations.)

Many variations of cooling were attempted in other centres. In 1959 one investigator described super cooling the heart alone, while lowering the temperature in the rest of the body. Heimbecker picked up this thread, and as early as 1960 was packing ice chips on the heart after cooling the rest of the patient's body. The ice chips, made of a saline solution, sufficed to arrest the action of the heart and opened a space of perhaps forty minutes for operating on defective valves (which takes much longer than stitching septal defects). Heimbecker's first operation on a human, on 18 October 1960, with ice chips plus bypass, permitted the repair of the aortic valve in a fifteen-year-old boy.[89] Heimbecker published on this research in 1962.[90] (Ice-chip cardioplegia came from Norman Shumway at Stanford.)

In the UK heat-exchanging devices to chill and rewarm the blood were used for heart surgery under hypothermia, most notably the apparatus designed by Charles Drew.[91] Goldman saw this device in action during his fellowship in Bristol with thoracic surgeon Ronald Belsey.[92]

Bypass does supplant hypothermia as the main modality of open-heart surgery. But it would be incorrect to think that hypothermia has vanished, and even today, patients' bodies – certainly their hearts – may be cooled in the course of temperature moderation for organ preservation. Scully said, "We take the temperature down to twenty-four to twenty-seven degrees, depending on what we're doing." The "cardioplegia" solution to nourish the heart goes in at around ten degrees.[93] Thus, even today, patients are cooled, and the memory of one of the great Toronto firsts lingers on.

Chapter Six

Homes

With advances in cardiovascular surgery occurring on every front, it was clear that major medical news was in the offing. And it is to Bigelow's credit as a leader that he never lost sight of this objective, not just the perfection of technical excellence, but the creation of a program that would shape the big hospital and seed the development of cardiac surgery in Canada. In April 1955, he asked Carl Burton of the Ontario Heart Foundation for "the establishment of a cardiovascular service at the Toronto General Hospital."[1] Bigelow was not one for loud horn blowing, but in approaching the trustees of the hospital for support, he did call attention to the accomplishments of the young program. In 1957 he told them, "Visitors – fairly steady stream of foreign surgeons, anaesthetists and physiologists visiting our laboratory since 1952." Articles published in major surgical journals since 1949: forty-two (thirty-nine of them co- or entirely authored by Bigelow); 18,000 requests for reprints had come in; there had been several major prizes (Peters, Lister); and the "First Gold Medal of the International Society of Surgery "for most important contribution to surgical science in the last ten years." Bigelow was able to accept only nine of twenty-six invitations from the United States to speak and only two of six from Europe and Great Britain. As for "firsts" in the world medical literature, he mentioned, of course, hypothermia and the pacemaker, and then came to the reason for boasting to the trustees of his triumphs: "[We] did not capitalize on the hypothermia concept by early clinical application. Part of the reason for this was the lack of investigative facilities which would have provided the surgical teams with congenital heart material for operation."[2]

In 1960, the first "cardiovascular surgery division" in Canada was formed at TGH.[3] (The university postgraduate course and the Cardiac Surgical Unit were set up in 1958.) The division had several components.

The Cardiovascular Investigation Unit

There were two "cardiovascular units" at TGH in the late 1950s and
60s. One was the Cardiovascular Investigation Unit, also called, con-
fusingly, the Cardiovascular Unit. It was established in 1956 and run
mainly by cardiologists with surgical assistance.[4] Investigation meant
mainly catheterization, studying the various pressures and lesions in
the heart before operation.

The other was the Cardiac Surgical Unit, also called the Cardiovascular Unit, founded in 1958, then acquiring a big new presence on the
eighth and nineth floors of the University Wing (Private Patients Pavilion) in 1961. The two units worked closely in collaboration between
surgeon Ray Heimbecker and cardiologist Ramsay Gunton in the 1950s.
Yet in fact only a couple of times a year did the cardiologists need to
call in the cardiac surgeons and (because many more of their patients
needed imaging) the cardiologists expressed a desire to be closer to
radiology than to cardiac surgery.[5] (Fred Kergin became professor of
surgery in 1957 and in 1960 he created the Division of Cardiovascular
Surgery under the leadership of Bigelow, as well as several other surgical divisions in those years.)

Based on a personal friendship between Bigelow and cardiologist
Bill Greenwood, the close collaboration between cardiology, a medical
subspecialty, and cardiac surgery went back a long way. But it made
intrinsic sense as well, because it was the cardiologists who conducted
the catheterizations that lay out the topography of the diseased heart.

This Story Begins in 1952

Efforts to found a cardiovascular unit go back to 1952, when Herbert
Pugsley, a chest specialist with a particular interest in tuberculosis,
and cardiologist Bill Greenwood proposed the formation of a "cardio-
respiratory investigation unit." They specified their space requirements
and estimated costs. A month later, Bigelow tacked on an addendum
indicating that cardiac surgery would also be involved in such a unit.
The group apparently never received a response from the hospital
administration ("no official answer," Bigelow noted), and the idea died.
It is interesting that the investigators wished a dedicated space at the
General for cardiac catheterization (at this point, cardiac catheterization was being done at the Wellesley Hospital), as well as for "routine
electrocardiography" and pulmonary-function tests. It is also interesting that Murray, who at this point was still Bigelow's boss, was not
involved in the plans.[6]

In January 1954, Bigelow, now in charge of cardiac surgery on Ward C, again proposed to Janes a unit for the "investigation of cardiovascular cases." Respirology was now out of the picture. It was exasperating to haul the patients back and forth to the Wellesley, often bringing these very sick patients "back in [one's] own car." At the General were badly needed, Bigelow said, facilities for angiocardiography: "In the last four months I have operated upon two patients with a preoperative diagnosis of [patent] ductus arteriosus, both of whom were catheterized and in each case the diagnosis was proven wrong." Proper angiocardiography could have diagnosed these patients before they were catheterized. Bigelow, as noted, sent the letter to Janes, who verbally approved it, then passed it along to Farquharson, the professor of medicine, where it died.[7] By the mid-1950s, cardiac surgery was in full blast at the General. But it was spread out all over the hospital, in four separate operating rooms, with no dedicated corps of nurses – and with the necessity of pushing these patients with desperate illnesses hither and yon. "Patients are in three or four hospital areas during this critical post-operative period," Bigelow said. Two dedicated operating rooms were urgently needed, plus an "intensive therapy unit" for post-operative care. (It would be, in fact, H. Barrie Fairley and his team of anesthetists who established this post-operative recovery room.[8])

A year later, in February 1955, Bigelow tried again. Cardiac work had been exploding, he told Janes. Since the beginning of heart surgery at the General, "over one thousand heart operations have been performed. It is one of the commonest operations in the hospital. Four years ago, we were operating on only four kinds of heart conditions, now it is fourteen." Ward C was becoming, essentially, a cardiovascular service. Bigelow wanted a full-time cardiac surgeon (this would be Ray Heimbecker) and a full-time cardiologist (this would be Ramsay Gunton) appointed. Bigelow was now calling this a "cardiovascular unit."[9] As late as May 1955, Bigelow was still ready to accept the idea of a cardiovascular clinic as part of a general surgical service: He and Heimbecker would look after the cardiac side, and Jim Key and another colleague would do the general surgery and help out on cardiovascular. Yet Professor Janes opposed the formation of a cardiovascular service combining investigation and surgery because, as Bigelow said later, "he did not wish to lose a division of general surgery." So the cardiovascular service would be limited to investigation.

Money got the wheels rolling. In June 1955, John T. Frame and John A. McFadyen made a donation, each in the amount of $17,500, "for the purpose of building an addition to the Toronto General Hospital to be used primarily for the investigation of surgical diseases of the heart and blood vessels. It is our request that future work in this unit be under the direction of Doctor W.G. Bigelow." The prose following "It is our request" was inserted specifically at Bigelow's request, who doubtless was mindful that non-earmarked donations to hospitals had a way of getting lost in general expense funds.[10] The Ontario Heart Foundation contributed funds for staff.

The unit, sustained by grants from the federal and provincial departments of health, opened informally in April 1956 on the site of a former greenhouse next to the Emergency Department; but it was mainly a catheterization unit. Bigelow did, to be sure, have a special interest in cardiac catheterization, and he had been present when Richard Bing at Hopkins conducted the first in 1947.[11] Investigators used the transthoracic technique of Viking Olov Björk of Uppsala, introduced in 1953,[12] to evaluate the mitral valve in particular.

This was a cardiology operation, but "in selected cases" the cardiovascular surgeons did "vascular surgery": grafts in the body and lower limbs. By September 1956 the unit had done sixty catheterizations.[13] Rounds on the unit were held to consider individual patients, with cardiologists, surgeons, and radiologists in attendance.[14]

A grand official opening of the unit (called colloquially "Bigelow's Bungalow") took place on 11 September 1956. As Goldman remarks, "This is probably the first example of recognizing the need of cardiologists and cardiac surgeons to be together." Many had offices elsewhere, of course, such as the Medical Arts Building at the corner of St. George and Bloor streets.[15]

Goldman's office was the cath lab itself. He later writes, "As a junior cardiac resident assigned to cardiology, John Evans let me do the diagnostic catheterization on his patients. My work space there then became my office in 1968 so for my first couple years on staff I was right with the cardiologists. I do recall Ray Heimbecker doing cardiac catheterization via the "shish kabob" method. Skewering the aorta and pulmonary arteries and left atrium via a needle inserted from above the sternal notch downwards and inwards. Days of Giants!!"[16]

By September 1957, left-sided cardiac catheterizations were routinely conducted in the new unit, as many, said one report, as at the Mayo Clinic. One journalist observed "cardiac cath" at the unit: Working carefully, two surgeons "forced the long needle into the women's anesthetized back. In a few minutes, when the needle had approached the heart, an X-ray machine was wheeled up to the operating table ... Then the lights were turned off, the patient was given barium to swallow, and the surgeons bent over the X-ray machine."

They were trying to guide the needle, pushed by a catheter, into the left ventricle of the heart in order to measure the pressure. "The catheter, hooked up to a cardiograph, was the line of communications through which the surgeons would find the information they were seeking. [Almost certainly one of these "surgeons" was a cardiologist.]

"For half an hour, while the air conditioning equipment hummed, the two doctors slowly, patiently pushed and pulled the wiry plastic tube, trying to get it to enter the left ventricle of the heart.

"A new catheter was tried in the hope that it might be more flexible. The painstaking probe continued.

"Finally, a doctor said, 'There it goes!' And the technician verified the fact. The needles [on the pressure manometer], faithfully recording blood pressure through the catheter, suddenly jumped. The needle had been placed in the left auricle. The catheter moving through it, had been forced through the heart valve into the left ventricle." Measurements were made.

The doctors asked the woman "if she was comfortable. After a short time, they removed the catheter. The operation was finished."[17]

Diagnostic Medicine

But this investigation unit was not what Bigelow desired. He told Professor Kergin peremptorily in November 1957 that he absolutely wanted a cardiovascular unit to move forward now. "Over the last five years I have finally lost faith in the effectiveness of the ordinary lines of communication which the head of a service must use to order to make the type of progress we hope to make. I have typed copies of five memoranda, which were submitted to the Heads of Surgery and Medicine since March 1952 [under Murray's nominal headship], outlining the need for a Cardiovascular Unit." And what had happened to these submissions? "After five years, when we finally established, with our own funds, an investigative unit, I discovered that the Cardiovascular Unit had never been discussed by the Medical Advisory Board and I have an unofficial opinion from the Board of Trustees that they were never really made aware of this." Bigelow was now steaming, and told Kergin that he would be giving him a detailed document. "[It] goes to you with the guarantee which you made me that you would give it your full support with your assurance that this would be presented strongly to the Medical Advisory Board and the Board of Trustees."[18]

Perhaps the memo had some effect. In 1958 this unit was upgraded. Ramsay Gunton was about to leave the General for private practice,

Bigelow said. So "Bill Greenwood and I made overtures to Dr. Janes and Prof. Farquharson requesting that the latter consider putting Ramsay Gunton on an adequate full-time salary so that he could be retained in the hospital and work together with Ray Heimbecker in developing [cardiac catheterization]." In 1958 a cardiovascular investigation unit was established with funds from one of their surgical patients ($45,000). "This Unit immediately became a meeting ground for medicine and surgery with combined efforts at introducing new catheter techniques." Indeed, that was the point. The unit created a physical space where Heimbecker and Gunton could "live side by side ... along with their research fellows ... [They] shared secretaries and had coffee together in this unit. Actually that in itself was a unifying force ... We had Gunton and Heimbecker scrub up together for the early left-heart catheterizations where needles were poked through the patient's back into the left atrium in order to get pressures on the left side of the heart. The presence of the surgeon ensured resuscitation expertise and I believe these were the first left heart catheterizations carried out in Canada. I actually brought the Bjork needle back with me from Stockholm to initiate this." On the unit, they also began joint rounds with the radiologists, surgeons, and cardiologists, "and very often the pulmonary people under Dr. Colin Wolf [sic: Woolf]."[19]

Gunton mused about some of the incredibly large hearts seen on X-ray, "If your heart is a big as your head, you're in trouble." This became known, half in jest, as "Gunton's sign."[20]

In 1973 a new Siemens-built image intensifier had replaced the old one, making direct visualization of the coronary arteries possible.) In 1974 the unit installed a new X-ray unit, the Cardoskop U, that Siemens had designed for them. The machine was about four times more powerful than previous imagers and permitted visualizing quite small blood vessels. Siemens used the Cardoskop U as a prototype and ushered numerous groups of visitors through the unit to show what the new machine could do. Harold Aldridge, co-director of the unit, said at the time of the official unveiling in October 1974, "This equipment is the best possible now available in Canada for our type of work."[21]

A fire in August 1980 closed down the old Bigelow Bungalow, destroying all the equipment. A new CVIU was opened in the John David Eaton Building in November 1980. By this time, a host of technical innovations permitted catheterization under subdued general lighting rather than under a dark-room lamp, as had previously been necessary. In June 1981 Leonard Schwartz and Harold Aldridge commenced percutaneous transluminal coronary angioplasty, using a balloon catheter to widen plugged coronary arteries.[22]

Doug Wigle

Ernest Douglas Wigle was Greenwood's successor as the cardiologist in charge of the unit. He was born in 1928, grew up in Windsor, Ontario, the second son of a surgeon, and graduated in Medicine as the gold medalist from the University of Toronto in 1953. At the University of Toronto he had been a varsity quarterback and retained those broad shoulders. He completed his training in cardiology in 1958, was a "senior research associate" of the Ontario Heart Foundation between 1963 and 1966 (meaning that they paid his salary), and took over the direction of the Cardiovascular Investigation Unit in 1964. He was director of the Division of Cardiology, a division of internal medicine, from 1972 until 1982.

As a teacher, he was known for the "Wigle look," directed at poorly organized house staff. As his obituarist noted in 2013, "No words were exchanged. Dr. Wigle simply cast his eyes toward the offending intern, managing to convey disdain, disappointment and impatience all at the same time." He was nonetheless a gifted teacher and trained many of today's leading cardiologists. "And as a surgeon, if you had Wigle's blessing," said Scully, "you were OK." He was also known as "the father of Canadian cardiology."[23]

Doug Wigle and Ramsay Gunton helped focus attention in 1962 on a new cardiac condition: subaortic valvular stenosis, meaning that the septum between the two pumping chambers has become thickened on left side, blocking the output from the heart (the extra work causing sudden death in otherwise healthy-appearing people).[24] Heimbecker looked after the surgical treatment: an incision of about an inch long and half an inch deep in the cardiac muscle, to permit it to give way. Because the thickened muscle is apparent only when the heart beats, it doesn't show up on X-ray and has to be visualized in cine X-ray films, a dye-carrying catheter touching the heart wall. The first patient with the diagnosis was Bigelow's, and Ramsay Gunton was looking after him. Bigelow said, "I felt there was something very bizarre about this man's history and findings and I twisted his [Gunton's] tail and almost demanded that he catheterize him, which he did with some reluctance. He was interested to find the picture of muscular subaortic stenosis, and that particular catheterization set off the later studies followed up by Doug Wigle."[25] By November 1967 the cardiac group had operated on more than seventy such patients, some from as far away as Oregon and Georgia.[26] Wigle made the General into a world centre for the study of hypertrophic cardiac myopathy and provided the missing key to many sudden, tragic deaths of athletic young men.

At the General, under the calming influence of Wigle, the rift that opened between US cardiologists and cardiac surgeons over the usefulness of coronary artery bypass never occurred.[27] Doug Wigle had a strong relationship with Bill Bigelow. "They cooperated, rather than fighting with each other," said Scully, "which was very important for the development of cardiac surgery at the General."

Perhaps the financial stakes in Canada's publicly funded system were lower than they were in the United States, where literally billions of dollars were involved in "CABG" (coronary artery bypass grafting, pronounced "cabbage"). Perhaps this fountain of cash in the United States broadened the indications to include patients who in Canada would not have been candidates – and thus made the Americans' results less impressive. In the United States, debates about verifying the effectiveness of bypass with randomly controlled trials were intense;[28] but at the General, at least, they were non-existent. The procedure clearly saved lives. There had not been randomly controlled trials about the effectiveness of penicillin, either.

Cardiovascular Surgical Unit

Surgery was separate from catheterization. This is a story that goes back to the early 1950s and Gordon Murray on Ward C (see chapter 1). Most Ward C patients, on the third floor of the College Wing, were vascular (aneurysms, etc.) or cardiac; the ward was also shared with the orthopedic service. These were all "public" patients. "Private vascular patients and all open-heart surgery patients were concentrated in the PPP with the beds on the 6th floor and the single OR on the 9th floor."[29] Open-heart surgical mortality was 20 per cent to 30 per cent. They could do only one or two operations per week because cleaning the oxygenator (the rotating disk design of Viking Bjoörk) was so time-consuming.[30]

Nobody was going to be too enthusiastic about a procedure with a mortality rate of 30 per cent. But this began to change with the introduction of pump operations in January 1958.

Professor Janes, as we know, had opposed the formation of a dedicated Cardiovascular Surgery Unit because, as Bigelow said, "he did not wish to lose a division of general surgery." (Bigelow commented sardonically in September 1957, "Within six months to a year it is likely there will not be enough general surgery left in the Third Division [where Ward C was] to train a general surgeon."[31])

But Janes's successor, Fred Kergin, was more open minded, and in the summer and fall of 1957 discussions began about how to set up a cardiac surgery unit. Bigelow told Kergin in August 1957 that he wanted it called a "Cardiovascular Service," rather than "the Third Division of General Surgery," because it would be easier to get money for it.[32] The concentration of cardiac surgery into one spot at the General began when Bigelow said that a dedicated space was needed, preferably the ninth floor operating room in the Private Patients Pavilion, where cardiac operations were already being done.[33] "It is requested that H.O.R. [the] Pavilion Operating Room be assigned for private and public heart lung pump operations and arrangements should be made for twenty-four hour nursing service in Private Operating Room Recovery Room."[34] (H.O.R. was the private operating room.) At its meeting of 21 November 1957, the Medical Advisory Board gave its approval for "the formation of a Cardiovascular Service on the 8th floor of the Private Patients' Pavilion and with separate operating room facilities and dedicated ICU services on the 9th floor."[35] The unit was born. (Yet the prized sixty-bed facility on the eighth floor almost slipped from their grasp as Ray Farquharson, head of medicine, insisted that some of those beds be reserved for psychiatry. But he lost out.[36])

It was not that the pump suddenly put an end to hypothermia. Indeed, even today many heart operations are conducted under cooling of the patient. Rather, the heart-lung pump and hypothermia were used simultaneously. In April 1960 Bigelow wrote a colleague, "We are doing most of our open heart work on the pump and we have been using a heat exchanger and body temperature of 30°C with our bypass. 48 of the last 54 bypass cases we have used hypothermia."[37] ("Bypass" meant at this point merely the heart-lung pump for different procedures, not necessarily "coronary artery bypass graft.")

Only in January 1962 did the new unit open. Among the first patients was Mrs. Wilfred Lace of the Toronto suburb Scarborough, who had a stenotic mitral valve from an earlier attack of rheumatic fever. She was said to have "a kind of preview of her operation because she worked at the hospital typing out reports of heart operations." On the unit she told a journalist, "I didn't mind that, I figured if all these people could go through it, so could I. Anyway, I had no choice, did I?"[38]

Acute Therapy Unit and the Big Move

There was one more thing. Bigelow very much wanted an "Acute Therapy Room," or "recovery room," where nurses and residents could closely observe the patients post-operatively. The cardiologists had had an intensive care unit since 1962, when Robert I. MacMillan and Kenneth W.G. Brown opened the first coronary cardiac care unit in the world for cardiology patients. Until 1965, said Bigelow this was "a specifically medical show."[39]

The surgeons' interest in an intensive care unit of their own went back a long way. In November 1957, as the new space on the eighth and ninth floors of the University Wing was being planned, Bigelow wrote to Jack Sharpe, the hospital superintendent, "I was looking for you Friday morning to improve our concept of 'communication.' There was an open heart surgical patient, post-operative, on the sixth floor who was in very bad shape. She died Friday afternoon, as a matter of fact, and I thought I would have liked you to see the type of patient I am talking about and the special problems that are involved. We have had two cases in the last two weeks, post-operative patients, that have died that may possibly have lived with more adequate post-operative care. I realize ... that this is a fairly new concept to you and I want to make sure that it is fully understood."[40]

Bigelow's philosophy was, as surgery chief Fred Kergin put it, "that the patient should spend about 24 hours in an ordinary recovery room [acute treatment room] and then go to their own bed in their own room, which should be in a specially staffed area with laboratory facilities at hand."[41]

Bigelow was determined. In January 1957 he wrote to R.M. Janes, who was just stepping down as head of surgery, that his people needed space of their very own, "such as you have already assigned to the neurosurgeons and the orthopedic surgeons. I would gather than the neurosurgical and orthopedic operating rooms are not available to other surgeons even though the rooms are not being used. I think this policy is good."[42] In September 1957, he told Fred Kergin, the new head of surgery, "We shall be doing pump operations in six or eight weeks."[43]

The Cardiovascular Service was officially constituted in September 1958. Getting patients required sharp elbows for a new service. For one thing, in Emergency the residents and consultants were simply not accustomed to seeing ruptured aneurysms or wounds of the heart as "cardiovascular." (One recalls that the term embraces such "vascular" problems as ruptured varicose veins and esophageal bleeding.) Accordingly, the Emergency doctors referred such patients to general surgery, not to cardiovascular surgery. Bigelow told Fred Kergin, "I have purposely refrained from making any specific overtures with the hope that cases which obviously should be treated by a cardiovascular service might automatically come our way." But this had not been happening.[44] (This was virtually the last time the cardiac surgeons would ever complain about lack of business – or at least not until the 1990s.)

Thus it was that in 1958 the cardiovascular people – including Don Wilson and Jim Key – began preparations to move from Ward C to the eighth floor of the Private Patients Pavilion and to the private operating rooms on the ninth floor. Bigelow called this move "the beginning of the cardiovascular service."[45] On another occasion, "With this move," said Bigelow, "the staff all agreed to confine their work to vascular surgery [meaning no more general surgery]. This was a voluntary move on our part since we felt that we had received a privilege in acquiring a geographical area for all our public and private patients."[46]

As the cardiac surgeons began pump operations early in 1958, they had a small, terribly inadequate room on the ninth floor of the Private Patients Pavilion to serve as a recovery room. Bigelow wanted this turned into an "acute therapy room," which meant merely "the addition of a night staff and a screen around one bed."[47] (The beginning of pump operations is discussed in chapter 8.)

By May 1961 the new cardiovascular operating rooms on the ninth floor of the Pavilion ("P9") had been completed. Key boasted to John Sharpe, hospital superintendent, "Largely through Dr. Bigelow's reputation, we have many visitors from other cardiovascular centres, and among the pleasures [of seeing them] will now be the added delight of 'showing off' our new operating theatres."[48] The "official opening" would take place in January 1962, with eighty-seven employees, seven of whom were cardiologists, given that catheterization was undertaken at the Cardiovascular Surgical Unit.[49] At this point the Acute Therapy Room numbered around four beds on the ninth floor, compared to the fifty otherwise available for cardiac patients on the eighth floor.

In 1966, lung surgery was expelled from its cardiac "home" and made into a new Division of Thoracic Surgery under F. Griffith ("Griff") Pearson. Janes as professor of surgery was said to have been suspicious that this unit "would operate on thoracic cases only after the more popular cardiovascular procedures were performed." Yet the separation turned out to be a wise move because the lung surgeons went on to make dramatic breakthroughs, such as early tracheal surgery.[50]

Many problems were associated with the growth of this unit. In the fall of 1967, the surgeons said of their budget: "There has been a marked increase in the admissions to the Acute Therapy Unit over the past year. With increasing frequency patients are being given mechanical ventilating assistance during the early postoperative period. All cardiopulmonary bypass patients have received this for the past three years. Its great effectiveness in enhancing patient survival has lead [sic] to the expansion of this treatment to closed heart procedures and major vascular procedures as well. But we have only 5 Bird ventilators for our

9 to 11 beds in Acute Therapy. Sometimes we have to borrow from other departments. We badly need to buy more ventilators."[51]

Further growth was needed. By 1968 plans had solidified to turn part of the eighth and ninth floors of the Private Patients Pavilion into a separate cardiovascular surgical unit with a dedicated intensive care unit on the ninth floor. In July 1968 Trimble, who was the point person on the project, told Bigelow, "Apparently the planning stage is being reached where the architects and planners need some relatively firm idea, within the next few months, as to what the total square space area of the whole intensive care unit is going to be ... Already it has increased markedly over the original plans and is now estimated to be approximately 60 beds."[52] (This was separate from the cardiologists' intensive care unit opened in 1962.) The cardiac surgeons ended up with four rooms on the ninth floor, a chest-opening room, a pacer room, and two ORs. One of these cardiac rooms was not used by other surgeons for private operations (unlike the ORs in the later Peter Munk Cardiac Centre, where, of course, there were no private operations but neither were there ORs dedicated solely to cardiac surgery).

Treatment became more comprehensive. In 1968 Jane C.D. Channell, a master of occupational therapy, initiated a program of occupational therapy for cardiac patients. She emphasized three elements: (1) "group work," giving patients a chance to discuss their fears with others and allowing them "to see that they are not alone in their concerns"; (2) "individual work ... building his confidence [and] showing him that he is capable of leading a normal life within the limits of his disability"; (3) "work assessment," determining how well the patient functions in the long recovery process.[53] The following year, 1969, Maureen Moody, the director of volunteers, organized a program of "diversional therapy" quite separate from "traditional occupational therapy, which has a definite rehabilitation emphasis," as Nancy Howard, the psychiatric social worker of the Cardiovascular Division explained. The emphasis was "on offering diversion to nonambulatory patients."[54] With these innovative new programs, the emphasis on general surgery of Ward C was being left behind.

Infection is a severe complication of cardiac surgery, and sharing with other services would have meant admitting infectious cases. In February 1960, a woman was admitted to Emergency "with proven gas gangrene of the uterus." The Emergency surgeons forbade her being operated there (because they didn't want gas gangrene contaminating their unit!), and the central block operating rooms rejected her as well. What to do? Send her to POR on the ninth floor, where only a resident was on duty that night. Happily, as Bigelow put it, "my Assistant

Resident, Dr. [Peter] Kuypers, interceded and Dr. [Terence] Doran [the gynecology resident] recognized the danger in this and was good enough to do the operation in one of the south wing operating rooms [that were still under construction]."[55] The poor woman's odyssey is probably not a sign of optimum patient care, but one can understand why the cardiac surgeons wanted their own space.

The cardiac surgeons rejected the rather odious distinction between (poor) public patients and (well-to-do) private patients. All patients, said Bigelow, received the same care, and all were "teaching patients," meaning that the two senior residents and the two junior (assistant) residents could learn from them. "The staff give the same degree of operating room supervision to the resident surgeon," he said, "based on the seriousness of the case and not on its category public or private ... An important psychological barrier is overcome by the grouping of public and private patients in the same geographical area," he said. (There were, technically speaking, in the Cardiovascular Surgery Division twenty-four public beds, sixteen private, and five "semi-private." With the occasional exception, there were no interns in the division.)[56] Yet, lest Bigelow be celebrated as the great champion of medical democracy, it was really because, as Kergin further summarized their conversation, "[Bigelow] thinks it quite impossible to reduplicate a set-up and have 2 areas of this type operating, one for private and one for public patients." Put the joint service in the old public Ward C? No. Bigelow does not "think it acceptable that relatives of private patients should have to struggle in through a public part of the hospital."[57] (The hospital bylaws stipulated that on the whole 50 per cent of the beds were private – billable by attending staff; and 50 per cent public – attended by the residents and called "university teaching beds." This inequitable system was abolished beginning with the Ontario Medical Services Insurance Plan of 1966, followed by the Ontario Health Insurance Plan – OHIP – of 1972. On the Cardiovascular Division, however, the public and private wards were adjacent and, ironically, in the hospital as a whole, it was the public patients who received more attentive care because these wards were thick with trainee nurses and students.[58])

A page was turned in November 1980 when the cardiac surgeons moved from the ninth floor of the University Wing (the former Private Patients Pavilion) to quarters in the new Eaton Wing.[59] So cardiac investigation and surgery received two serviceable new homes.

A third home, however, the basement of the Banting Institute, used for animal operations, remained a disaster. In 1959 Bigelow dilated on "the need for a Heart Laboratory" in the Banting Building. Conditions were notably cramped, and Bigelow routinely had to turn down fellows from elsewhere who wanted to come for research.[60] In December 1964, Bigelow said that since July, they had operated on 133 dogs, "which represents about three quarters of the large animal work that is done in the Banting Institute."[61] The cramped quarters in the Banting Institute became a matter of increasing vexation. In 1966 Bigelow complained to the chair of the Users' Committee, "The fact remains that after 19 years we are still in an unclean basement area attempting to carry out complicated [animal] surgery with long term survival studies."[62]

Thus, cardiac medicine remained sprawled across the two sides of College Street. In 1970 Charles Hollenberg had come from McGill to head the Department of Medicine in Toronto. Scarce had he unpacked his affairs than Bigelow asked him about progress in "bringing the cardiological and cardiovascular surgical beds together." "I think the most unfortunate aspect of this current arrangement is that it perpetuates the archaic two-tiered system of caring for patients ... The most forward looking units in the U.S.A. and particularly in the field of coronary artery disease arrange for joint care from 'day one.'" Previously, Hollenberg had promised to "give this matter top priority," but, alas, in 1973 as well, care remained divided.[63] It would remain divided until the opening of the Peter Munk Cardiac Centre in the new century.

Chapter Seven

The Pacemaker

Motto: "No procedure in modern medicine has aroused more controversial thought than the attempt to revive the dead."[1]

– Albert S. Hyman (1930)

What to do when the heart stops? A pressing need for cardiac pacing existed in the form of "Stokes-Adams attacks," or seizures, in which cardiac arrest and syncope occur periodically due to failure of the heart's normal pacing mechanism: the electrical conduction system of the heart. This form of "heart block" could easily end fatally, and was unmanageable medically. The pacemaker story is the history of urgent cardiac care.

Albert Hyman

In October 1930, Albert Hyman at the Brooklyn Naval Yard Hospital reported the first attempt, not at just restarting the stilled heart but at pacing: using an external stimulus to march its beat. Hyman recalled the desperateness of the dying patient, the "ill-defined attempts to do something to restore cardiac function. In the brief interval before complete surrender to death has taken place and before utter helplessness has seized those administering to the dying person, many random and badly executed procedures are invoked with the late minute hope of rescuing the stopped heart."[2]

Hyman said later, "We had one case here in this hospital, a retired engine room officer aged 76, with ECG evidence of complete atrial and ventricular dissociation. The atrial rate averaged 76 to 80 beats per minute, while the ventricular rate was 32. At 24 he became unconscious and no pulse could be felt at the wrist." He temporarily revived with an injection of epinephrine. "About 4 days ago, during a long period of Stokes-Adams (attack) [more or less complete heart block], he received a 30-minute application from the pacemaker, with a more or less prompt return to consciousness." The "pacemaker" was two needle electrodes that they inserted through the chest wall; the electrodes were connected to a hand-cranked DC current generator.

Then on 16 February 1942, Russell Burton-Opitz at Columbia convoked Hyman and the other surgeons involved in the Naval Yard pacemaker for a meeting at his laboratory. "We were discussing," said Burton-Opitz, "the extended possibilities of the Hyman pacemaker. While it is true that Dr. Hyman originally intended this instrument to be used as an emergency measure in reactivation of the stopped heart, we considered the concept of using it when dangerous rhythms occur before cardiac arrest develops."[3]

This discussion marked the beginning of the modern pacemaker concept. The conversation on the Hyman Artificial Pacemaker continued in February 1946 at a meeting of the New York Clinical Society, which Hyman attended. "Three patients from the First Medical service of the New York City Hospital were treated. All three were selected on the basis of advanced arteriosclerotic heart disease," with heart block. Again, the surgeons used the Hyman technique of inserting needle electrodes in the region of the right ventricle; two of the patients survived, achieving normal heart rhythm. None of this extraordinary research was ever published, and the world remained ignorant of it until Hyman communicated details to a colleague in 1972.[4]

John Callaghan

In the meantime, Bigelow in Toronto was recruiting his team. First on board was the young surgeon John C. Callaghan, a University of Toronto medical graduate in 1946. The son of a works manager of the Steel Company of Canada in Hamilton, John Callaghan had been treasurer of the University Medical Society, evidencing an interest in surgery. In 1948, accompanied by his young bride, he went to Aklavik in the Northwest Territories to practice medicine. There, he had his own brush with hypothermia. En route from Fort Good Hope to Arctic Red River, Callaghan's plane, piloted by Mike Zubko, crashed in bushland, about 1,200 miles northwest of Edmonton. In the bitter December cold, a First Nations member of the party made the grim trek back to Fort Good Hope to seek help. In the intervening three days, "Zubko and Dr. Callaghan huddled over a brush fire to keep warm in the icy desolation ... Today [December 8] they saw a ski-equipped aircraft drone overhead and they knew the Indian [sic] had succeeded."[5]

What was Callaghan doing in the Northwest Territories? He had wanted to train in surgery at TGH, and while waiting for acceptance he took this job "at the mouth of the Mackenzie River in the Arctic looking after Eskimos and Indians," as Bigelow put it. When Callaghan received word from Professor Janes, "indicating that he had been accepted for his surgical training and that his first year would be spent in the experimental laboratory working on a cardiovascular subject under Dr. Bigelow, his enthusiasm disappeared. Leaving this life to enter training in surgery was an acceptable decision but to leave it in order to work in some laboratory on animals was almost more than he could face. Because of this discouraging prospect he was so long in replying to Professor Janes's letter that he very nearly lost his appointment altogether. He entered the laboratory with something less than burning enthusiasm but immediately became involved."[6] On another occasion, Bigelow said, "Callaghan arrived in the laboratory reluctantly with zero interest in medical research. He was on fire within a month, and ended up a year of experiments in the pacemaker, hypothermia, diathermy rewarming, happy and fulfilled but with a bad nervous tic in one eye. One of my senior surgical colleagues at the General Hospital chastised me for working him too hard. Actually, Callaghan was 'fixed rate' and not 'adjustable.'" Callaghan was not just an assistant; he had actual charge of the pacemaker project, and the credit for its success is owed primarily to him and Jack Hopps. (Bigelow's time was taken up operating.)[7]

In 1955 Callaghan left Toronto to take a post as the founding member of the division of cardiac and thoracic surgery at the University of Edmonton, where in 1956 he performed the first pump open-heart operation in Canada.[8]

Jack Hopps

Everybody involved with the pacemaker project seems to have been dragged in reluctantly. Jack Hopps later told Bigelow, "I came to Toronto to assist with your rewarming project. I had ... just found my niche in life – the pasteurization of beer, with O'Keefe Brewery providing the raw material for my studies. I came to the Banting Institute with some reluctance!" (Hopps joked, "I told this story to the President of the U of Manitoba when they gave me my doctorate and he wondered whether it was too late to revoke the degree!"[9]) But Hopps, too, soon caught fire in the basement labs of the Banting Institute.

Hopps had arrived at exactly the right moment in the story. Bigelow said of Hopps's joining the team, "It is difficult to visualize the crude knowledge of electricity at the time ... We had Jack Hopps, a guy who was handpicked from N.R.C. [National Research Council] Ottawa. When he came to our lab he was at the cutting edge of knowledge. He found we had been using 'smoked drums' [to record the heartbeat] and he introduced us to a cathode ray oscillograph recording before they were available on the market (circa 1948)."[10]

Zero hour for pacemaker research came in November 1950 as Bigelow asked Hopps to get going on a project. Bigelow said he had been "talking to Callaghan about the problem of the pacemaker. We have finally decided, and I hope you will agree, that if we are ever to use the pacemaker clinically, we will have to have a simply operated portable machine which can operate on 25 cycles ... Would it be difficult for you to make up a simple thyratron stimulator (is that the correct term?) which will be set up for pacemaker stimulus with the minimum of variables. I would conceive perhaps of just varying the voltage or whatever else you think necessary."[11] They had a Grass stimulator, called a thyratron, in the lab to shock the heart back into action, but it wasn't a pacemaker. (The Grass Instrument Company in Quincy, Massachusetts, founded in 1935, was an important manufacturer of medical electronic equipment.)

Over the years, Hopps, though still resident in Ottawa and a member of the NRC, continued his involvement with electrical aspects of the Toronto program. Indeed, at the end, he benefited from them and ended up wearing a pacemaker himself.

Bigelow later told Dwight Harken, the cardiac surgeon in Philadelphia, "When we decided to develop a pacemaker in 1948 the only such instrument in the literature was that of courageous Hyman ... I guess no one imagined the scene we have today where half of one's buddies are wearing them – including Jack Hopps."[12]

The Pacemaker Story

It is 1949. We are in Room 64 of the Banting Institute on College Street, just across from the General Hospital. Trying to determine how deeply dogs could be cooled before their hearts stopped, Bigelow and Callaghan have been doing a series of experiments, taking the dogs down to 24°C or so. On this morning the dog was at 22°C; its heart was not expected to stop beating until 20°C, but then it stopped anyway and did not respond to cardiac massage.

"I looked at the heart," said Bigelow. "It was quiet, cool, pink, and the muscle was firm. It was of normal appearance in all respects. What was wrong with the little rascal?"

In frustration, as the morning's experiment had been ruined, Bigelow gave the dog's left ventricle a poke with the forceps. "There was an immediate and strong contraction that involved all chambers – and then it returned to standstill. I did it again with the same result ... I poked it regularly every second. It resembled a normal beating heart ... The technician-anesthetist said, 'Hey, I am getting a blood pressure here.' This mean that these were real contractions, that the heart was not only beating but forcibly expelling blood in the normal manner ... Our experimental animal was successfully resuscitated with manual cardiac massage while it was being rewarmed."[13]

Bigelow and Callaghan had discovered the principle of pacing. Or one might say they had revived it, because, as we saw, Albert Hyman at the Brooklyn Navy Yard, using a hand-cranked generator, had done the same thing. "John C. Callaghan and I, in an atmosphere of excitement and anticipation, sat in our dingy lab well into the night, and over many cups of coffee we discussed the prospects of an electric pacemaker for the heart."[14]

But creating a device for humans would require some engineering. The team had been working with Jack Hopps on a device for rewarming the dogs after hypothermia. Could Hopps help them again?[15] Bigelow went over to Ottawa to see B.G Ballard, the head of the electronics division of NRC and told him of the potential importance of their work. "Dr. Ballard listened attentively and acted promptly. He must have possessed a remarkable intuitive sense, because I had little to recommend me as an investigator." The NRC gave Hopps permission to travel back and forth between Ottawa and Toronto, and the team procured a Grass stimulator that could deliver periodic bursts of electrical current in any waveform, duration and frequency. But what waveform would the heart respond to?

"Hopps and Callaghan then commenced a careful and painstaking series of experiments to assess the electrical activity of a normal heart," to determine the appropriate waveform and duration of stimulation.[16] "The current should be low. With the heart exposed, the sinoauricular [atrial] node could be stimulated using an electrode at the tip of an insulated rod." It was just a single electrode, with the other "dispersive" electrode on the chest wall. (Electricity passes from a positive to a negative electrode.) Hopps created a catheter electrode that could be passed through the external jugular vein in the dog's neck into the heart near the sinoauricular node. This was the "intravenous approach." Then Hopps determined that both electrodes could fit into one catheter, creating the "bipolar electrode." Hopps thereupon returned to Ottawa, and with the help of technicians there created "an efficient portable pacemaker unit incorporating the desired electrical features with a specialized circuit."[17] Back in Toronto they started testing the unit, recording blood pressure and heart rate with a stylus that produced a tracing on a rotating drum of smoked paper.[18] (As we know, they did not yet have an oscilloscope.)

It worked. "At 20°C the heart stopped, the pacemaker was turned on at a rate optimum for that body temperature, and it immediately took control of cardiac action." It is just stunning to read these lines thirty years after they were written in 1984 and to realize that Bigelow, Callaghan, and Hopps were perfecting on dogs a device that would bring relief to, or indeed save the lives of, millions of humans around the globe whose hearts were beating poorly, irregularly, or not at all.

Bigelow later said, "To design the first pacemaker for humans at normal body temperature sounds simple and obvious in retrospect. Why was such a simple concept never developed before ... 1950? The explanation from the literature is simple. All previous experimental attempts at electrical and mechanical stimulation were carried out in cardiac standstill due to anoxia or drug toxicity ... Any contractile response was *not* expulsive. Our hypothermia standstill heart was fully oxygenated during a well-controlled experimental surgical procedure. It was perhaps the first time in history that such an opportunity had presented itself."[19]

Callaghan presented the results at a meeting of the American College of Surgeons in Boston on 23 October 1950. This was not the first outing of their findings, as the Toronto team had given a preliminary version of their results at a meeting of the American Surgical Association in Colorado Springs on 20 April 1950.[20] Yet it remained unmentioned in the press. Journalists, however, were present at the Boston meeting, and the press plunged into the story; the discovery became the object of a front-page account in the *New York Times*.[21] Several of the Toronto papers sent correspondents to Boston.[22]

Callaghan and Bigelow published a complete account of their findings on dogs and rabbits in July 1951, describing two approaches to the sino-atrial (S-A) node, which initiates the electrical current that flows across the Bundle of His and drives the heartbeat. One was "external," anchoring one electrode on the chest wall; the other was via an incision on the lining of the heart (pericardium). Here an incision just large enough to admit the electrode was made so that it was fixed against the sino-auricular node region. Alternatively, they went via the "transvenous" route: inserting the electrode into the right external jugular vein, through the superior vena cava (which drains the head and neck into the heart), with the stimulating tip in contact with the surface of the S-A node. They used a "Grass Thyratron physiologic stimulator." In eleven dogs cooled to a low temperature, the pacemaker controlled the action of a heart at standstill; at normal body temperature, stimulating the right vagal nerve had created standstill, whereupon the pacemaker produced "beats of good expulsive force." Indeed, in normal hearts the pacemaker could take over control of heart action "to increase or decrease the heart rate at will."[23] This was compelling.

At this point a Boston cardiologist named Paul Zoll enters the story.

The Zoll Imbroglio

Paul Zoll came to the Boston talk. Zoll, thirty-nine, was a not inconsiderable scientific figure. He had graduated in medicine from Harvard in 1936 and served as a cardiologist in the Army Medical Corps during the Second World War, writing, together with Dwight Harken (a very distinguished cardiac surgeon), a series of papers on using their fingers to remove foreign bodies in and around the heart. ("Foreign bodies" meant mortar fragments and other high-explosive shrapnel.) The two clinicians discovered that the heart could be entered with relative safety for the removal of these fragments, and of thirteen patients with intracardiac "missiles," they had zero deaths.[24] It is possible to see these events, as Goldman put it, as "the springboard for the surge of activity in the postwar years."[25] The point, however, is that Zoll was not a nobody who descended from the blue to expropriate the work of someone else.

After Callaghan's lecture, in October 1950 Zoll wrote to him, asking for information.[26] Callaghan later said, "I could tell he had done no work on the subject but was interested. I sent him all the details of the circuitry (what a naive fool). Bill was very annoyed he won the $50,000 [sic: $25,000 was the award] Lasker award considering the early work at the Banting."[27]

On 13 November 1952, Paul Zoll published an article in the *New England Journal of Medicine* claiming priority. They used a "thyratron physiologic stimulator" (a Grass stimulator)[28] and thanked Harvard pharmacologist Dr. Otto Krayer for making it available. One patient survived, one died. Zoll mentioned the Toronto machine as a possibility for the future and cited the Hopps-Bigelow 1951 paper.[29]

The Toronto team were convinced that Zoll had copied the device for his pacemaker from them. And Hopps and Callaghan had proof! Bigelow said later, "Actually, the pacemaker was a technical creation of the N.R.C. To establish proof that Zoll would use our circuity, Jack Hopps (N.R.C.) and Callaghan decided to submit it with a key omission. Sure enough there were requests for this missing circuitry from Zoll's team."[30]

The Toronto team believed implicitly that Zoll had applied for a patent. There is no evidence that he did, or that he or the Electrodyne Company ever were awarded one for a pacemaker.

Why the Canadians never received a patent is a bit of a mystery, because in February 1953 Hopps appeared at a hearing of the Committee on Patents of the NRC to discuss applying for a patent. Pattenson from the NRC pointed out that "the stimulator will restart a stopped heart and maintain beating until normal beating is resumed." This sounded pretty useful, and "the Chairman remarked that it seemed to him every major hospital on the continent would have use for one of these instruments." The Smith & Stone company had declared they didn't want to proceed with development, seeing little profit in it. But the committee recommended that "an application for a patent in the United States be proceeded with immediately," and that the question of a Canadian patent be pursued shortly.[31] None of these initiatives ever took place, however. By 1955 a Canadian machine was being produced by the Measurement Engineering Company, in Arnprior, Ontario, but under what patent arrangements is unclear.[32]

The bitterness of the Toronto group did not subside. Hopps wrote to Bigelow in 1953, "Dear Bill, on television a few nights ago I saw a film on cardiac research. Featured in this film was our friend, Dr. Paul Zoll, with his cardiac stimulator which he had pioneered on his own hook. It is imperative that we get our *Surgery* article out." Hopps closed his letter, "PS, The Son of a Bitch!"[33]

Zoll's role in all this remains a tenebrous one. In February 1953 he told Hopps that "the negative electrode of the output circuit be applied near the cardiac apex and the positive electrode at the distant point in the chest," thus revealing that he had not understood at all the Canadian "transvenous approach" of threading a bipolar electrode into a vein (the "transvenous approach" that the TGH group had described in their article). He said that the Electrodyne Company in Norwood, Massachusetts, was building a stimulator that he himself had designed. If Hopps wished further detail, he should apply directly to them. In the meantime, he would be pleased to have further details of the Toronto apparatus.[34]

For all his flattery of the Toronto group, Zoll, it must be said, was not keen to publicize their work. For example, his 1954 article on the pacemaker makes no mention of their work.[35]

Hopps later wrote Bigelow of these events: "Zoll received data on the original stimulator including circuit details ... from Rugg in November 1952. [Henry H. Rugg was an engineer at Smith & Stone Ltd. in Georgetown, Ontario.] About the same time, I provided John Callaghan with a circuit and other information in answer to a request from Zoll." (Hopps said that the Smith & Stone model was based on the circuit for the original stimulator.) "A photograph of the unit appeared in your July 1951 paper (*Annals of Surgery*), and the Zoll stimulator, which I saw on a television program in October 1953, was remarkably similar, even to the location of the controls and range switch." Hopps added, "I am afraid there is little to be gained from further recrimination now. It would just sound like sour grapes to belabour the point further. Albert Grass of Grass Instruments once told me that we were not the only victims of this gentleman's plagiarism."[36] And William Glenn, professor of surgery at Yale, told Bigelow on another occasion, "We, too have had our troubles with Zoll!"[37]

Zoll continued to haunt Bigelow's mind, such was the Toronto outrage about the supposed deceitfulness. In the mid-1950s the main commercial vendor of Hopps's stimulator-defibrillator was the Measurement Engineering Company in Arnprior, Ontario. But here Bigelow sensed trouble. "There is some confusion with regard to the amount of publicity that has been given the stimulator-defibrillator put out by Doctor Zoll in the United Sates," he told the company in 1955. "Actually, they have used Mr. Hopps' circuit for their machine but their stimulator is devised for external stimulation rather than stimulation within the heart. In order to avoid confusing the two machines, I would like to suggest that you sell this machine as the 'Hopps' Stimulator-Defibrillator."[38] Measurement Engineering disliked naming the device after Hopps, given that a number of people were involved in its development, and proposed "Canadian Stimulator-Defibrillator," which Bigelow accepted.[39]

What stands out here is the outrage of the Toronto group. Hopps said to Bigelow in March 1974, "There seems little that can be done about Zoll. The fact that he collected $25,000 for plagiarism [Lasker Award, 1973] is the final insult. However I imagine our reward awaits us in heaven."[40]

The argument between the Toronto group and Zoll threatened to become one of medicine's famous "priority disputes," turning on who was the first to discover something. Bigelow wrote an affronted note to Zoll in July 1964, and Zoll replied that he was "disturbed" by it. "You evidently feel that I did not properly acknowledge the assistance you and Dr. Callaghan gave me and did not adequately credit your previous work." But, Zoll said, the Electrodyne apparatus owed nothing to the Toronto model, and he himself had been busy "for a number of years on a clinically applicable technic of stimulating the ventricles electrically" before he heard the October 1950 lecture at the American College of Surgeons in Boston. As well, Zoll continued, his approach was different from the Toronto approach: He used two "electrodes placed externally on the chest wall," as opposed to the Toronto technique "of direct stimulation of the sino-atrial node" (via the jugular vein). He also doubted that the Toronto pacemaker would be useful in clinical emergencies of ventricular standstill (cardiac block).[41] (In fact, the Bigelow device stimulated the SA node, which is of no use in heart block.) Bigelow then assured Hopps that he didn't intend to take the matter any further, and that was that.[42]

To be clear, under Zoll's guidance Electrodyne did develop two separate devices of undoubted utility: one was a "cardiac pacemaker for ventricular standstill;" it was to be externally applied, in a closed chest and "provides an electric stimulation to which the heart responds with a ventricular contraction." The other device was a "cardiac defibrillator for ventricular fibrillation," for use in the open chest "to meet the emergency of cardiac fibrillation." The electrodes were to be "applied firmly to the surface of the heart." These devices could be sold separately, or in a combined form.[43]

One would think this *Akademikerstreit* (as the Germans say, a quarrel among profs about semicolons) couldn't possibly go on any longer, but it did! After Bernie Goldman excerpted in 1987 in a journal Bigelow's version of the discovery of the pacemaker, which Bigelow had originally given in *Cold Hearts* in 1984, Paul Zoll explicitly denied in a letter to the editor in November 1987 that he owed anything to the Toronto group. He said he had begun his experiments in 1950 using a "home-made pulse generator," then had switched to a Grass Physiological Stimulator after talking with Callaghan after the Boston lecture. He said that his engineer, evidently at Electrodyne, had designed a commercially successful pulse generator, devising the circuits independently of the Toronto group.[44] On the basis of documentation currently available to us, it is impossible to sort out these rival claims.[45]

"What do you think?" Bigelow asked Hopps. "After 36 years it really doesn't make much sense. I have avoided priority controversies all my life. Jack, you could answer this in a devastating manner by telling Zoll his engineer wrote requesting clarification of the circuit diagram (the part you omitted) … One other method would be to remind him how great he is … OR just disregard it."[46]

They disregarded it.[47]

The Pacemaker Evolves

After the Boston lecture in 1950, in Toronto the pacemaker continued to evolve. "In 1950," Hopps later said, "we used a very fundamental circuit in a simple defibrillator." They called it "model D1." Model D1 served for a year. This would have been the Grass stimulator. As Bigelow told Henry Swan, the professor of surgery at the University of Colorado, in January 1951, "We originally used a Grass model 3 C stimulator but later Mr. J.A. Hopps, the electrical engineer on our team, assembled the essential parts in a more compact device. This present model is small and quite mobile. It was developed by the National Research Council, and Smith and Stone Company, Georgetown, Ontario are constructing several small models which should be ready in the near future."[48]

This Hopps device would have been Model 2, which they sent out to Smith and Stone in February 1951 for production of a limited run of six units. Smith and Stone promised to charge them "not much more than the cost of production as they have made these more or less as a favour to us with no hope of profiting on the deal."[49]

There was a problem. As the dogs began to rewarm, their hearts often started fibrillating, meaning "an irregular squirming action to the heart … with no expulsive beat," as Bigelow put it. "The technique of shocking a heart which has become irregular (called defibrillation) is being developed with Mr. Hopps' help," Bigelow said in 1950.[50] But the pacemaker was ineffective in restarting hearts stilled at around 17°C. A defibrillator was needed to deliver a single sharp jolt of electricity. Independently of the pacemaker, Hopps constructed "a small machine for our use in defibrillating the heart [where] all we control is voltage and current." This was ready by October 1951.[51] Bigelow said that Hopps had "combined the pace-maker and defibrillator in one cabinet for the sake of simplicity of operation. Once we have developed cardiac standstill following defibrillation the electric pace-maker is then turned on and provided the heart is in good condition it usually stimulates beats." It had a timing circuit "for limiting shock duration."[52] This defibrillator-pacemaker, devised in October 1951, became "the Model 3 Stimulator-Defibrillator."[53]

At this point the combined pacemaker-defibrillator idea took wings. In July 1952 Bigelow wrote to Professor Janes, "I would imagine that there are three or four patients each year who die of cardiac arrest in the operating room that may be salvaged by prompt resuscitative methods and the use, if necessary of the two special procedures: electrical defibrillation for ventricular defibrillation and an artificial pacemaker for standstill of the heart." Bigelow observed that Mr. Hopps of the National Research Council had fashioned for the hospital a defibrillator and a pacemaker. "I shouldn't think that the cost would be more than two hundred to two hundred and fifty dollars for a combined unit." Mindful of the hospital's two-class system, Bigelow said that that they might keep one in the main building and another in the private operating room.[54]

The apparatus was thus by this time quite complex. But Bigelow had requested a "'nurse-proof, doctor-proof' simplified unit for operating room use."[55] A Model 4 was produced in February 1953, but their efforts at treatment of patients had already begun with Model 3. NRC's Model 4, a "clinical stimulator-defibrillator," remained in production with Measurement Engineering into the 1960s.[56]

In 1953 Hopps joined the Banting Building group full time, while retaining his appointment at the NRC, and there on College Street he would remain for many years.

Exasperated by his own inability to answer properly colleagues' inquiries about closed-chest defibrillation, in 1955 Bigelow said to Hopps, "I believe it is time that you devised an external stimulator such as Zoll has to apply to our stimulator-defibrillator. I have already have several requests for this."[57] Hopps went to work, and by 1962 (though perhaps earlier), Measurement Engineering Limited of Arnprior, Ontario, had produced a closed-chest defibrillator, "designed by the Medical Electronics Group of the Canadian National Research Council." It used "higher current pulses than are obtainable from defibrillators which are designed for open-chest defibrillation."[58] It is details at this level that illustrate the desperateness with which these devices were deployed: failure at closed-chest defibrillation meant death, and these defibrillators are the direct lineal ancestors of the defibrillating "paddles" currently in use in every hospital in the country. (Around 1959 the researchers had, in fact, gone over to paddles, and we find Alan Trimble, who looked after the unit's budget, ordering an extra pair in 1969 because "we have had constant breakdowns in the older paddles and it is essential to have an extra pair ... when coming off the heart-lung machine."[59])

First Use?

The story is that Boston cardiologist Paul Zoll was first to use the pacemaker clinically in 1952, as described earlier in this chapter. Even Bigelow accepted this story. But another version is possible.

In 1949 Callaghan may possibly have been the first to use the pace-maker on patients. He wrote in 1980, "In November or December of 1949, I had been requested by Dr. [Robert] Janes, then chief surgeon at the Toronto General Hospital, to attempt to resuscitate five surgical patients who were in cardiogenic shock following major surgery, by the insertion of a transvenous pacemaker through the jugular vein in the neck to the junction of the superior vena cava and right atrium [this is the sino-atrial node, or SA node]. I was unable to create controlled beats, and unfortunately, have been unable to trace these patients, now 30 years since the attempt, and some 12 years since the death of Dr. Janes."[60] This account suggests that the five patients survived.

But then, Callaghan had given a different version of this story in 1969, telling a US colleague that, under Bigelow's supervision, in the surgical recovery room of the Private Patients Pavilion, he had unsuccessfully used the pacemaker, stopping the catheter at the SA node. "Had we pushed our catheter ... into the ventricle we could conceivably have successfully captured cardiac action but unfortunately we were just two inches too high at this period." He didn't say, in this account, if the patients survived, merely that his efforts to pace them had been unsuc-cessful.[61] Callaghan added later, "Had I but tripped, fallen, coughed, pushed forward and in some way pushed the electrode into the ven-tricle through the tricuspid valve, I probably would have commenced transvenous pacing, ten years [before its US discoverers]."[62]

In 1964 Bigelow told an engineer at General Electric, "Doctor Zoll was the first to report using this in humans, although prior to this we had used it without success in the operating room. This was not reported."[63]

Is it possible that, out of courtesy, Callaghan said he had operated "under Bigelow's supervision," when in fact he had operated under Janes's instructions and on his own? Could it be that Bigelow thought the patients had died, because Callaghan simply had not told him that, despite the failed pacing, they had survived?

The question of stimulating hearts in standstill remained vexed. Big-elow thought there was no substitute for massaging the heart, and so negative had his experiences with the pacemaker-defibrillator been at TGH that he declared flatly in 1962, "If it is cardiac standstill [as opposed to fibrillation] then the defibrillator is of no use." (Only an EKG, he said, would tell whether the left ventricle was fibrillating or in standstill.)[64]

Wounded Pride

It gnawed at Bigelow that the Toronto group had never received suf-ficient credit from the Americans for pioneering the pacemaker. "Dear

Mike," he wrote to Houston heart surgeon Michael E. DeBakey in February 1974, "I am aware that you attach some importance to priorities in research and development in medicine recognizing, as I do, that these should be accurate and preserved in order to provide motivation of future research." Bigelow noted Callaghan's talk at the American College of Surgeons meeting in 1950. "Some of my friends with injured Canadian pride feel I have been remiss [in not claiming some pacemaker priority], but historically the individual who applies something clinically usually receives the plaudits. I do not expect you to do anything about this but I thought that I would like you, as an important representative of the cardiovascular scene, to know about the part we played."[65]

In reply DeBakey coolly stonewalled Bigelow: it was Zoll, he said, who had made the greater contribution to clinical care.[66] *Time* magazine ran a story on the Lasker Awards, stating, of course, that it was Zoll "who invented the device."[67] Callaghan saw the story as well as Bigelow's letter to DeBakey. He wrote back, "I don't think it will have any effect on Mike DeBakey, but I am sure you feel better and I know I do, knowing at least he [DeBakey] knows that Canadians played a role in this."[68]

A sense of injustice continued to worm at Bigelow. "It is quite understandable that you did not know this Canadian contribution because we have never spelled it out in any article," Bigelow told heart surgeon Harold Segall in 1989.[69] In a letter to R.E. Beamish, Winnipeg, Bigelow insisted we innovated "the first electrical artificial pacemaker for *clinical use*. The NRC duplicated as closely as possible the current that passes down the cardiac nerves. We were the first to put both electrodes in one catheter with a bipolar tip, thus eliminated the painful contraction of the 'indifferent' electrode on the chest wall ... We learned that it would not only start the heart but it would slow it and increase the rates, which had never been done before." In a postscript, Bigelow added, "Zoll unquestionably had the first successful human use in treating a patient with heart block via oesophagus. As our file of letters can show, he also unquestionably used our circuit with a *single* electrode. The indifferent electrode was contacting muscle and producing such pain it had to be discontinued. He did not read our article thoroughly!!"[70]

The Toronto group's record of pacemaker innovation stops here. The next development in the field would be Ake Senning's implantable pacemaker in 1959. But the group's exasperation with the Americans' refusal to recognize an important Canadian priority did not stop here.

Hopps later told Bigelow about giving a lecture in November 1991 at Lakeland Regional Medical Center. "At that meeting I was introduced by an enthusiastic neighbor as the developer of the pacemaker. The speaker coldly remarked that I should meet Wilson Greatbatch who was the real developer [implantable version in dog pacing 1958] and challenged me to meet with him on a planned visit to the hospital." But in fact Greatbatch was already familiar with Hopps, having been present at a meeting in Niagara Falls, NY, in 1987 of the US Alliance of Engineering in Medicine and Biology at which Hopps had been given "their Leadership Award for development of the pacemaker."[71]

And there were shocked laity! Miss Elizabeth Callow on Whitehall Road in Toronto wrote Bigelow in 1965, apropos a *Reader's Digest* article on history of the pacemaker that omitted any mention of Bigelow and Callaghan. "The Canadian reader is fed to the teeth with this sort of American oversight, so unjust is it."[72] Bigelow replied that "Doctor Callaghan and I in fact were the first people to develop an electrical artificial pacemaker designed for human use, and were the first to prove that heart beats produced by such a pacemaker were normal beats, and that this pacemaker could maintain normal blood pressure. We also showed that this pacemaker when applied to a normally beating heart would take over from the normal pacemaker [sic – normal heart]." He said, "This was reported at the Basic Science Forum, of the American College of Surgeons and printed in the Annals of Surgery, vol. 134 July 1951." Then came the supposed Zoll rip-off. "Doctor Zoll wrote us and asked for the electrical circuit and method of construction. He subsequently used this pacemaker circuit, increasing the voltage slightly, and had it patented. We have never done anything about this, nor have we even written Doctor Zoll. He is aware of this and most informed scientific articles on the pacemaker give us proper credit."[73] As stated, this Toronto outrage at a Zoll patent seems to have been delusional.

Bigelow was proud that this was a Canadian story. It's worth dwelling, he said in 1983, on "the role of dedicated Canadian research workers in the evolution of the pacemaker. Why? ... to assuage our inherent national sense of insecurity ... In spite of our government's efforts to provide perspective in the news, Canadians are often insufficiently aware of the input by their countrymen." He enumerated the Canadian contributions, the pacemaker itself, the intravenous catheter electrodes, the demonstration in dogs that the beats were expulsive, and so on. His list was a careful one because, he said, "a relatively new country needs a sense of national pride in order to mature in a normal manner."[74]

Yet this is not a simple national-pride story. For much as the Canadians resented being ignored by the Americans, the Toronto group owed their entire intellectual model, which emphasized research, to the Americans, rather than to the English, who emphasized clinical teaching rather than research.[75] On the adoption of the American model of research rather than the British model of teaching, Bigelow said, "Until recently Canadian medical schools ... have followed the lead of Britain and France and accepted their standards of excellence. Now the United States is the leader in most phases of medicine and ... this has been brought about by the rapid transition and heavy orientation to research. As other world leaders have done in the past, the Americans have set their standards of excellence in medicine and, as we have done in the past, there is little alternative but to try to meet them ... Thus the excellence of our medical schools would appear to depend in a large measure, upon the extent of research."[76]

"What a Period"

In retrospect the potential contribution of this research was enormous. But the practical contribution of the Toronto pacemaker in the years following its introduction was small, simply because it was too large for ambulatory use and the hospital patients that came under Bigelow's care were desperate cases. As he wrote to a colleague, H. Brodie Stephens, in San Francisco in 1954, "We have had this instrument in the operating room now for four years and have not had a satisfactory case upon which to try it. It seems that most of the hearts that develop standstill or refuse to revert to rhythm with massage and full oxygenation of the coronaries are either terminal hearts or there is something preventing adequate oxygenation of the myocardium."[77]

Bigelow did not, it must be said, appreciate the potential uses of the pacemaker. "Gentlemen," wrote one New Yorker in 1954, who hoped the pacemaker had now been developed "in cases of irregular heartbeats, to restore the heart's action to normal rhythm. I am 58 years of age and have had rheumatic fever about 19 years ago, and since then I have been under doctor's care ... I feel tired most of the time. Unfortunately, I have to work and travel to and from work, also climbing stairs. However, I am making the best of it but am very nearly interested to learn more about your pacemaker. Maybe it could be something for me." Could Bigelow possibly let him know if the pacemaker was available in New York City.[78]

Bigelow's reply was disappointing: "I am afraid that with our present knowledge of the electrical pacemaker it does not seem to have any place in the treatment of a condition which you appear to have. This is essentially designed for a heart that has stopped beating during an operation, and the pacemaker stimulates the heart to commence beating again." Other clinical applications for the bulky device were not envisaged. "I am sorry that I have such a pessimistic report to make."[79] Even as late as March 1956, Bigelow was unable to answer a colleague's question about the utility of the pacemaker in open-chest operations: "We have not had any particular success, nor have we had much opportunity to use the artificial pacemaker in humans."

But in animals, different story: "We have been able to use the pacemaker following cardiac standstill at low body temperatures, and leave the animal on the pacemaker while the chest is closed and the animal rewarmed to a temperature at which they automatically take over the pacemaker duties from the SA [sinoatrial] node. Animals have been carried on in this manner for thirty to forty minutes."[80]

Indeed, said Bigelow, the "external stimulator" of Paul Zoll was actually better "in certain medical cases of heart block where the heart is beating with an idioventricular rhythm and the patient not doing well. Here the [Zoll] stimulator steps up the heart rate and cardiac function by supplying a new sinus pacemaker, and if the condition is temporary, the patient is helped."[81] It speaks well of Bigelow's scientific objectivity that he would grant such a kudo to the hated Zoll.

Anyone who thought the Hobbs-Callaghan pacemaker a huge advancement in medical science had obviously not read Bigelow's letter to H. Keith Nancekivell, a surgeon in Fort William, Ontario: "Dear Keith: you realize that the pacemaker part of the defibrillator has very rare usage for occasional cases of heart block. It is of only temporary value there too and if you are thinking of the operating room I would advise you to get a straight forward defibrillator ... There are fewer dials and it is less confusing to the operating room staff to have a simple defibrillator."[82]

Yet the pacemaker was an enormous achievement, if only as a hint of promise of what could be done; it cried out for credit. Bigelow was a very modest man and advocated modesty as a requirement for the scientific mind. So he attributed a good deal of the credit in this story to Callaghan rather than dancing in the spotlight himself. In 1960 he told William Glenn at Yale, "I think that John Callaghan's physiological studies in which he showed that the rate could be slowed and increased, and blood pressure could be maintained, were the first physiological studies to be carried out ... All the work and most of the ideas [behind the pacemaker] were John Callaghan's."[83] At the time of an award in 1985 Bigelow said, "John Callaghan, the reluctant researcher, planned and carried out the major part of the pacemaker research."[84] On another occasion, he added that he now understood what Callaghan's real contribution was: "It was the first scientific attempt by bioelectronics engineering to accurately duplicate the electrical discharge that comes from the SA node with the development of circuitry and the eventual construction of a true pacemaker."[85] He rather pooh-poohed his own contribution: "I was in an experimental setting that had never before been available – an exposed hypothermic heart, in standstill, pink, firm and fully oxygenated, with ECG and blood pressure recordings. Poking with a probe produced a strong expulsive contraction. To evolve from that to the concept of the pacemaker did not require any great genius."[86]

How do we make discoveries in medicine? The pacemaker story is an interesting mixture of luck and science. It was luck that, in exasperation, Bigelow poked at the stilled heart of the overcooled dog. It was science that John Callaghan and Jack Hopps were able to conceive an electrical device that would pace the irregular, flagging heart at a steady, solid rhythm – although at the time they didn't realize at all that that was what they were doing. They conceived their invention as a means of restarting the silent heart – so again, luck and chance played at role. When the implantable pacemaker came along in 1959, the conceptual groundwork had been laid – in Toronto.

There was a lot going on at the time. The Bigelow group dropped the ball on the patent, but as Bigelow said, "It was ... a busy moment in the history of cardiac surgery with many distractions. We had just developed the first pacemaker (with NRC), our diathermy rewarming of hypothermic patients had proven successful. On the clinical front at this time the surgery of acquired heart disease was born along with that of peripheral vascular surgery ... What a period."[87]

PART TWO

Full Speed Ahead

Chapter Eight

Bypass

In open-heart surgery the interior of the heart is motionless, fully visible and clear of blood in order to repair internal lesions such as stenosed mitral valves and atrial septal defects. Yet the Toronto surgeons did perform, under hypothermia alone, more complex "blue baby" operations; and for Bigelow it was quite routine to undertake the "Blalock operation" under hypothermia – as, for example, for Elizabeth N. in May 1957 – hooking up the left subclavian artery to the left pulmonary artery. "The patient's condition was good throughout."[1] This was hypothermia, not the pump.

At the international level, in the early days an atmosphere of negativity pervaded cardiac medicine because of almost uniformly poor results. Yet breakthroughs began. In 1955 Walton Lillehei and Richard DeWall in Minnesota developed the first bubble oxygenator. Goldman said that this "had an explosive effect on the worldwide growth of open-heart surgery."[2] And it was in August 1956 that surgeons at Minnesota used a new pump (the Sigmamotor).

In 1955, John Callaghan, an alumnus of the basement of the Banting Building (and designer of the pacemaker), left Toronto for Alberta. And it was a year later, in September 1956, that Callaghan conducted Canada's first successful open-heart surgery at the University of Alberta Hospital.[3] He and his team had gone down to the University of Minnesota to watch Lillehei and DeWall perform open-heart surgery, and on their return they used the Lillehei-DeWall helical reservoir bubble oxygenator to surgically correct an atrial septal defect in ten-year-old Suzanne Beattie.[4] Callaghan was a retiring man, but his nursing team was so proud of his achievements that they "bought a personalized costume for their hero that was similar to Superman's outfit. The uniform featured a large red and yellow logo with an S on the front, and a red cape attached to his operating clothes."[5]

The Toronto part of the pump story began at the General in 1956, when Bigelow asked Heimbecker and Barrie Fairley in anesthesia to revive research on a heart-lung machine. Heimbecker and Fairley travelled to the Mayo Clinic and to Lillehei's group at the University of Minnesota in Minneapolis, and returned with a Lillehei-DeWall machine that they copied (with Heimbecker's modifications) and set up in the lab in the basement of the Banting Building. They then took the device across College Street to the Ward C operating room. By January 1957 they had done in the Banting basement "over a hundred animal experiments," using a "simple bubble oxygenator."[6] Meanwhile, the vogue for using monkey lungs to supply oxygen in bypass rose and fell with Bill Mustard.[7] The mortality was very high. George Trusler, then a resident at HSC, recalls, "Unfortunately, the monkey lungs became edematous and ceased to function after 15 or 20 minutes."[8] After a number of deaths, Mustard had his first surviving patient later in 1953. Artificial oxygenators offered a more practical alternative.

With Heimbecker's oxygenator ready, in November 1956 Bigelow asked the hospital administration to purchase two Sigmamotor pumps. He noted that "the University Hospital in Minneapolis have operated on 190 patients with this pump and it is being used regularly in many centres now including Johns Hopkins, The Mayo Clinic, Chicago and even Edmonton." Furthermore, "We are already building up a back log of patients awaiting operation with a pump oxygenator that cannot be treated by any other technique including hypothermia." This was no longer "research," and, Bigelow concluded, "I hope that the hospital will approve buying this." They should acquire it "as soon as possible."[9]

The bypass team honed their skills on dogs in the basement lab at the Banting. As Heimbecker told Murray in March 1957, "Enclosed is a little summary of the problems of extra corporeal circulation ... To bring you up to date, six adult patients [dogs are presumably meant] have now been operated upon, and all are well." Heimbecker then listed the six subjects, all of whom survived. "It is really remarkable to see a bloodless heart lying there motionless for 40–50 minutes, and then literally 'snap' back into activity."[10] (Unfortunately, by December 1957 it appeared that the real mortality rate among dogs was 51 per cent.[11])

So, the cardiac team was ready to go. On 10 January 1958, Bigelow told a correspondent, "I think we have found most of the major problems in hypothermia and this month we will be starting our pump cases."[12] Two days later, on 12 January the first pump operation in Eastern Canada took place. Heimbecker recalled, "The OR was electric that day." Present were Bigelow, Key, Wilson, and Heimbecker, plus Barry Fairley as anesthetist. Their patient, a twenty-five-year-old woman from Northern Ontario, had a large atrial septal defect ("the size of a silver dollar" in some accounts). The Red Cross provided twenty units of blood less than twenty-four-hours old. There was as yet no intensive care unit, so the surgeons themselves had to provide twenty-four-hour coverage. "Much to our delight the operation proceeded beautifully." The pump ran twenty-five minutes. The patient had a very smooth post-op course and was discharged on tenth day, to the "excitement and delight of the entire hospital." Maybe the "pump" was not "pie in the sky after all," Heimbecker said.[13] (On the end of Heimbecker's pump, see chapter 18.)

The pump at this point was for the repair of intracardiac defects, not for bypassing blocked coronary arteries. (Operating on the coronary arteries does count as "open-heart surgery.") In October 1958, Bigelow told Eric Nanson at the University of Saskatchewan that they were doing two pump cases a week, "with very satisfactory results on complicated atrial septal defects, mitral regurg [mitral valve regurgitation] and simple ventricular septal defects. We have had very unhappy results with our Tetralogys [sic] and for the moment I think we will set them aside. We are using the Cooley modification of the bubble oxygenator at present but I think we will probably switch into a disc fairly soon. This is very time consuming work as you know. Ray Heimbecker and I seem to be tied down by the amount of operating and the intense post-operative care that they require. It takes quite a team."[14] (In a bubble oxygenator the venous blood is pumped through a reservoir of oxygen, either directly or through a filter; in a rotating disk oxygenator, the extracorporeal venous blood passes through a series of rotating disks in a container of oxygen.)

Bigelow may have been pretty-facing what were apparently disastrous early results. According to a tabulation of Heimbecker's, on "14 October" (presumably 1958), of nineteen "pump" cases to date, there had been six deaths, one in a case of "mitral regurgitation." Two of the three tetralogies had died.[15] Note that the alternative to surgery was certain death.

I January 1959 Bigelow performed what he said was the first mitral valve operation on the pump, adjusting the ring about the valve. (Tightening the mitral annulus for regurgitation must have been meant.) It was, for this female patient, the first of a series of heart operations, but Bigelow wrote on her chart, "Probably the first open heart mitral valve operation."[16]

Bypass changed a number of things: operating room times, for example. The typical bypass operation took about four hours. The demand was such that the division tried to schedule two bypass operations a day, in each of the two operating rooms on "POR" (an OR on the Private Patients Pavilion). The procedures would start, as always, around eight o'clock in the morning. Four o'clock in the afternoon was the conventional closing time for the ORs. The problem, said Bigelow, is that "we are increasingly finding ourselves in the situation that the first operation is over by 12:30 or 1:00 and we are unable to start the second case for fear of running overtime." This was wasteful because it "leaves the operating rooms lying idle all afternoon," and was upsetting to the patients whose surgeries were postponed or cancelled as a consequence. The solution was to extend the OR time to six o'clock in the evening.[17] This does not sound like a big deal, but it was.

Once the patient was hooked up to the pump for over an hour, the bubble oxygenator became unsatisfactory, as it traumatized the blood and had a tendency to pump the anti-foaming mixture, which was necessary for its use, into the brain.[18] Baird later said, "The greatest nightmares that I still have are of the early open-heart surgery, with the pump, because the use of the early pumps defibrinated the blood, so it would stay nice and fluid while you were operating but you couldn't get it to clot afterwards. A major cause of death was post-operative hemorrhage in the early 60s."[19] Thus, for such lengthy procedures as total valve replacements, attention now turned to disk oxygenators.

The pump meant that space dedicated to cardiac surgery was also necessary. (See chapter 6.) Bigelow said in September 1957, arguing for a special cardiac-surgery facility on floors eight and nine of the Private Patients Pavilion, "No special operating room and hospital facilities have been requested in the past for ordinary heart and great vessel surgery but this field of open heart surgery, which is rapidly expanding, does require special space, equipment, and staff. Most of the better centers in the United States have already met this problem."[20] (He often used this argument on hospital administrators keen not to be left behind the United States.)

In the coming five years, the cardiac surgeons at the General operated on aortic stenosis and a host of other cardiac conditions. (Aortic aneurysms in the abdomen belonged to the general surgeons and, later, the vascular surgeons – although the cardiac surgeons continued to do abdominal aortic aneurysms until the 1980s.) It was an unbelievably exciting time. After 1953, "[Bill] was soon joined by Don Wilson and shortly thereafter by Jim Key and Ray Heimbecker," Baird said. "These are the five men whom I deeply revere as my teachers. When I first worked on Ward "C' as a junior intern in 1954, they were still doing varicose veins and gallbladders. That didn't last long."[21] (The east side of the College Wing, where Ward C was located, was surgical; the west side, medical.)

There was, however, a bit of ill will. As Baird reports, "At that time only Bill Bigelow and Ray Heimbecker were allowed to operate with the pump. Don Wilson could not accept this situation and made plans to leave the Toronto General Hospital for the Toronto Western Hospital." In 1959, Wilson moved to the Western, and in 1964 Baird joined him.[22] In years ahead, Wilson and Baird built a huge cardiovascular service with a heart-lung pump at the Western – a service that Tirone David then ramped up even more powerfully (but let's not get ahead of our story).

By October 1961, four bypass teams had been formed at the General: one led by Bigelow himself, the others by Baird, Herbert Basian, and Heimbecker; with Bigelow doing two pumps a week, the others one. Bigelow urgently demanded a big increase in space to increase the number of bypass operations.[23]

Don Wilson

Born in 1917 in Saskatoon, Saskatchewan, Donald Richards Wilson grew up in a home that valued education. His father was a teacher, and both his grandfathers were ministers. He attended Nutana Collegiate Institute in Saskatoon, then the University of Saskatchewan to study the first years of medicine for a BA degree. This is interesting: Don Wilson was from Saskatchewan, Bill Bigelow from Manitoba, and Ray Heimbecker from Alberta. Wilson said later, "We were known as the Western group."[24]

In 1939 Wilson progressed to Toronto, where in 1942 he completed a medical degree. At University of Toronto, he played intramural basketball. He later said that he had "no great driving ambition to be a doctor" but his mother wanted him to be a minister or a physician, so he chose medicine.[25]

Wilson served in the Royal Canadian Army Military Corps from 1942 to 1946, and it was at a Canadian base in the UK that "Kager" Wightman, his commanding officer and later head of medicine, tried to persuade him to go into internal medicine. Yet Wilson returned to Calgary after the war, planning to be a family physician. He then got a call from Professor Gallie inviting him into the surgical program at University of Toronto. He won his surgical fellowship in 1950, then spent half a year in Britain and Sweden before returning to the General – and to the Wellesley Hospital, which then was a kind of surgical Ward 4 of the General.

Thus, Wilson began his surgical experience "with the excitement of Gordon Murray and Bill Bigelow," as John Evans – later University of Toronto president – put it. "Since Gordon Murray was heavily engaged in heart surgery and other types of surgery with private patients and Bigelow was working on hypothermia in the Banting, Donald Wilson had all of Ward C to himself for his surgical experience."[26] It was in these years that Wilson started to become interested in cardiovascular surgery. He said later, "Uncle Bill brought his hypothermia to the clinical side and I helped him do every original case he did on the hypothermia routine ... Bill and I were first and then Jim Key came along."[27]

But what is of interest here is that, after leaving the General in a moment of irritation, in 1958 he founded cardiovascular surgery at the Western, becoming in addition surgeon-in-chief at that hospital in 1966.[28] In 1959 Wilson organized the Cardiovascular Society, which met at the General six times a year.[29] As we shall see, it was under Don Wilson's aegis that the first heart transplant in Toronto was done (see chapter 9). Wilson later became professor of surgery in Toronto and chair of the Department of Surgery, as well as president of the Royal College of Physicians and Surgeons of Canada and was a figure of great distinction in Canadian medicine.

Coronary Artery Bypass Grafting (CABG)

Bypass surgery – circumventing a blocked coronary artery with a piece of vein – began with Argentinian surgeon René Favaloro at the Cleveland Clinic in May 1967. On pump, the surgeons bypassed the blocked artery with a piece of vein, permitting oxygenated blood in the aorta to flow into the coronary arteries beyond the area of stenosis or blockage, thereby restoring oxygenated blood flow to the ischemic myocardium (heart muscle). In Toronto the operation was often referred to as aortocoronary bypass.

Bypass surgery in Toronto began in March 1969, on a patient with stable angina (pain on exertion but not usually at rest). Baird later said, "None of us realized what a massive change in cardiac surgery had begun." Soon the cardiac surgeons were so busy they had to discontinue peripheral vascular and abdominal aortic surgery. By December 1972 they had done one hundred procedures for stable angina alone, with a 2.5 per cent mortality rate.[30]

The late 1960s and early 1970s offered the picture of a cardiac surgery service in full technological transformation. In 1968 no aortocoronary bypass operations were done, and 52 Vineberg single internal mammary implants were carried out. As we saw above, aortocoronary bypass began in 1969: 14 operations. The Vineberg single-sided operation fell from 52 to 12.[31] By 1971 aortocoronary bypass had risen to 198, the Vineberg internal mammary procedure (single or double) had fallen to 22. The Cardiovascular Unit in "Bigelow's Bungalow" was used mainly for catheterization; all "pumps" – well over 400 altogether – were still done on the ninth floor of what was now the University Wing. And the Pacemaker Clinic was in full swing with almost 300 procedures (new insertions and battery changes together).[32] Perhaps out of discretion, to spare Bigelow's feelings, statistics on operations conducted solely under hypothermia were not tabulated, but there could not have been many.

By November 1973 the Toronto surgeons had performed bypass surgery on just over one thousand patients, the great majority for "unstable angina" as a result of blocked coronary arteries. Eighty-two per cent of the patients were men; without hypothermia, the average period of arrest in bypass was thirty minutes; with hypothermia, sixty minutes. Eighty-seven of the patients got the Vineberg procedure, not the standard aortocoronary bypass.[33]

The advent of aortocoronary bypass changed much of the work of the cardiologists and surgeons. Said Harold Aldridge, associate director of the Cardiovascular Unit, in 1971, "With the advent of saphenous aortocoronary bypass surgery, many patients who were turned down for evaluation are now being investigated [catheterized]; even such patients as were considered for cardiac transplantation now fall into the category in whom aortocoronary bypass surgery can be carried out. This means that we are investigating a higher risk group than previously, and it therefore follows that the mortality for procedures within the Cardiac Unit may well rise."[34]

Bigelow saw a giant wall of patients advancing for bypass. In May 1971 he told hospital executive director James A. McNab, "Aortocoronary by-pass has become available in the last two to three years for the treatment of patients with coronary heart diseases. A vein graft is used to bring blood directly from the main aorta into the coronary artery by-passing around the coronary artery obstruction. The results are quite dramatic. Ninety per cent obtain relief with a mortality rate of only 5%. Ninety-two of these operations have been performed since the new year, which is more than we performed in the previous two years as an index of the upsurge of the interest in this procedure. Certainly the number of people in the population who would benefit from an improvement of the blood supply to the heart is staggering."[35]

At the beginning of the 1970s, an American surgeon named George Green began using the left internal mammary artery rather than the saphenous vein for coronary bypass.[36] The tougher artery better withstood the higher pressures on the arterial side than did the vein. We shall not follow this story in Toronto, but readers will want to know that left internal mammary artery or bilateral internal mammary arteries have become the gold standard of bypass in the last decades.

In the early days, the surgeons hedged a bit on the mortality rate. Rather than reporting overall mortality, they said in 1974 that in patients with "good or fair left ventricular function," it was only 2.7 per cent; and for the last two hundred patients overall mortality was only 1.8 per cent.[37] The mortality picture then improved steadily. In 1981, 2,400 Toronto patients received bypass operations, with an average of 98 per cent surviving. Bernie Goldman said that in 1982 and 1983 the "mortality rate for coronary bypass procedures was only 0.9 per cent or one in a hundred" – down from 30 per cent in the 1970s.[38]

A Vast Reservoir of Cardiac Disease

Despite these challenging odds, patients now came literally hurtling into the OR, so great was the buildup of jaw pain, chest pain, arm pain, and other prognosticators of crippling, fatal coronary artery problems. Ontario turned out to be a vast reservoir of cardiac disease, and now that relief was available in bypass, the demand on the service was overwhelming. In June 1965 Bigelow, desperate for more operating-room time, wrote to W.R. Harris, chair of the OR committee, "The total number of open heart operations is increased by 42% in 1965, and the total of all cardiovascular operations of all types is up 39% in 1965. I think you will admit this is an incredible increase in operating load, and each week we have many cases left over that do not have booking time."[39]

Who might be left over? Ray Heimbecker told Bigelow in May 1965, "At the moment there are four patients that I know of in hospital who are waiting urgent or semi-emergency pump procedures." All were aortic valve replacements. There was Mr. O. "[who] has been urgently waiting for four and a half weeks. Mr. E. for over four weeks. Mrs. S. for almost four weeks and Mrs. H. for five weeks."

"All of these patients ... were considered too ill to be discharged and re-admitted." But the pump itself was "totally booked up to early July."[40]

Waiting could mean an unfavourable outcome. Some cardiac problems in particular had quite a short time between the onset of symptoms and death. In angina patients, for example, there was a 15 per cent mortality rate per year after the surgeon had seen them.[41] (Stenosis of the aortic valve and abdominal aortic aneurysms are discussed elsewhere.)

Under these circumstances, being put on a five-month waiting list was really cutting things very finely.

In Bigelow's numerous requests for a unitary cardiac unit (see chapter 6), there was an underlying theme: the waiting times justified a cardiovascular unit. Said Bigelow in 1964, "[At present] a patient destined for open heart surgery [has] to await three months for his admission to hospital for investigation, following which he is booked for surgery which cannot be done at this time, and will involve a two to three month wait again before surgery is available. Many of the valvular lesions and practically all of the aortic valve surgery cannot wait this long. This requires an urgent admission for investigation." But, said Bigelow, when the patient is admitted, the catheterization is often delayed several days. But if the Cardiovascular Division had its own beds, on its own unit, all could be done with much greater dispatch.[42] Expanding the cardiac surgery unit on the Private Patients Pavilion, floors eight and nine, was discussed continually. There was extensive planning in 1967 about the location of the nurses' station, the patients' rooms, the doctors' offices and so forth.[43]

Alan Trimble noted in October 1966 of "the present problems with the Urgent List and even more, of the problems of admitting pump patients. At present we cannot get beds for elective admissions, and this includes elective pump bookings, despite plenty of space available in the pump book, until March 1st of next year ... There are a certain number of aortics and mitrals [valves] that just can't sit this long, and what the solution is, I don't know."[44] Nature, in a sense, offered the solution: in 1965 Bigelow threw up his hands: "I have reached the stage where [waiting] is past being a service problem and it almost appears to be a hospital responsibility to get some of these patients in, in view of the deaths we are having while on the waiting list."[45]

Demand was soaring. In 1967 Heimbecker noted a huge increase in volumes of open-heart surgery, from 93 in 1961 to 163 in 1967. "What is even more important, however, is the type of case has changed considerably. The open heart repair today is usually much more complicated." In 1961, there were only 47 cardiac valve patients, 120 in 1967. "It is this type of lesion which requires a much more sophisticated system of pump heads and tubing. In aortic valve replacement for instance, we require three arterial lines, five pumping heads, as well as the usual system of venous return, suction return etc. Thus the pumping equipment and management is three or four times as complicated as it is for a straightforward congenital heart repair." (This was regarding the need for a third pump technician.)[46] By 1968 approximately one-third of the cardiac patients were on pump (in the first six months, 101 of 325).[47]

The above were valve and septum operations. But it was in the area of coronary artery disease that the reservoir of illness in the population was enormous. Changes were needed. "As the field expands," Heimbecker quizzed Bigelow in December 1970, "specially that of coronary artery disease, are we going to ask for a larger unit; do we need more beds and therefore do we need expanded operating room area – perhaps a third pump room? ... We seem to be reaching 300 pumps or more for this year." Heimbecker added in a handwritten postscript: "(1) Anaesthetic room needed to expedite our operating day; (2) Need of third pump room clear as with emerging [emergency] pumps in CBOR [Centre Block Operating Room] recently."[48]

The pressure on the unit for new admissions became ever more intense as the news spread that cardiac surgery could offer new hope to the many languishing heart patients. "I think a [great] problem is our volume load as it now stands," Al Trimble told Bigelow in 1971. "I think we all realize this is not seasonal but I think it is putting a terrific strain on the resident staff, nurses etc, and unless we take immediate action everybody is going to crack up."[49]

So, how to deal with this increased demand? In a big hospital this is not so simple. Can we increase the number of operations on the ninth floor, Jim Key, in Bigelow's absence, asked the head nurse Joan Breakey. But Breakey told Key that a heavier patient load was just impossible – "not for lack of nursing staff – but because she – at present – has to spend most of the morning trying to get patients accepted either on the eighth floor or the floor from which they have been bed-spaced and make room for the day's OR cases." (Bed-spacing means finding a bed any place for chronic patients who can't be discharged home or to community-based facilities but for whom active treatment has stopped.) "But not only does she run into trouble trying to get patients back to a bed-spaced ward, but, of course, their [own cardiac] patients (one or two days post-pump or major post-op) are not suitable for transfer to say wards like 2 G.B., where the nurses know nothing about post op acute heart care and the residents are just too much out of touch and too far away. It is obvious therefore," Key concluded, "that our prime need is more ward beds first and foremost if we are to try and continue the present turn-over rate because this is the primary bottle-neck."[50]

Research Begins on "Cardiac Protection"

Stopping the heart completely during bypass ("anoxic arrest") had considerable advantages for the surgeon, now able to operate on "a quiet, bloodless field in a flaccid heart," as the Toronto team, led by

Goldman, reported in 1971. Yet after more than half-hour or so of "cross-clamping" – clamping off the ascending aorta so that blood no longer flows into the coronary arteries – the anoxia risked damaging the heart muscle. An alternative was the more cumbersome technique of "continuous perfusion" of the coronary arteries. After comparing the two techniques in dog and human hearts, the Toronto team found that anoxia lasting more than twenty minutes was deleterious to the dog heart. The human heart could apparently tolerate longer periods of anoxia, but after around forty-five minutes at normal temperatures ("normothermia"), the team recommended nonetheless that coronary artery perfusion be commenced.[51] The issue of "cardiac protection" continued to preoccupy Toronto researchers for the next several decades, as Richard Weisel became the chief player.

Bypass Becomes Routine

There was no arguing with success. By 1980 aortocoronary bypass had become so routine that Eddie Keshen, who for twenty years had played handball at the downtown Jewish Community Centre with his pal Jack Kwinter, was thinking about getting one. Kwinter and Keshen had started playing handball one day around one o'clock and stopped around five, as Kwinter won 21–17. He thereupon had a heart attack. He later quipped, "It was worth it." But it wasn't quite worth it, because he did not recover spontaneously from the apparently mild attack but started to go downhill. His cardiologist, Brian Gilbert, sent him to Bernie Goldman. Kwinter had "one artery completely blocked and another was on the verge," he said.

On 11 April 1980, Kwinter had the surgery and two weeks later was back at work. "I feel terrific, 100 percent," Kwinter said, "If someone asked me if I had ever been seriously sick in my life, I'd tell them no." Keshen found his newly invigorated handball buddy an even tougher opponent, and thought that he might need a bypass himself.[52] Bypass surgery had thus become routine.

But there is routine and routine. By the year 2000, coronary artery bypass surgery had become a routine procedure on an international basis. Yet the Canadian rate was lower than in many other places. A study in 1997 contrasting CABG for Ontario and New York state found the New York rate 1.8 times greater than the Ontario rate. Whereas in New York state, the procedure tended to be performed on older women and patients over age seventy-five who'd had heart attacks (myocardial infarcts), in Ontario the procedure was used before an actual heart attack: more often for blockages in the left anterior descending artery ("left main disease"), for other forms of severe coronary artery disease, and for left ventricular dysfunction (which may have been caused by a previous heart attack).[53] There was also some indication that the medical methods of cardiology were just as effective in the management of patients with "stable" angina.[54]

Even at the present, the debate continues: percutaneous coronary intervention via a catheter in the groin versus bypass surgery? It is not hard to stack the deck. Just try asking a patient, "Which would you prefer: a huge incision in your chest and two weeks in hospital, or a small incision in your groin and discharge the next day?" For patients, this is not a difficult choice. Yet the cardiologists' stents in the coronary arteries tend to clog up. Redos are necessary. The surgeon's fix may last for decades, or forever. Your choice.

Chapter Nine

Moving On

As Bigelow eased back, his early colleagues and students started to come on line. This is basically why Toronto edged past Montreal as Canada's premier heart centre: Bigelow's students were so productive.

Heart Transplantation: First Wave

Following the success of Christiaan Barnard in transplanting hearts in South Africa in 1967, heart transplantation was on everyone's lips. Not all were thrilled. John Callaghan, who had left Toronto for Edmonton, predicted in January 1968 the imminent death of Barnard's patient and roundly criticized the operation,[1] yet the patient, Philip Blaiberg, lived for nineteen months. Montreal surgeon Pierre René Grondin performed the first heart transplant in Canada on 30 May 1968, at the Montreal Heart Institute; by October 1968 he had conducted six, three of whom remained alive.[2]

Could Toronto be far behind? Bill Drucker, who was the university chair of surgery, wanted to make sure it wasn't. Heart transplant was now a very hot potato thrown into Drucker's lap. In 1967, Drucker had become professor of surgery. Baird said, "Bill had tough political sledding in Toronto. In his first year he had to publicly deny Gordon Murray's claim that he had developed an operation which could cure paraplegia."[3] In May 1968 Drucker noted that heart transplantation was creating "world-wide interest." Therefore, the Toronto hospitals must move forward in a "coordinate[d] manner." "In view of the magnitude of this job, I have asked that Dr. William [sic] Bigelow, the Director of the Cardiovascular Surgical Services, take full responsibility for the organization and implementation of the clinical and laboratory program for heart transplantation." He was sure that everyone would cooperate with Bigelow.[4]

Goldman recalls, "After Barnard's transplant in December 1967, Bigelow corralled me in Bristol and made suggestions for my stay in Boston – make side trips to Palo Alto and Houston to learn about their transplant programs, which I did in the Winter of '68."[5]

But there was a problem. The four Toronto hospitals, which had just formed the Inter-Hospital Cardiovascular Surgical Committee, were unable to agree on who would first perform the procedure (although Drucker insisted in the press that there was perfect comity).[6] At St. Michael's, the surgeons were said to be "keen to go ahead." The Western argued for its deep reservoir of experience in kidney transplants. And at the General, "[the] surgeons feel their hospital has the most extensive background in other forms of open heart surgery." (An article by Joan Hollobon, the medical columnist for the *Globe and Mail*, pointing out these rivalries stirred up much irritation among the surgeons, who definitely did not want this washing displayed publicly.[7])

Thus, the nod went to the Western. Why not the General? Ron Baird later said, "Bill Bigelow was then Canada's most famous cardiac surgeon and head of the largest unit in the city. However, he was in his mid-fifties, and his unit was in a period in which staff relations were very unsettled. He was barely on speaking terms with Prof. Drucker. No one at TGH was expert in transplant immunology; they had no animal experience in cardiac transplantation [this was false], and their clinical renal transplant program was in the doldrums. At TWH we had the first and the largest renal transplant program in Canada, and a core of excellent immunologists. [Ontario's first successful kidney transplant had been conducted at the Western on 31 January 1966, under the aegis of George deVeber.] Our cardiac surgery program was smaller than TGH but was growing faster. Don Wilson and I were close colleagues and had excellent relations with Prof Drucker ... [The feeling at TWH was that] it was time for us to show what we could do."[8] (It was also helpful for the Western that Wilson was able to use the prospect of doing heart transplants as a spur to fundraising.[9] Indeed, in December 1967, Wilson strengthened the hospital's hand by announcing plans for a heart transplant centre.[10])

Yet, despite this pushback, Bigelow was not shy about suggesting that the General be considered the dominant hospital in Toronto. He said in 1967 of the structuring of cardiovascular services in Metro, "It is felt that one hospital should be authorized and supported as a central cardiovascular unit. It should serve, in adult surgery, as the major training area and be expected to explore many of the new ideas and techniques ... An example is the planned provision of immune chemist[ry] at the Banting Institute attached to our Cardiovascular Laboratory whose services could be used by other University teams."[11]

Baird and Bigelow visited the Montreal Heart Institute and then travelled with Al Trimble to Houston to watch DeBakey. Baird said of the politics of this, "Don Wilson, Ray Heimbecker and the surgeons at SMH were rather pointedly excluded from these trips. In September 1968, there was a rather acrimonious meeting of the cardiologists and cardiac surgeons at TGH and TWH in which Bill stated that he and Al [Trimble] planned to perform the first transplant. Ray would take the pictures and Don and I would observe. The delegation from TWH did not agree. Don Wilson acquired Bill Drucker's blessing to proceed at TWH."[12]

In view of the acrimony, Drucker was at pains to make sure that everyone played nice. On 11 October he sent out a memo pleading for unity. "I do hope that we may succeed in establishing this project as a model of a 'University based' activity of the Department of Surgery."[13] But Bigelow was sooner resentful than pliant. He responded to the Drucker memo, "I have visited the Toronto Western with Donald Wilson and I did not encounter any specific research program that has been planned in relation to the operation of heart transplantation."[14] Thus Bigelow dismissed the Western's claim of a carefully prepared program (although at this point both hospitals had set aside dedicated operating rooms for heart transplant).

It wasn't that Wilson did an end run around Bigelow. On Saturday, 19 October, at 4 a.m. Bigelow phoned Drucker in his Montreal hotel room and said they had a donor. It was Bigelow who suggested that the donor "should be sent to Western Hospital, rather than be retained at Toronto General" (where he would have donated his kidneys). Drucker consented.[15] Goldman said, "I obtained the heart at TGH and rushed it over in a cold basin to the TWH." Then Baird and Wilson transplanted it. (Officially, Don Wilson led the team.[16]) At the Western, said Goldman, "Ron Baird graciously insisted we all scrub in and place a stitch or two to make the combined effort a 'pan University event.'"[17] Kidney transplant specialist George deVeber assisted. The operation, on Pietro Ongaro, age forty-two, was a complete success and a sensation in Toronto.[18] After the operation a tired-looking Don Wilson came down to meet the thirty reporters and photographers who had gathered in a dining room. He expressed surprise at all the media attention. "You're news now," said a reporter.[19] (This impromptu press conference contravened completely Bigelow's recommendations to Drucker for carefully managed press relations.[20])

The patient survived in relatively good health for seven months but then died rather suddenly from rejection.[21]

A second transplant patient at the Western, Henry Taylor, age forty-five, died a week after the operation. Yet the kidneys and the eyes from the body of the donor, a lad of twenty, brightened the lives of other patients.[22]

Metro Toronto's third heart transplant took place at TGH on 13 November 1968. There, all was in readiness. "Bernie [Goldman] had been assigned to preservation of the donor [heart] while Trimble organized the recipient's operation. Key and Heimbecker also participated. The heart of Jerry Shanahan, twenty-three, whose pickup truck had overturned near Barrie, was transplanted into the chest of Alfred Gagnier, fifty-four, a father of nine and former milkman from Belle River, Ontario.[23] The operation lasted forty-nine minutes, and "The heart began beating immediately after an electric shock, and generated a blood pressure reading of 120 to 140."[24] The *Globe and Mail* ran a photo of a beaming Gagnier, who unfortunately stroked shortly thereafter and died a week later.

Metro's fourth transplant was performed at St. Michael's Hospital on 17 November 1968 by Clare Baker and James Yao. The story is that Bigelow wanted another shot at transplant and wasn't keen that St. Mike's was moving ahead on this. So, as Goldman recalls, "Bigelow called over to Clare [Baker], because he knew they were going to do a transplant, and he said 'Clare, this should be a pan-university thing, and it should be done at the General, because we have the resources and the backup.' Clare is reported to have said 'Well thanks for calling Bill, but I've got to get to the OR, our patient has just arrived.'"[25]

The patient was Charles Perrin Johnston, an engineer, and the operation was a stunning success. He didn't need a respirator, and his wife, a head nurse at St. Michael's hospital, and Bigelow were able to chat with him the following day.[26] Two years later, in 1970, he was playing cribbage with Father Edward Madigan, the parish priest at St. Monica's Church on Broadway Avenue and the second St. Mike's cardiac transplant patient; this operation, as well, was also a great success.[27] (Johnston's new heart was such a success that he began jogging two miles a day, but had to give it up "because so many people came to watch him."[28]) Madigan lived for almost a decade and, said Baird, "was one of the world's longest survivors from this era of transplantation."[29] Yet the record of the 1968 wave of transplants was discouraging: there had been four transplants with one survivor. Cardiac transplant was almost abandoned in Toronto.

But not quite abandoned. When, in April 1969, Ron Baird conducted Toronto's fifth heart transplant, Bigelow, "who had taught all of [the surgeons]" and Clare Baker – animosities now forgotten – stood side by side looking on.[30]

Yet that was almost the end of it. Why did they give up so easily? Other early cardiac procedures were accompanied by horrendous mortalities, yet not abandoned. Bigelow said in 1969 that "if the heart transplant death rate is too high the operation may become discredited in the minds of the public and the general practitioner. [The early valve and septum operations weren't discredited because they were not followed so avidly in the press.] A family doctor might then fail to send a suitable candidate to a heart surgeon, so that people who could benefit might end up being denied the operation."[31] (So unseemly had the inter-hospital infighting been about these transplants that in December 1968 Bigelow asked Drucker to stop referring to him as "Chairman of the Inter-Hospital Cardiovascular Surgical Committee and that the importance of this position be de-emphasized ... This position has not been associated with authority as to where or when heart transplants should be done."[32])

As early as January 1969, some of the cardiologists were in revolt about the transplant deaths. What to do? Bigelow justified continuing the cardiac transplant program in this manner: "Future heart transplants are considered experimental," he said in a closely circulated memo. "We are doing them to accumulate scientific knowledge. It must be emphasized ... that it requires human material for its fulfilment."[33] Today, a bioethics committee would blink in disbelief at such lines.

By 1972 there had been seven cardiac transplants in Toronto, with three survivors, all from St. Michael's Hospital.[34] It was these successful transplants that really put St. Mike's on the cardiac surgery map, said Goldman later. He ranked the General number 1, the Western number 2. "And number 3, which we didn't even accept, was St. Michael's. It was just out there – until the transplant."[35]

Enthusiasm at the General for heart transplants definitely cooled. Meanwhile, transplant lists were still being kept, but none were being done – not because the surgeons were demoralized but because of an absence of donor hearts. By February 1971, all twelve patients awaiting heart transplants at St. Michael's Hospital had died on the list; twelve others had died at the General.[36]

Parenthetically, it will not have escaped readers that the names of the transplant patients and the donors were bandied freely about in the press. For physicians accustomed to patient confidentiality, this caused a certain discomfort, as well as discouraging families of future donors, who might not wish to see the identity of a departed loved one – particularly one whose death had been, in a sense, pre-arranged – displayed in the

public prints. (The donor, of course, dies as the heart is "harvested.")
So in May 1970 the Inter-Hospital Cardiovascular Surgical Committee decided "that this Committee would like to carry out future heart
transplants without any publicity and this would apply particularly to
publicity regarding the donor." Bigelow was to contact the newspapers,
and indeed acceptance had already been obtained from the *Telegram*.[37]
Such was the enthusiasm of the press for cardiac stories, however, that
this request was not always honoured.

The Intra-Aortic Balloon Pump Assist
(IABP, "Counter Pulsation")

On 4 August 1970, Joseph M., age forty-six, came into the hospital with
symptoms of a severe heart attack. He died ten days later. He actually
didn't have a chance. He had a history of heart attacks, and now all
three of his major vessels were almost completely blocked. At autopsy,
the pathologist noted "old occlusions" in various vessels and "recent
thrombotic occlusions in the left anterior descending coronary artery
and circumflex coronary artery. These had produced a large, recent
anteroseptal infarct and a recent posterior septal infarct."[38] (Septal
infarcts occur in the walls between the chambers.)

Bigelow reflected in September 1970 to pathologist Malcolm Silver,
who had conducted the autopsy, "From the description of your autopsy
report, he sounds as if he were in the group of patients whom they
recognize as having about 100% mortality rate. We are interested in
attempting to salvage these patients." Joseph M. had not undergone
surgery because the mortality of attempting even catheterization on
these patients was horrendous. "Our project for the next year or two,"
Bigelow told Silver, "is to have a safe and efficient method of circulatory support" for the sake of buying time so that the patients could be
properly investigated for surgery without dying on a gurney en route
to the catheter lab.[39]

The background is this: some patients, said a TGH report from around
1971, are admitted to hospital with "pre-infarction angina, meaning
they have a good chance of developing a heart attack with a 50 per cent
mortality." Other patients, like Joseph M., are admitted with frank heart
attacks. Those likely to die are patients "in shock or who have serious abnormalities in heart rate or rhythm." These patients need at once
emergency "mechanical support of the circulation, cardiac catheterization and surgical treatment."[40]

OK – what's the problem? The problem at the General in the 1970s
was that "the Coronary Care Unit, Cardiovascular Investigation Unit

and Cardiovascular Operating Rooms exist in diverse areas of the hospital. It is impossible," said Bigelow, "to suggest that any success at managing these patients surgically could be expected if they were on circulatory support in the Coronary Care Unit, transferred down elevators and halls to the Investigation Unit for the catheterization and then subsequently transferred to the Operating Room."[41]

So, how to stabilize them while they're awaiting care? The solution was to instal a portable "balloon support system" in the acute therapy unit of the cardiac surgery area (called "POR," after the former Patients Private Pavilion). Balloon support was a form of "supportive circulation while the doctors attempt to determine what part surgery might play in treating the patients ... The balloon is attached to the end of a catheter. Every time the heart fills the balloon opens, and when the heart beats, the balloon closes. The purpose of the circulatory support is to keep the patient alive while an x-ray can be taken to see whether surgery is indicated."[42] (When the balloon fills, it forces the blood back into the coronary arteries, letting them resupply the heart muscle. Note that this is not "balloon angioplasty," or using a balloon to clear plaque in coronary arteries, which German radiologist and cardiologist Andreas Grüntzig introduced in Zurich in 1977.[43]) The catheter was inserted in the aorta via the femoral artery (in the groin).

In June 1971 Ray Heimbecker went down to Pittsburgh to attend a heart association meeting and told Bill Greenwood on returning, "As a result of the recently reported series from the MGH Hospital [Massachusetts General] in Boston it would appear that there is a very worthwhile future in aortic balloon support of the circulation in patients in cardiogenic shock." (Joseph M. had died in cardiogenic shock: the heart simply stops pumping after sustaining so much damage.) At the Massachusetts General there had been "14 cases with balloon support followed by emergency coronary bypass ... Our own facilities would probably involve some 24 patients a year who are in cardiogenic shock on admission to our Coronary Care Unit."[44]

As senior resident, Scully put in the first twenty balloons with an aortic balloon pump (to rest the heart in cardiogenic shock) "to see if they would work, and they did." It was actually Goldman who brought the concept back from his own stay at Harvard, but it was Scully who installed the first ones. Used before the operation, the intra-aortic balloon pump (IABP) had the advantage of assuring the blood supply to the heart in patients who'd had heart attacks and were at imminent risk of dying: it maintained "pulsatile" (heartbeat-like) blood flow to the heart muscle in patients "with left ventricular dysfunction and minimal cardiac reserve [who] cannot afford to lose any more myocardial tissue." As the investigators reported in 1976, preoperative use of the pump increased survival of their high-risk patients to 88 per cent.[45] The IABP could also be used during the operation on patients who had trouble coming off the pump.

In June 1973 Bernie Goldman wrote to surgeon-in-chief Bob Mustard (not Bill Mustard, the cardiac surgeon at the Hospital for Sick Children) about a new program for inserting a catheter with an expansible balloon at the end of it to keep heart-attack patients alive while major surgery could be organized for them. Complicated approvals for something like this were necessary.[46] The big hospital and the provincial Ministry of Health were nothing if not bureaucratic.

Bigelow was irritated that Goldman had rather jumped the gun on this. There were all kinds of budgetary sensitivities involved. Bigelow back-pedalled to the administration and said, oh, really, this program has been discussed since January and the Budget Committee has "approved in principle the establishment of this program."[47] This may have been a fib.

The balloon catheter service was set to go as of 1 July 1973, when Hugh Scully, who in February had gone down to the Massachusetts General in Boston to learn the balloon techniques, returned to Toronto. Scully, who had been back and forth to Boston for two years, would be the senior resident in charge, assisted by resident John Gunstensen.[48] The Massachusetts General served as the lode star for balloon surgery: by February 1973 the Boston hospital had five balloon support pumps going; Bigelow observed that "to-date they have operated upon nearly 70 patients with a survival of over 80%. Nearly all of these patients would have died without this emergency management ... The Toronto General Hospital can be considered one of the senior regional centres for cardiac surgery in Canada ... Because of the heavy patient demand it is essential that these deficiencies be corrected."[49]

Indeed, the IABP turned out to be so useful that the division over-spent its budget in 1974 by about $17,000. Could Bernie Goldman possibly present a request for a supplement to the TGH Research Foundation? "This is a sensitive political area," Bigelow told him, "and the manner of presentation should probably be discussed."[50]

The residents in cardiology loved the balloon work because it got them involved on the invasive side; the nurses on the cardiac surgery acute treatment unit were equally thrilled; they had, Goldman said, "no fear of the pump console and there have been really no nursing problems at all." The problem lay in the acceptance of the procedure by a calcified hospital administration and the provincial bean counters. Bigelow would have to make some kind of presentation to them. He asked Goldman for an overview of the balloon pump patients.

The overview showed various outcomes. Some efforts had failed outright: "Patient B.L., 35, with LAD [left anterior descending artery] and circumflex [artery] bypass grafts. Massive infarct on table and balloon assist instituted relatively late and without any effect."

In other cases, the surgeons simply could not get the balloon catheter into the blood vessel. For example, there was "a patient with true infarction angina in whom the balloon simply would not pass through the buckled iliac artery and showed a kink pattern in the aorta." Outcome: fatal.

Or the balloon salvage was successful, but the patient died anyway: Patient A.G., age forty-eight, male, "three weeks post myocardial infarction. Repeated VT [ventricular tachycardia] and VF [ventricular fibrillation], gross failure, renal failure, cardiogenic shock. Balloon support reversed shock and controlled rhythm and allowed pulmonary and renal stabilization. Selective coronary angios and ventriculogram were performed using balloon support. Tolerated despite VF." But the patient developed a huge aneurysm on the wall of the left ventricle, and "although patient came off CPB [cardiopulmonary bypass] well on balloon, arrested just prior to Recovery Room transfer."

Yet the balloon success stories became ever more numerous. Patient G.B., age fifty-seven, male "with severe aortic stenosis, Grade IV ventricle, high LVEDP [left ventricular end-diastolic pressure] and triple coronary disease. Turned down at Rounds for surgery. Balloon pump instituted with induction [of anesthesia], through CPB and postoperative. Patient did well."[51] An apparently hopeless patient had been rescued through an act of surgical courage, despite the risk of making the mortality statistics look awful.

Cardiology also got a balloon pump for its Coronary Care Unit, under the direction of Al Adelman. If these patients required further cardiac procedures, they would, as we know, be moved to the ninth floor of the University Wing for care under Scully and Goldman.[52]

By the time of a *Toronto Star* story on the balloon pump in February 1975, the statistics were looking pretty good. Said Bigelow, "We have used the pump 88 times in the past 16 months with great success. On 33 patients with dangerous impending heart attacks, 32 survived ... [Many] of these people were in their 40s."[53] The balloon pump became the standard procedure for patients in cardiogenic shock, and more commonly, for those in unstable angina unresponsive to treatment, for patients with left main coronary stenosis and for those with poor left-ventricular function. It also became the standard tool for weaning some patients from bypass – and, said Goldman in 2018 – "still is!"[54]

Mortality

Motto: "If you can't handle people dying, you shouldn't be in cardiac surgery."[55]
                                          – Nurse Linda Harris, 2018

Bernie Goldman remembered that his wife once had to go see a very senior physician about something. "And I said, ooh, you mean the one whose mother-in-law I killed? I remember going out and telling him and his wife that the operation went beautifully. And then she arrested in the ICU and I had to go back out. So, you know, a) don't go out too soon, and b) send a resident."[56] (Scully always informed the family himself.)

Goldman said of the senior staff in the 1970s, who were always going off to their places in Collingwood – there were, of course, no cell phones – "They had built this insulation around themselves. Just like Bill Mustard, who I spent over a year with, couldn't speak to families, because he'd gone downstairs too many times to say, 'Your child is dead.'"

Lynda Mickleborough, part of the generation who *never* went away if their patients were in any danger at all, said to Goldman, "Do you think part of that, Bernie, may have been the difference between when they started cardiac surgery and when you started cardiac surgery? When they started, the mortality was so high, there was a fatalism built into it. Like you do the operation, either the patient's going to sail through or they're not. And when you came along, mortality is like 3 per cent or less." When Mickleborough herself came along, mortality was 1 per cent. Paradoxically, she almost never went away on weekends, just in case something should happen.[57]

(Goldman said, "Bigelow could never understand why I didn't have a place in Collingwood. And the invitation to join the Osler Ski Club. Because he said, 'There's two other Jewish men there' [laughter]."[58])

Surgeon Robert J. Cusimano ("R.J.") remembered every death. He would walk out to give the family the news. "It wasn't a surprise that he died, it was a risky thing," he told a journalist. "But what was a surprise was the family – how grateful they were. I am not saying everybody is thankful when someone dies. People are angry – and they should be. But I have been taken by how people react to a bad outcome, where they are almost consoling to me."[59]

Deaths on the table were demoralizing for cardiac surgeons. Dwight Harken, who initiated mitral valve operations in 1948, said, "Six of my first 10 patients died. This was so devastating that with the tenth patient and sixth death, I left the operating theater, insisting that I would never do another heart operation. I went home and to bed." (He reconsidered after a cardiologist drove to his home and insisted he must continue.)[60]

In Toronto, deaths on the table were frequent enough that a special protocol was required to deal with them. In normal discharges, the resident would write a note to the family doctor "including an assessment of the degree of success of the operation and what his future is." But "death on the table" was different. In 1960 Bigelow reminded resident Wolf Sapirstein, "Some of the final notes on patients that died are rather peremptory and should not be forwarded to the doctor without a proper covering letter." Could you, Wolf, please "telephone the doctor after a death, or write him, or both."[61] This was still not enough. In 1967 Bigelow insisted, "Operative notes should be written by the staff man and final notes, in such cases, should be dictated by the *Senior Resident* and should not be sent out to the local doctor until countersigned by the staff man."[62] Thus, an extra degree of gravitas in death was warranted.

How long to massage the heart in conditions of standstill? When could you stop? In August 1951 Bigelow wrote Robert M. Hosler, a Cleveland cardiac surgeon, "Regarding your resuscitation … what is the longest time which you have applied cardiac massage in the presence of complete standstill and no irregular isolated ventricular beat? – and yet obtained a return of cardiac function. I am asking this question to help me determine how long one should carry out massage before considering it hopeless, what is your criterion to discontinue the massage."[63] (Hosler's reply has not been preserved.) The operative notes from these years often contain the concluding comment, "Attempts at resuscitation were finally given up." (Less frequently do they say, "The patient died on the table.")

What to do with anxious and grieving relatives? Relatives who were smitten with news of a loved one's death needed someplace to compose themselves. The "sun room" on the eighth floor was the customary waiting area and a bit public. So in November 1971 Peter Tink, the hospital chaplain, asked Bigelow if a vacant office nearby might not serve this function. "It would be ideal if this could be furnished with some type of temporary sleeping accommodation, as well as a room with a telephone which can be used in emergency situations."[64] The nursing supervisor, Judy Wass, added that we need "this area as a quiet room for bereaved relatives; it is necessary at the present time to utilize either my office or the lecture room for this purpose and the atmosphere is not conducive to comfort."[65]

How often were such facilities actually required? Quite often. The situation was not so rosy in the operating rooms of the ninth floor. In 1968, for 714 admissions to the Cardiovascular Unit, there were 54 deaths, a rate of 7.6 per cent. Neurosurgery, also a high-mortality service, had a mortality of 6.8 per cent.[66] The reason for these high rates in both services is obvious: these were very sick patients with life-threatening brain and heart conditions. The mortality rate of valve replacements in 1970 and 1971 was 9.5 per cent: 21 deaths out of 220 patients operated on, mainly for mitral valve "splits" (commissurotomies) and aortic and mitral valve replacements. Of the 19 patients who'd had previous valve replacements and now had developed complications ("usually salvage cases with heart failure with infection"), mortality for second valve replacements was now 31.6 per cent.[67] These were the "higher risk group" – and Tirone David's acclaim today is based on his success with patients in this group (see chapter 20).

Mortality drops off quite rapidly, but the early figures were quite terrifying. Why was it so high? We have to remember that these surgeons were pioneers: They were carefully feeling their way across terrain that was entirely unexplored. George Trusler, speaking of early operations at the Children's Hospital for ventricular septal defects (mortality of 30 per cent), said, "We didn't know where the bundle of His was [a small muscle band that carries the electrical current that makes the heart chambers contract]. We didn't know exactly, and it was some years before we got a really precise idea of where it was. And that would cause a heart block, and in the early years, we didn't have implantable pacemakers, so if it was a permanent heart block it was – a child was going to die, yeah."[68]

Then the mortality picture began to improve. In 1969 Al Trimble told the director of the hospital, "Quite frankly I think because our open heart surgery is going so well now with very few early complications such as renal, cerebral, respiratory that used to be so frequent, that many of these open heart cases are almost easier to handle than some of the older aneurysms [of the aorta] and vascular surgery. Certainly this is the impression of the Nursing Department."[69]

In May 1971 Bigelow, explaining to executive director McNab why private donations were sometimes necessary, said "The field is advancing so rapidly that last year's budget doesn't always reflect this year's needs. We have been a tremendous success." Cardiovascular diseases now represented 25 per cent of admissions to the entire hospital. In bypass, for example, "The results are quite dramatic. Ninety percent obtain relief with a mortality rate of only 5%."[70] By 1984 the deaths had become few. Said the General's *Annual Report*, "As the largest cardiac surgery centre in Canada, TGH performed over 1000 open-heart procedures during the year." Overall survival was now at 96.5 per cent.

"Survival for aortic valve replacement was 99%, while for mitral valve repair it was 100%."[71]

Yet in cardiac surgery, unlike obstetrics or pediatrics, there are deeply chilling notes. On the occasion of Bigelow's retirement in 1977, Jim Key said, "Heart surgery, in the early days was a unique blend of crowning success and desperate failure. This has been true of many fields of surgical endeavour but in cardiac surgery, when the patient's heart stops – everything else seems to stop and it's very lonely and cold."[72]

Over the years, the risks of cardiac surgery declined steadily. Yet the risk didn't vanish. For patients needing emergency bypass surgery, the overall mortality was 8.1 per cent in the years 1990 to 2009. The figure, however, is deceptive. For patients who arrived in congestive heart failure, the mortality was 18.9 per cent (compared to 4.3 per cent in patients without congestive failure); for patients who needed cardiac support (called low cardiac output syndrome) in the intensive care unit, the mortality was 25.4 per cent (compared to 2.5 per cent of the patients who didn't need support).[73] So congestive failure and the subsequent need for support were highly lethal conditions; the other patients getting bypass grafts who arrived from the ER actually did quite well. They would have reason to be grateful.

Grateful Patients

Men and women pulled back from the brink of death by cardiac surgery were often grateful, for sure, and some were in a position to express their gratitude by supporting the hospital. The situation, for a hospital that prided itself on supplying all that was medically necessary, was not without ambiguity. Yet there was an avalanche of new admissions, and all kinds of new equipment suddenly became necessary. In bypass operations for example, in 5 to 10 per cent of the cases the grafted artery did not become patent. In 1971 a new flowmeter had just come onto the market that made it possible to check during the operation if the vessel was open. The TGH surgeons wanted one, yet it hadn't been in the year's budget. Then there were all the battery replacements and new pacemaker operations. "These two operations [bypass and pacemaker] are *new* operations putting a real strain on existing facilities," Bigelow emphasized to McNab in May 1971. "Many of them are urgent or emergencies, and the demand for this work reflects the confidence that the public and referring doctors have in our General Hospital service." Thus, a flowmeter was urgently needed but it wasn't in the budget.[74]

In the late spring of 1971, as Trimble later put it, a "voluntary group of grateful Jewish patients got together in their private campaign to get funds to purchase us a Flowmeter. This resulted in a certain degree of embarrassment and I know that they have all been thanked."[75] (In their enthusiasm, one of the donors contacted Brian Magee, who happened to be on the board of the hospital, who naturally asked what was going on that the hospital itself couldn't pay for this vital equipment.) The donors, twelve in number, had all been animated by Al ——, owner of —— Electric Company, and each contributed $500. Al —— said in a cover letter simply, "When this equipment is installed, I would appreciate the opportunity of meeting with you and seeing same."[76] In circularizing his friends at the Forest Hill Lions Club, Al —— noted, "This cause is very close to my heart. If not for this type of surgery, I would not be here today."[77]

Looking back over much of this work in 1973, Bigelow made an interesting point about bioethics, one with which many bioethicists will disagree – that sometimes it is necessary to expose patients to risk in order to make scientific advances. "I am only too well aware, as you know," he told Bill Greenwood, "of the individual risk that the patients produce by investigative procedures. My feeling is that in the past in this hospital we have possibly erred on the side of being too conservative in recommending the initial investigation for patients, although these decisions have all been made with the best interest of the patient at heart." Bigelow referred rather chillingly to his experience at Johns Hopkins Hospital with Richard Bing, the founder of cardiac catheterization: "We had patients die of air embolism and many other complications, but Bing's work paved the way for the whole field of cardiac catheterization. History is full of these incidents and I think if a unit such as ours decides they are going to function without taking a calculated risk for the benefit of medical science, then we will never be a great unit."[78] Today, this would be actively debated.

Another World

In April 1973 the director of TGH sent out a notice to "all staff doctors and house staff" that smoking in the operating room area was henceforth forbidden.[79] People had been smoking around the operating rooms! To us, this seems inconceivable, but they lived in a different world.

It was a much more formal world than ours. Bigelow's residents and fellows all called him "Dr. Bigelow." (He called them by their first names, of course.)

Goldman was astonished when, beginning a rotation in Boston, "I walked into the Mass General and I was introduced to 'Gerry.' 'Hi,

I'm Gerry.'" And who was Gerry? "He was the chief of heart surgery, and the chief of surgery at the Mass General and chairman of surgery at Harvard University. He was W. Gerald Austen."

In other ways, Bigelow's world is quite familiar, and he shares across the decades the same commitment to patient welfare and the same scientific curiosity that we have. He was a much more fluent writer than is customary today in the email space – although he invariably wrote the possessive "its" as "it's." And indeed, these pages have offered a quite favourable image of Bill Bigelow, who ranks among the founders of cardiac surgery and was undoubtedly one of Canada's medical greats.

Toronto medicine in the 1960s was no longer what it had been in the 1940s. The UK was no longer the holy grail, a destination that had to be included in the training of every academic physician. Bigelow was quite aware of this. "Until recently," he said in 1964, "Canadian medical schools and Canadian medical men have followed the lead of Britain and France and accepted their standards of excellence. Now the United States is the leader in most phases of medicine and it would appear that this has been brought about by a rapid transition and heavy orientation to research ... The Americans have set their standards of excellence in medicine and, as we have done in the past, there is little alternative but to try to meet them. These standards are based, among other things, on the amount and excellence of research in the university."[80] And, of course, philanthropy.

Yet in other ways, the Faculty of Medicine and the General were another world, quite unlike the big American research factories. A man like Bigelow, what was he worth? He would have been worth a lot at a US campus, which is why the Department of Surgery lost so many of its stars. But Bigelow was a big Canadian nationalist, and his salary reflected a meanness of circumstances typical more of Canada in the Depression than fast-lane science. Since 1968, he had been "geographical full-time," a full member of the hospital and university teaching and research faculty, to use the hospital jargon; in 1969 he received $25,000 from the University of Toronto, and he was entitled to earn an additional $30,000 or so that his total allowed income was $60,000. Anything he might have garnered above and beyond that went into a group fund and was dispensed for research and education purposes by a Finance Committee.[81] (Bigelow, with his modest compensation, was quite disgruntled when he found out how much Heimbecker was earning.)

So from a certain perspective Bigelow and his contemporaries were courageous people struggling to do right.

It must not, however, be thought that Bigelow was a latter-day Gandhi. A hint of bigotry peeked through the Upper Canadian graciousness. His recommendation for resident B., of South Asian origin, said, "My only reservation about Dr. B. is because of his ethnic origin, he does not have the aggressiveness or the ability to manage, organize and direct an important and active division or department in cardiovascular surgery. However, I may be mistaken."[82]

This is not to point the finger specifically at Bigelow. The entire upper-middle-class culture was biased against people who didn't "fit in." The Royal Jubilee Hospital in Victoria, British Columbia, it was bruited, was having trouble getting its cardiac surgery program off the ground. How's that? "I believe," said Bigelow, "they have an Asiatic Indian who they would prefer not to have involved in any proposed open-heart unit."[83]

And here is a surgeon at the Peterborough Clinic, petitioning Bigelow in 1964 to send a recent trainee to Peterborough: "We would like to have, naturally, the kind of person who fits in. I think Anglo-Saxon is probably a necessary qualification for this group."[84]

In November 1962 John Coles in London, Ontario, responded to Bigelow's request about recruiting residents by saying, "The only person that we have here that could at all fill this post, Bill, would be Nick Gergely. He is an extremely capable technical surgeon, but because of his racial background, you would probably want to take him on as an assistant resident first until your staff had a chance to see his work." The "race" in question here was Hungarian. The comment is an astonishing testimonial to the provincialism of these men.[85]

These surgeons lived in a climate immersed in anti-Semitism. Right up until the 1960s it verged on impossible for a Jew to enrol in a specialist training program at the General. This indeed is the reason Mount Sinai Hospital was founded. And it is no surprise to find some of the cardiac surgeons tinged with anti-Semitism, though they usually refrained from flagrant displays.

In the last half of 1963, Bigelow went away on leave and left Jim Key in charge of the service. On Bigelow's return, Key reported to him how things had gone. Pretty well, and Dr. S. who had a Jewish surname, had done exceptionally well as an intern: "I think he has everything and will make a superb doctor."

Dr. B., however – who also had a Jewish surname – was a different story. "Although of the same ethnic group, he is as unlike Dr. S. as day from night. His verbosity covers up his lack of perspicacity. He is brash, has an eye for the dramatic ... I think he is out to be a very successful surgeon (especially dollar-wise) and I am sure he will be. I don't think he is Teaching Hospital stature."[86] Jim Key may not have been a flagrant anti-Semite, but he clearly harboured bigoted stereotypes and had no reservations about expressing them to his chief.

How about Bigelow? Was he anti-Semitic? There certainly is no smoking gun here, but one exchange with Bill Drucker, head of surgery, raises an eyebrow. Drucker said to Bigelow about a recent conversation they had had, "Your comments regarding Bernie Goldman concern me a bit, because I do feel that he has the motivation and is now acquiring the education that will equip him to be a most productive member of our developing scientific establishment." Drucker said that Bigelow would agree that such people were needed. So, what was the problem with Goldman? "I am most anxious," Drucker told Bigelow, "that our judgements not be clouded by considerations of such immutable factors as race, religion or place of birth, but rather depend upon evaluation of [talent]."[87] Bigelow must have made some kind of slighting comment about Goldman's Jewishness. Much later, Bigelow was interviewed by Israeli heart surgeon Daniel Goor for Goor's (very worthwhile) book on the history of cardiac surgery. In April 1992 Bigelow explained to Goor his earlier reluctance to be interviewed: "I'll admit that initially I was not anxious to be interviewed by you. You sounded aggressive in your letters." Goor, who of course was Jewish, sounded aggressive? This is a classic anti-Semitic slur against Jews, and I have not seen Bigelow use the term "aggressive" elsewhere in his voluminous correspondence.

Toronto was, in a sense, a world unto itself. There was not a huge interest in learning from other services. Nonetheless, when in 1968 Bernie Goldman went on a tour of other cardiac surgery units – notably Denton Cooley's in Houston and Norman Shumway's in Stanford, he returned with some insights that highlight the carefulness and painstaking attention to detail of the Toronto service. In the northeastern United States the "meticulous" British approach to surgery prevailed, "stitch, by stitch, by stitch surgery, as compared to the southwest and west of America that was boom-boom-boom-boom-boom."[88]

In Houston, Goldman was astonished at the high throughput. "Cooley has done up to 9 pumps in one day." He always had two operating rooms going and sometimes three, doing all the surgery himself. The team "open and close" the chest, "while Cooley moves about with the pump anesthetist." (This is in contrast to the cardiac service of the National Institutes of Health in Bethesda, Maryland, where a languid service managed to squeeze in one pump a day.[89])

In Cooley's shop, Goldman continued, speed and efficiency were the watchwords in the pumps. "There is usually 1–2 pump technicians per case. Since the only part of their pump that requires cleaning is a small heat exchanger, it takes them no time to discard and set up the next case ... One doesn't see cases on the OR list like homograft valves, Vinebergs, endarterectomies, vein grafts etc since they take so much time."

At Stanford, "The essence here is to reduce everything to utter simplicity: no monitoring of anything except the CVP [central venous pressure] and the EKG [electrocardiogram], not even a urinary catheter." And then the astonishing: "Shumway's resident is 2 yrs. out of internship and does about 70% of the surgery alone, has put in over 100 valves so far and has yet to do his general surgery! This kid started a mitral valve at 7:30 sharp and had the patient out of the room by 10:15. I don't know where Shumway was all that time, but the resident did such a slick job on the pump that I thought he was another staff man ... I'm not sure what all this proves except that you can train a chimpanzee to operate. But this seems to go along with the slick, flip, jaunty air of the team there."[90] These are the last words one would choose to characterize the cardiovascular service in Toronto.

Adé

Bigelow retired in 1977.

Pioneers often smear a bit of Vaseline on the lens, and so it is forgivable if this particular group of pioneers saw themselves as struggling against odds. "Little more than 30 years ago, all the heart surgeons in the world knew one another," said Bigelow in 1985 (in a journalist's paraphrase). Then he continued in his own voice, "There were only two or three dozen of us. We had a common bond. We each knew what the other fellow went through. We all had to convert cardiologists who didn't believe you could operate on a heart, we had to convince hospitals to give us space to work, we had to argue for research money and a place to set up a lab."[91] Struggle against the recalcitrant cardiologists, struggle against the bean counters.

Yet the story ended in triumph. Bigelow was very aware of being part of one of medicine's great narratives, not that he placed himself at all in its centre. In 1975, two years before his retirement, he said, "I am personally convinced that there are very few examples, in the last 50 years of medicine, where an important specialty has received so many contributions from one single University, and principally from one hospital (the University of Toronto, and the Toronto General Hospital)."[92]

Still, as we try to weigh these achievements in balance, it is important to remember that in the 1960s it was Montreal and not Toronto that was seen as the Canadian centre of cardiac surgery. John Wedge, professor of surgery in Toronto from 1992 to 2002, later said, "With the history of cardiac surgery here, I wouldn't call them ahead. There were some pretty dominant characters like Tony Dobell [at the Royal Victoria Hospital]. Tony had a big international reputation."[93] And the Francophone Institut de Cardiologie (Montreal Heart) was *the* dominant player in the Canadian world in CABG, using the left internal mammary artery for the bypass graft. Later, of course, Toronto did forge ahead as the premier Canadian centre and among the topmost in the world.

There are layers and layers in Bigelow's sudden retirement. One was that his wife Ruth was increasingly unwell, and he needed to attend more to her. There were also internal political issues in the Department of Surgery. Further was his growing alienation from Al Trimble, whom he regarded almost as a son. Goldman had an insider's view: "Al broke his ankle and then his results began to tumble, and his behaviour began to tumble [Trimble had a bit of a drinking problem], and he was asked to step aside. And I think that was so hard on Bill. It just – I think by '77 he just walked away – walked away. You know, he retired without ever showing up."[94]

Bigelow stepped down in June 1977. In his letter of resignation he expressed regret at leaving "one of the great hospitals in the world."[95] Bigelow loved the General. And if one conclusion may be drawn from a work of this nature it is that great institutions are built when their leaders love them. Why was it important to "maintain a strong Toronto General Hospital?" he asked a colleague rhetorically in 1968. "I feel that Canada must have one hospital that can compete with the best in the United States, and there is no reason why it should not be Toronto General Hospital ... This is not just foolish pride, it is a very practical means of retaining the best brains seeking the finest post-graduate training in our country."[96] In 1968 McGill was just losing its primacy, and Toronto was emerging as the great medical academic powerhouse of the late twentieth century. In this project, the Big Hospital, as it was called, played a key role.

Chapter Ten

The Pacemaker Clinic

In 1960 a group of American investigators, including Wilson Greatbach in Buffalo, developed an implantable pacemaker that overcame the problems of the non-transportable, cumbersome Toronto device. This opened a new chapter in the pacemaker story.

In January 1961, Samuel Lasky at Electrodyne came up to Toronto to show Bigelow and the other surgeons and anesthetists one of their new implantable transistorized pacemakers.[1] Mr. F.F. was admitted on 21 February 1962 with complete heart block (Stokes-Adams attack), the pacemaker was inserted on 20 March, and the patient was discharged two weeks later. The cardiologist was Bill Greenwood; Bigelow, the surgeon.[2] A new era had begun.

In June 1963, Bigelow, Trimble, and Heimbecker presented a paper on "the implantable cardiac pacemaker" at a meeting of the Canadian Medical Association. The TGH was now using a miniature transistorized model entirely within the chest, "about the size of an old fashioned pocket watch," which eliminated the wires-through-the-skin format of the early models. To date, nineteen patients had been operated on: eight of them with complete heart block, and eleven with varying degrees of block. The division had begun with the Electrodyne pacemaker, then moved over to the model made by Medtronic, because of its longer useful life of five years with the mercury battery. They'd had one death, in the youngest patient in the series, age forty-nine, who had evidence of progressive coronary artery disease.[3]

At this point, Bernie Goldman entered the pacemaker scene. In 1967 he and Whit Firor described inserting a technically superior transvenous pacemaker, emphasizing "the importance of performing it under fluoroscopic guidance in a *proper surgical operating suite*."[4] But not every community cardiologist installing pacemakers was capable of this kind of exacting technique, and the drums began to beat for establishing a special pacemaker clinic at the General.

Goldman Helps Found the Pacemaker Clinic

Given publicity by the media, the pacemaker moved quickly from the doctors' world into the patients'. Grateful patients were heard in the media, such as seventy-five-year-old A.C. McCollum of Toronto, an Anglican archdeacon and one of the first Canadians to receive a pacemaker. "I had to do it or die," he said. "It was even a question of whether I'd survive the three weeks until they could make a pacemaker to my requirements. But it's worked out fine. I've only been to the doctor once since I had it put in. It sticks out my back a bit, but it doesn't bother me."[5] Archdeacon McCollum's account resonated widely.

Cardiology eagerly reached out to the surgeon colleagues, and in 1969, Doug Wigle, in charge of the Cardiovascular Investigation Unit, told Goldman that "the follow-up of patients with pacemakers is becoming a horrendous one and one that requires immediate attention by the surgical and medical cardiovascular people at this hospital." Goldman apparently had already proposed organizing a clinic. Wigle said, "You have my wholehearted support for putting this whole matter on a firm and scientific basis."[6]

What triggered the formation of a pacemaker clinic was a letter later in November 1969 from Bill Greenwood, chief of cardiology to Jim Key, then chair of the Medical Staff Association, proposing the formation of a pacemaker clinic. "At the present time, I believe there are some 300 patients who have had pacemakers put in in the last two years ... These patients should ... have electrocardiograms taken and probably have certain special electronic tests done to see about the efficacy of their existing pacemaker. I feel they should be seen about four times, a year, which would mean that there would be at least 1,000 visits a year and if you divide this by 50 weeks it would means something of the order of 30 patients to be followed in a week." This demanded a specialized clinic with a staff of its own. Cardiologist Ed Noble would direct it on the medical side.[7]

On the surgical side, the cardiac team at the General began to be inundated with pacemaker patients who needed their batteries replaced, whose devices had failed, or who had encountered some other technical ennui. Goldman describes a "constant stream of failing pacemakers." There were stories of elderly patients being held until 2 a.m. in the emergency room – competing with the fractured hips and wrists – for a simple battery-pack replacement.[8]

Goldman signalled to Bigelow that there was a real problem with patients not getting their pacemakers updated in a timely manner. As Bigelow recalled the story, he said: "Bernie, what do you think about the mortality that you recently reported from our emergency pacemaker failures?"

GOLDMAN: It is a real worry.
BIGELOW: Do you think we have a responsibility to this group of patients?
GOLDMAN: I sincerely think we do.
BIGELOW: I would like to ask you a great favour. I know you are busy, and I know the administrative hassles are not an attractive prospect, but would you consider setting up a pacemaker follow-up clinic?

"Bernie's face fell," said Bigelow later. "He thought for a while, then said: 'That's a hell of a thing to ask someone to do – but I believe if we are to accept proper responsibility it should be done. Okay, I'll do it.'"[9]

In December 1969 Goldman was sent to Montefiore Hospital in New York's Bronx to see how a pacemaker service might be organized. Seymour Furman, who directed the clinic there, had said in a letter to Goldman, "The implantation of 150 cardiac pacemakers is not only a problem at the time of the implantation but a time bomb sitting in the community ready to explode time after time after time. With a passage of time you will find that the patients are returning to you, often on an emergency basis for pulse generator replacement or for other complications of implanted pacing." Goldman was welcome to come down and observe, Furman said.[10] And Bigelow suggested that Goldman take along a cardiologist, as "I gather Bill Greenwood [head of cardiology] has doubts about the current appointment [plans]."[11]

In March 1970 Jim Key asked Griff Pearson, the chair of the OR Committee of the hospital, for permission to turn one of the cardiovascular operating rooms into a pacemaker operating room. The justification was "that many cases have to be done at the end of the day or at night; the difficulty of having all the required types of pacemaker available and the necessity often of someone having to run up to P.O.R. to get some vital part."[12] In November 1970, Goldman announced the formation of a pacemaker clinic as "mandatory."[13]

Goldman was thirty-four at the time he took over the surgical side of the pacemaker clinic. (David MacGregor took over part of the research side.) Goldman had graduated in medicine from Toronto in 1960 and, as we have seen, completed the postgraduate training course in cardiac surgery in 1967. He had the reputation of being bright, energetic, and quick on his feet – and at this writing he looks back upon this often-terrible time, in which he lost his father in misadventure, with ironical good humour.

Goldman, the surgical director, and cardiologist Ed Noble launched the TGH Pacemaker Centre in 1970. Goldman said, "[Prior to 1970] we were entering a period of chaos. We had too many emergency admissions, too many unpredicted failures, too much unnecessary morbidity ... Dr. Noble and I lifted these patients out of private practice, and asked them to come to an out-patient clinic for ambulatory care. [In short order] there wasn't one patient that we didn't know about and that wasn't being followed up. We've cut down our emergency admission rate to virtually nil."[14] The pacemaker clinic would have its own operating room. Goldman added that this was a necessity because "temporary" pacemakers were being left in much too long owing to a shortage of operating-room time.[15]

Things did not go smoothly. In March 1972, Goldman told Bigelow of his exasperation in delays in setting up the pacemaker clinic: "I really am a little bit tired of the whole hassle regarding pacemakers – and perhaps that is why I am on vacation now as you read this note. The hospital's budget committee has caused endless hassles, and we need all these authorizations from various department heads. Frankly, I am quite disappointed at this complete lack of enthusiasm and ability to move quickly."[16] He might well have had in mind thoracic surgeon Griff Pearson's dubiety about giving the pacers yet another operating room: shortage of nurses, et cetera. Pearson said, "At the moment, I am doubtful about the possibility of a further re-arrangement of various Divisional or Departmental times on the regular schedule."[17]

Hospital executive director James A. McNab finger-waggled at Goldman that unfortunately the pacemaker program had been featured "on national television ... while in fact all of the proper lines of communication and priorities of approval have not been observed."[18] So, the hospital rebuked him for courting publicity when it was in fact the Ontario Heart Foundation that allowed the media in.

And then, in 1972, the cardiologists wanted to set up their own pacemaker clinic and to incorporate Goldman's little operation. Goldman didn't know anything about this until Eileen Strike, the director of the nursing service, told him, "This [cardiology] brief is under review, and will have implications with regard to your request [for a dedicated nurse]."[19]

Simultaneously in 1972, the physicians and patients together founded a pacemaker club, which in time grew to hundreds of members.

There was more change: nuclear pacing was on its way, and in January 1972, the General ordered five of them.[20] On 8 October 1973

Goldman installed Canada's first nuclear pacemaker – in thirty-two-year-old Torontonian Jack Tootill. "As soon as Jack Tootill woke up," reported journalist Joan Hollobon, "within minutes of getting off the operating table ... he was given a glass of champagne from a bottle that had been cooling in an ice-filled bedpan." Tootill had worn conventional pacemakers since 1965 and since then had had one replacement. "I heard about the plutonium pacer when it was first used in France about three years ago," said Tootill, "and it seemed like a great idea for someone my age."[21] This turned out happily for Tootill, a bit less happily for Goldman: "October 1973. On Thanksgiving Day, I put a nuclear pacemaker in him. I got hell, doing an elective procedure on Thanksgiving, and having it publicized. 'First nuclear pacemaker in Canada, Dr. Goldman said yesterday.' Fake news. We declared it as a semi-emergency, but you're not supposed to do that."[22] "The patient is still alive and pacing to this day," he said in 2009.[23]

Goldman emerged as the public advocate for pacing. The benefits were enormous, the costs manageable. Yet the province pulled back from establishing the network of pacemaker clinics. Goldman said in January 1972 that for older patients "it is a hardship ... to travel to a university centre for routine checks ... simply because local doctors are unfamiliar with the management of pacer patients."[24] He added that because the Ontario Medical Association had recently dropped its reimbursements for pacemaker work, "the doctors' enthusiasm dropped with it." Goldman said, in a journalist's paraphrase, that "there should be a network of clinics in such places as Thunder Bay ... [Elderly patients] 'are forced to go mucking around the province,' travelling for hours by bus or train to get care that could be given at their local hospital."[25] Goldman, according to journalist Hollobon, "always noted for outspokenness," said that if you had questions about funding shortfalls for pacing, you should "direct your question to Mr. Frank Miller (Ontario Health Minister)."[26]

A Whole Pacemaker Network

By 1974 the Pacemaker Clinic at the General was overwhelmed to the extent that Goldman and Noble recommended a network of provincial centres to take the load off.[27] By 1978 the Pacemaker Clinic at TGH was implanting more than two hundred units a year, virtually all using the transvenous route – through a short incision in the anterior chest wall just below the collar bone exposing the vein leading to the superior vena cava in the heart – rather than the "myocardial." The surgery was done with a local anesthetic and involved, on the average, a three-day hospital stay. Indications for pacing spanned a range from complete heart block involving the bundle of His (35 per cent) to "sinus arrest" involving the sino-atrial and intra-atrial areas (11 per cent); other indications accounted for the remainder. Complications at the clinic were few; the commonest reason for a visit was replacement of the mercury batteries, which tended to last about thirty-four months; by 1978 the clinic had gone over to much longer-lasting and reliable lithium batteries (telephone follow-up changed from weekly to once every three months). The new patients' average age was sixty-nine.[28]

In 1980, David MacGregor became surgical head of the pacemaker clinic. MacGregor, who was forty-three, graduated from medical school in Toronto in 1962 and finished training in cardiovascular surgery in 1970. He had a longstanding interest in biomedical technology and pacing in particular. The issue was how to make the pacemaker more sensitive to the electrical activity of the heart. It was known that in hip transplantation, the bone grafted quickly onto artificial hips with porous, or crenellated, metal parts. MacGregor reasoned that a pacemaker with porous metal electrodes might fix in place more firmly and offer an expanded surface for sensing the heart's electrical activity ("P waves"). In 1979, he and co-workers, including Scully, demonstrated in dogs that this technical modification fulfilled the hopes of the investigators;[29] MacGregor went on to propose a porous no-clot heart valve, and after he left Toronto in 1981 to become vice-president for research – later president – of the Cordis Corporation in Miami, he presided over a whole series of innovations in pacing, heart valves, and ventricular assistance. With MacGregor's leaving for the United States in 1981, Goldman became once again head of the pacemaker clinic.

In retrospect, Goldman is the central figure in the history of clinical pacing in Canada. He was a founding member of the North American Society of Cardiac Pacing and Electrophysiology and its third president; he laced Canada into the huge developing interest in the United States in this technique. He also created a province-wide telephone follow-up network to augment the new pacemaker clinic at TGH.

This is very gratifying: making a difference. The cardiac surgeons on "Hospital Row" (University Avenue) in Toronto really did make a difference in people's lives. In 1995 the surgeons at the Hospital for Sick Children implanted a pacemaker in twelve-year-old Andrea Jones. But her mother learned from "The Pacemaker News" that it was Bigelow at the General who had invented it. So Andrea wrote to Bigelow, "I had to get a pacemaker because I had heart attacks after I did physical exercise. I kept on collapsing. I'm glad that somebody as smart as you could invent something as clever as the pacemaker because it does save people's lives. This morning I was running with my dog in the park." She went to camp and was "able to do anything like climbing ropes, canoeing and lots of running and I don't get out of breath any more." She passed her swimming test. Her mother added in a separate note, "Yesterday she raced home from school flaunting her ribbon for the long distance race at her school's track and field event. 'Sixth place' did not daunt her as it was her first ribbon ever!" Andrea wanted to meet Bigelow.[30]

Chapter Eleven

Ron Baird

On Baird's watch, cardiac transplantation was perfected. It is difficult now to appreciate how miraculous this seemed at the time. OR Nurse Leda Parente described the first time she saw a heart transplant: "You take a cold, dark, grey muscle, it comes in a container, it's just in a bowl. You take it out, the surgeons prepare it, sew, sew, sew, put it on. It sits there, everybody looks for a minute. It starts to get pink, and all of a sudden we start to see a little movement, and next thing it's beating like this. Everybody stands there. And every time I saw it, it's like the first time. You go, 'Wow, look at that.'"[1] On Baird's watch, it was magic.

Baird's Life

Ronald James Baird was born in Toronto in 1930 at the Toronto Western Hospital, as were his siblings and children. His father loaded freight cars for CPR, as he did himself, working to earn money in high school. Ron attended Runnymede Public School and Humberside Collegiate, where he was an honours student and gifted athlete. Religion was an important value in his family: they were members of a sect-like Protestant "assembly" called the Plymouth Brethren, a fundamentalist group that placed absolute primacy on scriptural text. He abandoned this in later life.

Ron entered and worked his way through medical school in Toronto. When short of cash, he would evidently (according to his wife, Fern) "ask the Dean for money." (Comment: Just try this if you are not an outstanding student!) He graduated as the Cody Gold Medalist in 1954 and completed his junior internship at TGH.

He was invited by Robert Janes to join the Gallie postgraduate surgical program. During his "basic science year" he wound up working in Bigelow's lab in the basement of the Banting Building, leading to his love of laboratory studies and an invitation to enter the exciting new field of cardiovascular surgery.

Fern said, "This was one thing he learned from Bigelow, a reverence for research. The lab was the area he found most rewarding – the idea of doing research to make something work in the OR or at the bedside." Baird earned a BSc (Med.) in 1956 from his laboratory studies. He successfully maintained research grant support for twenty-one years and was appointed university director of research from 1972 until 1987.

Baird trained in general surgery under Fred Kergin but was in awe of Gordon Murray, saying while a junior surgical resident in 1956, "I was amazed to read Gordon Murray's report of the successful insertion of a homograft aortic valve into the descending thoracic aorta." He worked for Murray as a junior and then senior resident from 1957 to 1959.

Baird then completed his cardiovascular and thoracic training under Bill Bigelow, Bill Mustard, and Fred Kergin. His mentors were Bigelow, Mustard, and in particular Gordon Murray. He was a pallbearer at Murray's funeral.

Baird's 1959 fellowship from the Royal College of Physicians and Surgeons of Canada in general surgery was followed in 1964 by one of the first fellowships in cardiovascular and thoracic surgery. He earned a master of surgery degree in 1965. Other awards in surgery included the Roscoe Graham Award (1960), the Lister Prize (1964), and the prestigious Medal in Surgery from the Royal College in 1969. He became a fellow of the American College of Surgery in 1961.

An interviewer later asked Baird how he became interested in vascular and cardiac surgery. He said of the early 1950s, "That's when it all happened: the first open-heart surgeries, the first valve surgeries, the first vascular surgeries of any note. It was quite obvious that this was an opening field, so I trained in general surgery but the people I was training with were swinging themselves to vascular and cardiac. My first [fellowship] exam was in general surgery but ... I immediately started, first mainly vascular, and then as the pump developed and eventually with coronary bypass I got pushed more and more to cardiac."[2]

In June 1960, in the newly founded "Cardiovascular Surgery Division" at TGH, Baird became "the first surgeon invited to join the staff as a specifically designated 'Cardiovascular' surgeon."[3] In 1964 Al Trimble was also appointed to staff as a CV surgeon. Apparently, Bigelow suggested to Ron that he should consider moving to Queen's University.[4] With the support of Fred Kergin, then chair of surgery at the university, he accepted an invitation from Don Wilson to stay in Toronto and move to the Toronto Western Hospital. Initially disappointed about leaving the General and reluctant to go to TWH, he quickly found that the move provided a real opportunity.

At TWH he found a service treating mainly vascular problems, always of great interest to him. He and Wilson set out to increase cardiac services. "Within a few years Don and I built the largest vascular, and the second largest cardiac surgical service in Canada." He was appointed head of cardiovascular surgery at TWH from 1972 to 1977, while Don Wilson was appointed chair of surgery at the university from 1972 to 1982.

Nonetheless, Baird retained an interest in the vascular side, and at the Western he was heavily involved in it. Lynda Mickleborough said, "I think his first love was vascular. I think cardiac became important for him – and he was very competent at it – but I don't think it was ever his first love."[5]

Hugh Scully recalls, "When I was senior resident and Bryce Taylor was junior resident in general surgery at TWH in 1969, we would occasionally get urgent calls from Lois Dwan, the very competent head nurse of the ORs, asking if Bryce and I could start an operation on a patient with abdominal aortic aneurysm because Dr. Baird was delayed, and they could not locate his fellow. When he did join us, Ron was always gracious with his helpful suggestions and praise."[6]

Academically, Ron Baird progressed rapidly from assistant professor in 1964 to associate professor in 1968 and a full professor of surgery in 1972.

He was well known as an innovative vascular surgeon and a pioneer in the early days of adult cardiac surgery, in the evolution of coronary valve remodelling and replacement, and heart transplant surgery. He was an exceptional teacher of the craft of cardiovascular surgery and was greatly admired and respected as a mentor to generations of residents and international fellows from many different countries. Ron was the author of many peer-reviewed papers in both vascular and cardiac surgery, numerous abstracts, book chapters, and editorials. He was an invited speaker at numerous international cardiovascular meetings, travelling widely and always enhancing the reputation and quality of cardiovascular surgery at the Toronto General and Western hospitals.

In his quiet way, Ron Baird was a remarkable leader. He served on the Council of the Society of University Surgeons, the board and governors of the American College of Surgeons, and the Council for Cardiovascular Surgery with the American Heart Association. He was president of the North American chapter of the International Society for Vascular Surgery, president of the Canadian Society of Thoracic and Cardiovascular Surgery, and was one of only four cardiovascular surgeons elected president of the Canadian Cardiovascular Surgery (CCS) over seventy-two years. (The other three, all trained in Toronto, were Bill Bigelow, Wilbert Keon, and Hugh Scully.) Ron Baird was active in virtually all of the top societies in cardiology, cardiac, and vascular surgery.

It is interesting to note whom Baird later acknowledged as "his teachers": Murray, Bigelow, Mustard, Wilson – which makes perfect sense, given when he came into the system – but also Key and Heimbecker.[7] He clearly saw himself as being on the receiving end of a long and distinguished tradition of cardiac surgery in Toronto. People told Baird that he talked and walked like Bigelow. "However, nobody ever told me that I looked like him, which would have pleased me even more, because, of course, he was as handsome as a movie star."[8]

Working together with Don Wilson, who was known as a very kind man, Baird was truly happy at the Western. It was with trepidation that he accepted the position as chief of cardiac surgery at the General when Bigelow retired in 1977. The decision to leave the Western was, said Baird, "difficult and emotional … Ironically, within the subsequent twelve years the entire division of which I was so proud would be forcibly closed and combined with that at the General during the 'merger' of the TGH and TWH. I had not realized that the thirteen years at the TWH were to be the happiest and most productive of my life."[9]

In 1977, as stated, Baird succeeded Bigelow as chief of cardiovascular surgery at TGH and head of the University Division. When Baird returned to the General, he joined Jim Key, Bernie Goldman, and Hugh Scully. Tirone David at the time was a senior fellow. Alan Trimble "was ill and had stopped practicing." Jim Key retired three years later, in 1981. Bigelow invited David to Toronto; in 1978 Baird appointed him to staff. Baird recruited Richard Weisel in 1979 and, in 1981, Lynda Mickleborough, the first female cardiac surgeon in the story (see chapter 12). This was the second generation, the founding generation having largely passed from the scene.

What was Baird like as a teacher? Mickleborough said, "Some people teach more at arm's length, and some people teach more directly. Ron was more of an arm's length. He found it easier to give people responsibility on their own, and that's the way he taught. It was great to be his resident. You learned a lot. You were the decision maker and sometimes you weren't sure, but that's what you did, and most of the time it worked out okay. People could bloom, they could achieve, they could aspire, and I think that was great."[10]

Baird resigned as chief of cardiac surgery at the TGH and as university chair of cardiovascular surgery in 1988 at the completion of his terms. He closed his office and retired from independent surgical

practice in 1994. He complained of feeling disturbed by the politics raging around him. Even so, Baird continued to stay as a kind of senior
assistant and mentor to residents and fellows until 2002. "It was a wise
move and I was more content with my life," he later said."[11]

At a personal level, Baird, like Bigelow, was universally liked and
praised for being, as head nurse Linda Harris put it, "a lovely man,
very thoughtful, very caring and attentive to people's needs, people's
concerns, and to describe him in one word, a gentleman." Nursing
supervisor Marion Ryujin recalled, "Rounds every day, saw every single patient. All the staff respected that. He was very much one who
wanted to bring the team and recognize the nurses' input, so we would
have to go around with him. He never went by himself to talk to the
patients."[12]

Ron Baird was a renaissance man, keenly interested in nature, science, history (particularly historic figures and great battles), and international travel. He kept himself fit with regular exercise sessions at the
YMCA, and like Jim Key, was an elegant dresser. (He had a standing
account at the upscale Perry's Menswear on Bloor Street.) He had a
wide circle of friends outside of medicine and greatly enjoyed bridge
and bon-vivant companionship at the Toronto York Club.

Ron was devoted to his family. Fern, his wife, was his greatest champion and supporter. With their three children, their children's respective
spouses, and grandchildren, there were many happy family gatherings
at their farm close to Toronto and their Bahamian retreat in Hope Town.

Baird's Work

In the 1960s and 1970s, Baird pioneered several areas of cardiac and
vascular surgery. In May 1961 while visiting a colleague's lab at
St. Vincent's Hospital in Cleveland, he made a side trip to the Cleveland
Clinic to chat with another friend. "Thus I happened to be present dur-
ing Mason Sones' historical first visualisation of the effectiveness of the
'mammary artery implant' or 'Vineberg' operation: both patients at the
Cleveland Clinic that day had received their operations in Canada; one
by Arthur Vineberg in Montreal, the other by Bill Bigelow in Toronto."
This happenstance encounter prompted Baird to further improve the
Vineberg operation.[13] In 1969 he received the Medal in Surgery of the
Royal College for his work on why the internal mammary artery stays
patent.[14] Baird said with pride, "This was the first Royal College Medal
ever awarded to a Toronto surgeon who was not on the staff at TGH."[15]

Baird prided himself on introducing to Canada in 1961, together
with the cardiac surgical team, the technique for relieving aortic-valve

incompetence called "bicuspidization" that Thomas Starzl at North-western University had introduced in 1959.[16] Yet the results of reduc-ing the aortic valve to two leaflets were not brilliant, and of the nine patients who underwent the procedure between 1961 and 1963, "the operation was less satisfactory in permanently correcting the incompe-tence."[17] The procedure was not pursued in Toronto, but the experience is interesting as an example of cardiac surgery led by someone other than Bigelow.

Baird had a strong interest in peripheral vascular surgery, and felt as comfortable with the popliteal artery (in the pit of the knee) and the blood supply to the esophagus (which develops bleeding varices in alcoholism) as with the heart. His interests included the liver as well, and in 1964 Baird apparently did the surgical work (in dogs) on isolat-ing segments of the hepatic veins with balloons to visualize the drain-age of the hepatic lobes (of clear utility in studying liver disease). The resulting paper by Baird and colleagues laid the foundation of hepatic venography.[18] In 1970 Baird devised a new operation transplanting the reversed saphenous vein to link at the top (proximally) to the common femoral artery and at the bottom (distally) to the arteries of the ankle and foot. This restored circulation to patients with gangrene of the foot owing to diabetes.[19] In 1977, Baird reported a saphenous vein graft he had performed two years earlier going from the ascending aorta, down through the diaphragm then passing in the subcutaneous fascia to link up with the femoral arteries.[20] It became known as "the Baird opera-tion" and was widely copied internationally.

These procedures were a solution to the problem of "the ischemic leg." Baird told an interviewer, "I think diabetes was certainly part of it, and the person lying there on the bed with a gangrenous foot, or his toe that wouldn't heal, or his heel that wouldn't heal, was a terrible prob-lem. They couldn't go home. You just kept chopping off a little more, all the way up. There was obviously a great need to fix them … My main claim to fame is that I did the longest saphenous vein graft recorded when I did it down below the ankle one time."[21]

But it was not copied so much in Toronto. Why? The reason is inter-esting. In other centres, many cardiac surgeons still did vascular work and felt at ease entering the chest (to get to the ascending aorta). But, said Baird, "none of the vascular surgeons in Toronto have performed this operation. Because they do not enter the chest, they are afraid of the ascending aorta. Similarly, because they do not use the heart-lung pump, they have avoided its help in surgery for aneurysms and dis-sections [a tear in the wall] of the descending thoracic aorta to the great detriment of their results." This was, said Baird, a consequence of the separation of cardiac from vascular surgery that occurred in the early 1980s (see "Vascular Surgery" and "The Vascular Division" later in this chapter).[22]

Baird was involved in the cardiac protection research begun by Goldman and colleagues in 1971. By 1977, Richard Weisel as senior resident and research fellow of the Canadian Heart Foundation was in charge of the cardiac protection file. And in that year, Baird, Weisel, Goldman, and colleagues demonstrated that infusing the coronary circulation with a solution of cold potassium reduced damage ("cold potassium cardioplegia" was the term). In a definitive paper the following year, 1978, they reported, "that cardiac hypothermia to a mean temperature of 22°C/min, and the infusion of multiple doses of the cardioplegic solution, significantly improved myocardial preservation."[23] It was in 1979 that Weisel joined the staff and became a champion of basic-science research in the division.

In his retirement Baird posted an ingenuous question: "Why has the human heart become so remarkably easy to operate on?" he asked puckishly in 1995. (The heart is not at all easy to operate on.) "It is close to the surface," he said, "not deep in a hole, like the kidney. It holds sutures well and is easy to sew, unlike the liver or the brain. It is a clean organ, not contaminated by micro-organisms, unlike the bowel or the lung."[24] Indeed, the Baird years in this story mark the transition of cardiac surgery from the "heroic" era of Murray and Bigelow to the routine procedures that prevail today.

The "Vast Reservoir": Part 2

As bypass became common and new techniques opened up, such as balloon angioplasty and clot-dissolving drugs, the vast reservoir of needy patients became even larger. In 1982 there were 2,200 adult open-heart operations in Metro Toronto, more than half of which were coronary bypass. The Metro Toronto District Health Council recommended that a new cardiac surgery unit be opened at Sunnybrook and that the unit at the Western be expanded. Baird said that the General's heart surgeons "are getting very tired" and could only stay on top of the waiting list by operating on weekends and evenings.[25]

A waiting-list crisis engulfed the province. In June 1987 Jim Morocco of Niagara Falls, thirty-six years old and father of two, died while on the waiting list at the General. At the time of his catheterization, he was discovered to have a heart "the size of a football." He was very much out of breath and had signs of heart failure. Yet according to his internist, Jim made the mistake of asking to go home rather than waiting in hospital for the procedure. "You cannot be classified urgent any more, once you've gone home," said the internist (who declined to have his name used). While at home, Morocco died in his sleep, lying next to his wife in bed. His mother made a huge stink about her son not being properly looked after, and in June 1988, a year after Morocco's death, the province announced a big new funding program for heart patients and the opening of a new cardiac unit at Sunnybrook (that Bernie Goldman would head).[26] (But see the "Sunnybrook," later in this chapter, for more on the death of another waiting-list patient, Charles Coleman, as the immediate trigger.)

Heart Transplantation: Second Wave

At dawn on 7 March 1985, Tirone David and nephrologist Carl Cardella, who was head of transplant surgery at the Western, boarded an air ambulance at the Toronto Island airport. A donor had become available in London, Ontario. At 6:04 a.m. in London, the team began the operation to remove the donor's heart. "It took 10 minutes," said a journalist. "The doctors instantly put the heart in an ice-bucket to keep it cool and prevent it from beating." The team now had four hours, the time a heart can live outside the body.

"The trip to the London airport was 10 minutes. The pilot had the engine running, and immediately took off for the 35 minute flight."

By 7:10 a.m. the team had landed in Toronto and had a police convoy from the island airport up Bathurst Street to the Western. "The police cleared the roads."

At 7:15 a.m. the doctors began the transplant operation. With thirteen team members in the OR, Tirone David "did his magic." "By 9:45 a.m. the heart transplant had been completed." Toronto's heart transplant program, the first in ten years, had resumed.[27]

What had changed? In 1981, cyclosporine became available, diminishing the body's rejection response, and it was on 18 April 1981 that Heimbecker, now in London, used cyclosporine to conducted a heart transplant; the patient survived for twelve years.[28] (The story of cyclosporine's actual arrival in Toronto in 1982 or 1983 is not widely known. Graham Peck from Cambridge University was doing a fellowship in Toronto in general surgery, and, as Richard Reznick recalls, "Graham had stolen some cyclosporine A from Roy Calne's lab at Cambridge where he had worked and he thought we should do some small bowel implants on dogs and try the cyclosporine out ... Anyhow, we did twenty-one dogs during my six months of research and we were the first to have dogs survive after a small bowel transplant."[29])

"By 1983," said Baird, "it was obvious that transplants would have to start again in Toronto. Since I was then in charge of the cardiac program in the city, I [wanted] TWH chosen as the single center for the second round of transplantation." The Western was Baird's former hospital; he was now head of the Cardiovascular Surgery Division at the General and the university.[30]

In March 1985 Tirone David transplanted a new heart at Toronto Western Hospital into Tayeb Khan, age thirty-seven, a cab driver (trained in Pakistan as a computer programmer); Khan left the hospital a happy man. "I can't believe myself how changed I am," he said.[31] David told the press he hoped that the Western would become Toronto's centre for heart transplants.[32]

It was in these early heart transplants that David exhibited the technical brilliance for which he became celebrated. By the second heart transplant at the Western, he had reduced the operative time from eight hours to ninety-five minutes. (He removed the heart from a donor at Sunnybrook and accompanied it on the ten-kilometre trip to the Western.)[33]

Baird noted that Tirone David and Chris Feindel soon had an excellent series. But internal medicine under Cardella had a key role. Feindel said later, "Once the organ was in, Carl Cardella took over the immunosuppression. Then the cardiologist Paul Daly took over and did the repeated biopsies you had to do to see if the heart was being rejected or not." When the services merged in 1989, the transplant program finally came to TGH. "All roads run to Rome," said Baird.[34]

Despite the availability of cyclosporine, observers recall that the antirejection drug used in this second wave of cardiac transplants was a compound that Cardella himself had developed, and that was produced in a lab at the Western, called RATS – Rabbit Anti-Thymocyte Serum. It was thought to be virtually as effective as cyclosporine. Cardella had used it in kidney transplants with good results. But it remained a kind of Toronto secret because Health Canada in Ottawa had never approved it, and RATS was discontinued in 2001 after an officious junior pharmacist at UHN noted that it had no official approval.[35]

Vascular Surgery

As the cardiovascular surgeons plunged into cardiac surgery in the early 1970s, they began to leave "vascular" surgery – on peripheral blood vessels – behind. The general picture is this: Cardiac surgeons were initially trained as general surgeons, and that included such vascular operations as gangrenous feet ("dead feet") and clotted popliteal

arteries. Abdominal aortic aneurysms were a grave "vascular" complication, and Toronto had a tradition of operating on them. But times were
changing. The cardiac surgeons, facing an avalanche of heart disease,
were growing increasingly impatient with the peripheral vascular procedures, and the general surgeons were just itching to take them over.
In 1971, Bruce Tovee, head of general surgery, offered Bernie Goldman
a new vascular service at the General, in the event that Bigelow didn't
keep him on in cardiac.[36] But Bigelow retained Goldman.

Bigelow was not really ready psychologically to surrender these
pieces of turf, and when the general surgeons tried to move into creating portocaval shunts around the diseased livers of alcoholics, he
kicked back. It was around 1970 that Bernard Langer, just about to
become head of general surgery at the General, wanted to move into
shunts, and asked Jim Key to show him exactly how they were done.
Key, "always a gentleman," gladly obliged. But apparently Key cleared
it with Bigelow first (who was not yet head of Ward C but was acting like it). Bernie Langer later said, "Bigelow was really pissed off."
But for the other cardiovascular surgeons, it wasn't such a big deal.
Bernie Goldman added, "It was ridiculous that we were looking after
jaundiced, hepatic coma patients who still had some esophageal bleeding … We were beginning to need all our resources for coronary and
valvular surgery. So it just happened, and it was so logical that most of
us just shrugged our shoulders, although we could feel the whittling
away on the horizon."[37]

The Vascular Division

As Baird said, "The longstanding combination of cardiac and vascular surgery on one service was no longer working well at TGH." He
had the "largest vascular surgery practice in Canada," but the residents
were losing interest in vascular and wanted to focus on cardiac. "In
1981, Don Wilson, Griff Pearson, and I acted to form a separate division for 'Vascular Surgery' at TGH and the University, both headed by
my former student, Wayne Johnston."[38] The cardiac surgeons, who had
once done popliteal arteries, esophageal varices, and abdominal aortic
aneurysms, now confined themselves to the heart and the vessels that
immediately connected to it (the "great vessels").

Johnston, who headed the service, had been recruited by Langer into
the Division of General Surgery, but from the get-go his interest was
vascular. Langer was intent upon building the subspecialties of general
surgery, such as colorectal surgery and cancer surgery, and identified
the need for a vascular division as well. Langer's formulation: "The

impetus to start vascular surgery as a subspecialty in general surgery was mine, but starting the division was his." (Johnston said that he coaxed Langer to this conclusion.) Ron Baird was said to have been "bitter" about this loss but there was little he could do.[39]

Thus, it was Johnston who actually pioneered vascular surgery, setting up the Vascular Division in 1981. "You know, send me all your gangrenous feet and whatever." Scully and Goldman were already doing vascular work, though amid the bypasses they weren't particularly interested in it. "And one of the concerns we had," said Scully, "was if we're going to be doing amputations and gangrenous limbs, and if those patients then came back into the cardiac intensive care unit, there was potential for cross-infection."[40]

Johnston persuaded the Royal College to set up an exam in it, then took the exam himself several years later. (Q: "Is this the way they normally do things at the Royal College?" A: "No.")

Johnston himself acknowledged Don Wilson and Ron Baird as teachers and became, as the first Canadian president of the Society of Vascular Surgeons, a distinguished figure within the specialty. In Toronto he opened up peripheral angioplasty and organized a Canada-wide data bank of abdominal aneurysm operations, said to be the world's largest prospective series.[41]

Yet all did not go well. By 2004 the Division of Vascular Surgery suffered from not being considered a hospital "priority program," and did not have access to the pricey "endografts" (stents inserted from inside the aorta) that were transforming the field in the United States.[42] Some of these problems were solved in 2006, when the new chair, Thomas Lindsay, took over and the Ministry of Health agreed to fund state-of-the-art stent grafting in the treatment of aneurysms, permitting vascular surgeons the use of less invasive techniques. "This was a big win for academic vascular surgery," said Lindsay. "It injected new energy into the specialty and created a sense of excitement for the team. It was also transformative for vascular surgery in Toronto."[43]

Yet the cardiac surgeons remained the tough guys on the block. Scully said, "Cardiac surgeons were the surgeons that the others called when they got into critical trouble with major vessel bleeding." Goldman said, "We were still the big guys. They would call a vascular surgeon for the groin, but they sure as hell would call us for something in the chest while they're doing an esophageal operation." Scully added, "If the lung surgeons got into trouble with the great vessels, they would call one of us. If doing major abdominal surgery and they got into one of the major vessels, they might call a vascular surgeon, but they were equally likely to call one of us to help."[44]

Sunnybrook

By 1970, two hospitals had been left out of the open-heart surgery picture: the Wellesley, which did not even have a cardiac investigation unit,
and Sunnybrook, which did. Sunnybrook, located in the north end of
the city, was keen to acquire a surgical unit as well, to avoid shipping its
investigation patients downtown. In December 1969 Sunnybrook formally petitioned the Inter-Hospital Cardiovascular Surgical Committee
for surgical status. They wanted Ray Heimbecker to come out and head
the unit.[45]

At this point very few aortocoronary bypass procedures were being
done, and the business from repairing septal defects and valves was
not overwhelming. In January 1970, the committee asked if there was
enough business to justify a fourth cardiac surgery centre in Toronto.
Clearly, there was not, but Bigelow did ask if "demands of ... of [car-
diac] surgery may change with the advent of aorto-coronary bypass."[46]
The comment was prescient: in the vast sea of cardiac pathology out
there, a wave was gathering.

It was in 1967 that surgeons at the Cleveland Clinic began doing aortocoronary bypass, especially in cases of acute myocardial infarction
with left ventricular failure. The Cleveland surgeons had good luck
with this, but their article in 1971 reporting the findings[47] touched off a
crisis at Sunnybrook. "We feel particularly disadvantaged and helpless
in dealing with some of these cases in our Coronary Unit here at Sunnybrook," Arthur Chisholm, chief of the Cardiovascular Division, told
Doug Wigle in March 1972.[48] This set off the chain of events leading to
the establishment in 1989 of a cardiac surgery division at Sunnybrook
with Goldman at its head. But it was a rather long chain: almost thirty
years.

It was actually the death in October 1988 of yet another cardiac
patient on the wait list at St. Michael's Hospital, Charles Coleman, that
triggered the opening of the cardiac unit at Sunnybrook. Coleman's
surgery had been postponed eleven times "because," as the *Toronto
Star* stated, "of a shortage of critical care hospital beds." (The newspaper tartly observed that other questions seemed more important for
Ontario Health Minister Elinor Caplan than critical care heart surgery,
such as "whether Ontarians should shop on Sunday."[49]) The publicity
surrounding this death lit a fire under the provincial government, and
the new cardiac unit at Sunnybrook would shortly open.

As noted, by this time there was increasing concern along with the
negative press about unacceptably long waiting lists for coronary artery
surgery in Ontario. Reference has already been made to the initiative

created by Bernie Goldman and cardiologist Ron Baigrie to address this at TGH.

The wait list crisis also resulted in the formation of the Cardiac Care Network of Ontario (CCNO) in 1998. The provincial Ministry of Health and Long-Term Care brought together a leading cardiac care specialist (cardiologist or surgeon) from each of the cardiac care centres in Ontario along with hospital executives, community-based family physicians, nursing leaders, and senior ministry personnel to create an integrated triage and evaluation system for heart patients in Ontario. Hugh Scully was appointed as a founding member of this organization from TGH.

A triage grid for emergent, urgent, semi-urgent, and elective cardiac patients was developed. Evaluation of time from onset of symptoms to cardiologic consultation, subsequent assessment of cardiac function (including ventricular function and coronary artery angiography), time to referral for cardiac surgery, and time to surgery was documented for each patient by teams appointed in each hospital.

The surgical results for each patient were recorded: mortality, morbidity (such as peri-operative bleeding), wound infection, peri-operative myocardial infarct [heart attack] or stroke, length of stay in ICU and hospital prior to discharge (either to home or to a long-term care facility), and readmission to hospital for related complications. Information about the results for each surgeon and each cardiac surgical service was collected on an annual basis. In a peer-to-peer process, the validity of the results was checked annually. Failure to report accurately led to Ministry of Health funding penalties applied to the hospital in the subsequent year and internal review of any surgeon thus involved.

All of these data were meticulously recorded and analysed by the Institute for Clinical Evaluative Sciences based at Sunnybrook Health Sciences Centre, brilliantly led by David Naylor (later dean of medicine and president of the University of Toronto) and Jack Tu.

With this transparent attention to detail, there was a dramatic improvement in all waiting times, surgical mortality, peri-operative complications, length of stay and readmission rates in all Ontario cardiac hospitals. Many millions of dollars were saved, allowing for further investment and improvement in all areas of healthcare. The end result was that the outcomes of coronary artery surgery in Ontario were as good or better than any other cardiac service in the world.

The Ontario model received international acclaim in peer-reviewed presentations and articles in premier scientific journals in Canada, the United States, South America, the UK, Europe, and Asia. Hugh Scully personally presented across Canada, in the United States, and in South America. From this work and collaboration with Merril Knudtson, a leading interventional cardiologist and scientist from Calgary, he published a major 1995 guideline document in the *Canadian Journal of Cardiology*, "Indications for and Access to (coronary) Revascularization."[50] In 2002 he gave additional addresses on evidence-based planning of cardiac services before the Society of Cardiothoracic Surgeons in the United States and the 20th South American Conference on Cardiac Surgery and Cardiology.

The CCNO has since broadened its scope. Currently, the recording and evaluation of heart valve surgery is being led very competently by Chris Feindel of TGH/UHN. In 2016 it merged with the Ontario Stroke Network, and the following year the combined organization was renamed CorHealth Ontario.

Heart Surgeons and Lung Transplants

The Department of Surgery led the world in lung transplants. In 1968, Griff Pearson helped create a Division of Thoracic Surgery, separate from the Division of Cardiac Surgery. This was good news for science in lung transplantation because, Shaf Keshavjee later said, "you had people who focused on thoracic surgery as opposed to cardiac surgery, and weren't doing it as an add-on case or a less important part of their practice." Yet he added, "Lung transplant couldn't have happened by thoracic surgeons alone without cardiac surgery. These guys used to sleep in the hallway outside, while Joel [Cooper] and Tom Todd and those guys tried to put a lung in."[51]

Keshavjee came soon to appreciate the importance of bypass, given that all the early lung transplants were done on pump. Thoracic surgeons weren't trained for that, so he resolved to master it: "The future of thoracic surgery means I as a thoracic surgeon, whether I'm going to do transplants or high end oncologic surgery, you need to understand cardiac surgery, be comfortable with the pump."[52]

Indeed, Scully recalled of those days that he and Joel Cooper went to the lab to practise operating on cows. "We did that successfully. In those days, there wasn't a Bob Ginsberg or an Alec Patterson [later lung surgeons], who were very superior technical surgeons. I got involved in the first series of lung transplants because a cardiac surgeon is able to work with fragile vessels. In order to sew up the pulmonary artery and the atrium after we connected them, we did the heart at the same time."[53]

Scully later said of this time, "There was no one who could successfully sew the pulmonary arteries and atrium. Tirone [David] had backed out. It was my job in the OR to work with the perfusion team and mediate and assist Joel Cooper."[54]

Thus, from 1982 cardiac surgery participated in the early lung transplants. In September 1988, Patterson, Goldman, and Bill Williams closed a patent ductus arteriosus in an adult woman with severe pulmonary hypertension, who also got a single lung transplant. Goldman said that "[we] provided cardiopulmonary support with total bypass as they created the multiple anastomoses necessary to 'retro-fit' the double lung in situ … Steven Fremes, then a senior resident in cardiovascular surgery, published [in 1990] on the first combined congenital heart repair and single lung transplant.[55] Bill Williams and I scrubbed … on a young woman with a PDA (patent ductus arteriosus) that had produced pulmonary hypertension from the significant and long-standing left to right shunt [blood coming into the lungs at high pressure]. The shunt had reversed [meaning that unoxygenated blood was now being pumped into the aorta], and she was breathless and cyanotic. No one knew if a transplanted lung could tolerate the high pressure that would ensue due to the remaining lung. She underwent closure of the large PDA through the opened pulmonary artery and subsequent single left lung transplant on cardiopulmonary bypass. Thankfully she did well … and three decades later was still alive."[56]

The double-lung-heart transplant was pioneered in Canada at University Hospital in London. New Yorker Morton Levine received the first double-lung-heart transplant in Toronto on 25 June 1984. Levine, who had been in the soundproofing business, had severely damaged lungs from working with asbestos, and before the operation he had been hooked to an oxygen tank around the clock. Heavily sedated after the operation, he was said to have spent his sixtieth birthday – "and U.S. Independence Day in a big fog." Still, reporters and photographers crowded round the hospital for this historic event.[57]

In November 1986, Toronto became the first centre in North America to perform a double-lung transplant *without* transplanting the heart as well. The team was led by Joel Cooper at the General and Sinai hospitals, who in November 1983 had carried out the world's first successful single-lung transplant. Since then, the Toronto team had done six other single-lung transplants, as well as seven single-lung-and-heart transplants. But transplanting the lungs without the heart was technically more difficult, and this was news. Bernie Goldman came in on the cardiac side, and over the course of the next five hours, the lung surgeons – Joel Cooper, Alec Patterson, and Griff Pearson – did the lungs. They made a midline incision in the chest of the female patient, forty-three, to remove the lungs. The new lungs, along with the donor's right atrium, were then lowered into place. The donor's right atrium was then attached to the patient's left atrium, and the great vessels reconnected. (The donor's lungs and atrium were transported in a Lear jet from a provincial Ontario town to the General.) "The operation went very well," said Cooper. "Dr. Patterson and I were pleased that it went so smoothly this first time."[58]

A Very Early Assist Device

In 1983 Hugh Scully was doing a mitral and aortic valve replacement on Mrs. Natalia Kowal, who had suffered rheumatic fever as a child. She had been on the heart-lung machine for over three hours, and when they took her off bypass, the heart refused to restart. What to do? The surgeons determined there was *right* ventricular heart failure – much less common than left failure – owing to a constricted right coronary artery.

"There is a sequence of things we do," said Scully in a later interview with medical journalist Joan Hollobon. "The first is to try to protect the left heart by putting in a device called an intra-aortic balloon pump." The balloon pump, as we know, protects the left ventricle by pushing blood back up the aorta and into the coronary arteries.

Mrs. Kowal's heart began fibrillating, which would usually be the antecedent to death. Scully started massaging her heart with his hand. Now what?

It happened just then that Scully's resident, surgeon Robert Kormos, was doing dog research using an assist device that didn't aerate the blood, not a heart-lung pump. It just pumped blood with a small rotor from one chamber or vessel to another. To give the right ventricle a chance to rest, Scully and Kormos attached one end of the pump to the right atrium (where the cavae were delivering venous blood to the heart), the other end to her pulmonary artery, which carries blood from the right ventricle to the lung. The lungs then oxygenated the blood and pumped it into the left ventricle.

"We had absolutely nothing to lose by trying it," said Scully, "because everything was lost already – and we had developed the knowledge in the laboratory." Kormos later added, "This pump is particularly useful in a patient after surgery because you don't have to keep the patient heparinized, avoiding a lot of bleeding and oozing from all the raw surfaces."

As soon as the pump was switched on, Mrs. Kowal's blood pressure rose to normal and all her rhythm problems disappeared. Scully meanwhile was in constant touch with doctors at the Cleveland Clinic who had already used the assist device, and it turned out that the Toronto surgeons had taken, untutored, all the right steps. The surgery began on Wednesday, and by Saturday "it was clear Mrs. Kowal's heart was improving – it was trying to compete with the pump, so that her blood pressure began to fluctuate." They reduced the pump flow and took her back to the OR, closing her chest, which up to then had the two big tubes of the assist device running in and out of it. They took her off the aortic balloon. Up to this point, the two Toronto surgeons had had little sleep. The family had been hovering anxiously. They, too, had had little sleep. The surgeons learned that Mrs. Kowal had been "a vital and active woman with no other major systems in failure." The immense effort had paid off. Mrs. Kowal's cardiologist, Harry Rakowski, described the pioneering effort as "a surgical tour de force – this is a situation where she was effectively dead in the operating room. This has saved her life so far." This was the first such right-heart assist device employed in Canada.[59]

Baird Knows the Score

It was Baird's last year at the Western. In 1977 he did an aortocoronary bypass on Huw Pritchard, a chemistry professor at York University. A roommate of Pritchard's predicted the graft wouldn't hold up. But it did for the next fifteen years, despite Pritchard's needing two further angioplasties. Finally, in 1992, at age sixty-four, after two cardiac arrests, it was clear that Pritchard needed a redo. He was flown by helicopter from his home in Orangeville to the heli-pad of the General, where it was Baird, now close to retirement, who operated on him again. "It was very difficult surgery," Baird told the family, "and he might not make it."

But happily he did make it, and in 2015, twenty years later, Pritchard was busy "building clocks and computers." Pritchard was not quite sure what he would say to Baird if he met him. But Baird, whose roots reached back into evangelical pietism, knew the score: "Surgeons do the cutting and God does the healing," he said.[60]

Chapter Twelve

The Damaged Heart

With the arrival of Heather Ross, who ultimately became head of cardiology, and with Vivek Rao as the head of cardiac surgery, the focal point of interest in the division became heart failure: when the damaged heart finally gives up. Here the first major player is Lynda Mickleborough, who was also the first female cardiac surgeon in Canada. But she preferred to be known for her not-inconsiderable achievements rather than as "the first" anything.

Lynda Mickleborough

If there is one thing you can say about Lynda Mickleborough it is that in Toronto she never felt oppressed by male prejudices against women. "I was one of the boys," she said.

Tough as nails, she became one of the stars of the division. "TGH was ahead of the curve on women cardiovascular surgeons," said Goldman. "Lynda Mickleborough was a highly regarded McGill trainee [who] retired after a remarkable twenty-plus-year career with seminal contributions on arrhythmia surgery on bad hearts. She was tough and spent long hours in the OR with these cases. She was considered a real prize catch from Montreal."[1]

There is a long list of star cardiac surgeons, such as Bill Bigelow, Ray Heimbecker, Don Wilson, and Gordon Murray, who grew up on the Prairies, and Lynda Mickleborough is one of them.

Born in 1947, she was raised on a farm in rural Saskatchewan, north of Regina, and attended a one-room schoolhouse for grades one to eight. She later said that being raised on a farm, compared to such high rollers as Scully, was an advantage rather than a disadvantage. "Because I had nowhere to go but up. I didn't want to be a farm wife, I knew that from a very early age. In school there was one teacher, there were thirty pupils in every different grade, so if you didn't make yourself learn, you wouldn't get anywhere."[2]

Then it was on to high school in Regina. "In grade 12 I had very good marks. I had a couple of very good teachers who suggested that medicine might be a good thing to do, because I liked science but I also liked people. Maybe that would work out. So I applied for a scholarship to McGill and I got it." It was a full ride, and so she went east to McGill, where she did four years of science and four years of medicine.

"I loved it. The only course I didn't do well in was calculus. I loved the physical chemistry, I loved everything else, but I hated calculus." She gained a BSc, then graduated in medicine in 1973 with the second highest marks in her class. She trained in the general surgery program at the Royal Victoria Hospital, winning in her first year the prize in surgery and the prize in psychiatry. "It was a very weird combination, but anyway."

How did she opt for cardiac surgery? "In my first year as a surgical intern I did a rotation with Tony Dobell, and one day on the ward I recognized that a patient was really in trouble. I went to the OR, even though I was an intern, and said, 'Dr. Dobell, you've got to come and see this guy because something's going wrong, I don't know what it is.' And he came, and the man was tamponading [blood from the ruptured heart pouring into the pericardium], and Dobell and I took him to the OR and relieved his tamponade. That's the day I decided to do cardiac surgery."

She did some research on dogs, creating infarcts and looking at electrocardiographic changes. "It taught me how to do research." It was an arduous schedule, "Running a lab. Ten o'clock at night, checking on your dog to see if it's alive or dead."

Then she took her American board examination in 1979 and afterwards came to Toronto at age thirty-three in 1980 as a fellow. "I did not want to be somewhere where English was a second language, and Toronto to me seemed the best centre at that time in Canada." At the end of the year they offered her a job.

"We wanted her here," interjected Scully.

MICKLEBOROUGH: You didn't know that before I came.

SCULLY: You wouldn't have had the invitation were that not the case.

Thus, Mickleborough arrived at Toronto as a star. Goldman said, "When she was a clinical fellow here, she was like Joan of Arc being brought into Paris. We had this blonde dynamo who was the queen of the McGill program. Tony Dobell and Lloyd McLean, I mean the references they had for her. When she was coming to Toronto, *we* were more pleased than she was, and her year as a clinical fellow was remarkable in terms of her capacity, her intelligence, her ability to work with other people ... [especially] some very strange people in electrophysiology – at that time electrophysiology was still a little woo-woo."[3]

Mickleborough established herself as a specialist in the heart damaged by previous infarcts. The backstory here begins with Murray and Heimbecker. Heimbecker, as previously mentioned, was Bigelow's colleague, not his student. But it would be fair to consider him as Gordon Murray's student, and in 1967 Heimbecker turned to a procedure – "emergency infarctectomy" – for which in 1947 Murray had laid the theoretical basis (see chapter 1). (Murray was listed as a coauthor of the 1967 article on the topic.[4]) The operation was perfected in calves and involved, said a journalist paraphrasing Heimbecker "excising a full thickness of the heart muscle." Heimbecker said it was "like cutting a piece out of a pie." A newspaper account described a fifty-six-year-old patient "operated upon as a last resort ... A piece of the lower chambers, the size of a filet mignon, was cut out. The wall between the left and right ventricle was repaired with Teflon and the heart muscle was sewn together again." The patient died a month later of causes "unrelated to his heart."[5] According to a report in 1968, two of four infarctectomy patients had survived.[6] By the time Heimbecker gave a talk to the Canadian Club at the Royal York Hotel in February 1970, he and Jim Key had performed twenty-five such operations at the Toronto General; a similar number had also been done at St. Michael's Hospital and the Western.[7] The procedure then rested for a while.

Mickleborough's research career in Toronto began with "the arrhythmia game," she said. "At the time we were in the forefront. We had a mapping system that was used intraoperatively." Beginning in the mid-1980s, Mickleborough and cardiologist Eugene Downar ran a series of experiments to "map" patterns of damage to the ventricles from previous heart attacks, and then to ablate the damaged tissue through electric shocks, delivered with a wired balloon, in order to make the tissue electrically silent (and thus incapable of interfering with the heartbeat). The balloon could be threaded into the heart on a catheter, which eliminated the need to open the heart surgically to deal with scarring. This research was pioneered on dogs, then used on a series of patients, with some significant long-term results.[8] The research stimulated work in many centres on using balloons to explore and ablate the damaged myocardium of the ventricles. The idea was to cut out the scar. The mapping system was a clever idea for dealing with dysrhythmias, but it was overtaken by defibrillators. Yet the goal of ablating (cutting out) the dead tissue in the ventricle from previous attacks remained an objective.

Goldman said, "When Lynda took on those cases of ventricular arrhythmia, I was a kind of pacemaker/defibrillator technician. I kept shunning away from it, thanking God that she was taking on these six and seven and eight-hour cases of high-risk bad hearts with arrhythmias, the combination of a bad heart and a bad rhythm."[9] The issue here: How do you control irregular heartbeats in the months and years following a heart attack? The muscle of the left ventricle has been damaged and is extremely vulnerable to failure.

There was, as we know, a Toronto tradition of "infarctectomy," beginning with Murray and running through Heimbecker. Yet that was for acute infarcts. Mickleborough's procedure was for *chronic* ventricular dysfunction.

How do you know what tissue to cut out? "It was experience. And I got the experience doing the mapping. So for years I was the only one talking about that and remember at the AATS [American Association of Thoracic Surgeons] one year [Texas heart surgeon] Denton Cooley got up and said, 'Why are you talking about this? We solved this problem years ago.'" He was talking about aneurysms. But several people said, to the contrary, it hadn't been solved years ago. "This is really neat," they said.

Mickleborough said, "I'm talking about the patient who has an infarct and then five, six years later is going into heart failure or is having angina. And when you do the ventriculogram, instead of having an ejection fraction of 40 or 50 per cent, they have an ejection fraction of 15 per cent, and instead of being *this* size, their heart is **this size**." They would be transplant candidates – if a transplant were available.

Thus, in the late 1980s Mickleborough went beyond an old idea of Ray Heimbecker's, cutting away the portion of the wall of the left ventricle damaged in a heart attack. Heimbecker had only one survivor in five attempts, and the procedure was allowed to languish.[10] Then in 1992, Mickleborough and Downar reported results for undertaking scar excision and ventricular remodelling in repairing the chronic ventricle.[11] Of the fifty-four consecutive patients, 72 per cent survived the operation, with six late deaths.

Mickleborough said, "Having had the ten years' experience with these patients, I realized that the ventricular architecture was important. And that there were a lot of patients who had lousy hearts, but I felt some of them would benefit from what I called the remodelling of the heart. Sometimes there's a clear aneurysm – no brainer. Your take the aneurysm out – no problem. But a lot of these patients were sort of in-between, with lousy ventricles; it wasn't working very well, it wasn't a well-defined, clear-cut small aneurysm. It was a more global dysfunction. But I felt that by bringing the volume of the heart down, taking out some of the thin, scarred area, you could actually help them live longer because the residual chamber would function better, and you also did the bypasses." So this was Mickleborough's big innovation: "remodelling" the heart.

Did It Work Out?

"It worked out. A lot of our patients were cured, and many of them lived for ten years, with lousy, lousy hearts, bypasses, and whatever." If the primary problem was arrhythmia, the defibrillator was a better choice. "So then I start doing more and more patients with poor ventricles. For years I was the only one presenting this at the meetings."

In her twenty-two years in the division, Mickleborough racked up fourteen grants totalling $1.5 million (not including the $16 million for the STICH [Surgical Therapy for Ischemic Congestive Heart Failure] trial, for which she was the chief investigator). Teresa ("Terry") Kieser trained under her and recalled, "I was always a little intimidated by her – she seemed so confident and not influenced by what other people thought. There was a little envy too – she was where I wanted to be. The thing I most wanted to emulate was her 'no nonsense – take no prisoners attitude.'"[12]

Mickleborough's swan song, in a sense, was a paper she delivered at the American Association for Thoracic Surgery in May 2003 – she retired that year – giving results of 285 left ventricular reconstructions she had performed at TGH between 1983 and 2002. At five years, 82 per cent of these patients were still alive, 97 per cent had not experienced sudden death, and the ejection fraction had increased by 10 per cent.[13] Mickleborough's work actually anticipated much later "surgical ventricular modelling," although she was not given credit for it – an old story!

As for women as cardiac patients, it was Mickleborough whose research put the lie to the myth that bypass surgery was more dangerous for women. Leading a team of investigators, she looked at records for 1,132 male and 355 female bypass patients. It turned out there was no difference in mortality from the operation. The women had been sicker than the men at the time of the operation and had fewer complications afterwards. The study concluded, "Concern over increased operative mortality in women should not bias referral patterns for angiography and coronary bypass graft surgery."[14] As Mickleborough told a newspaper reporter, "Women, just because they're women, aren't at higher risk. But women are more willing to put up with the symptoms ... A man complaining of chest pains would be sent home from work, where a woman will 'typically sit down and have a cup of coffee' and ignore her symptoms."[15]

In a sense the Mickleborough story confirms the adage that, in the early days, women had to be tough to get ahead. "Her clinical results, especially in coronary bypass surgery, were excellent," said Rao, "and probably the best in the division. She and Tirone – and I was witness to a lot of this – butted heads a lot, and I don't think Tirone really promoted her to the extent that he should have."[16]

Goldman added, "We used to say, 'Lynda wore army boots': she clomped into the OR, literally, butting heads with everybody. She was a tough lady. Tough in terms of survival, and tough in terms of the amount of work she was doing – with long, long cases. And she was a mother as well as a wife and surgeon."[17]

Discrimination because she was a woman? She was emphatic that that didn't happen among the Toronto cardiac surgeons. But elsewhere? In Montreal, "there was one cardiac surgeon, who, when he was writing my evaluation, put in 'good little seamstress.'"

But she stressed that women surgeons had to be just as stand-up as male surgeons. "My basic premise is you're a surgeon first, and whether you're male or female, you should be trained the same way, judged the same way. I don't believe you can be a cardiac surgeon and take three years off to have children. Because you're going to lose your technical skills, your expertise, so being a woman in cardiac surgery is not something I would recommend. You're going to have to make sacrifices. You're not going to have the life perhaps that you had hoped."

Why is her name not more widely known? Rao said he talked about "the Mickleborough repair," but said this phase had not been picked up in the literature. Mickleborough, too, suffered from "the Canadian disease" – modesty. Rao said, "Lynda was never one to go up there and market herself to the same degree as some other surgeons. She was recognized as one of the leading ventricular surgeons. [The US leaders] would recognize Lynda's contributions wholeheartedly."

> Q: If she had been a man, do you think the outcome would have been a bit different here in terms of celebrity?
> RAO: I don't know if it was a gender thing or just her personality.[18]

When asked if her remodelling procedure was innovative and had the priority over others in the field, Mickleborough shrugged and said, "What priority?" There was rarely anything new in medicine.

Goldman intervened and said that her procedure was "seminally important."

Was Mickleborough's own assessment of her achievement realistic – or the "Canadian modesty disease"? She allowed that her procedure was not really for aneurysms, which is what Vincent Dor in Monaco and surgeons elsewhere were treating. "I was trying to push it into people who didn't have clear-cut aneurysms but had huge hearts." It was not an "attractive procedure," in that it demanded long operations on very high-risk patients and had a mortality of 8 per cent. "It's just not attractive because it's bloody hard work and if you hadn't slid into it over ten years you'd never be there."

Yet she saved many lives. Goldman said, "She took on these cases that none of us had had enough experience with. Nor did we have the knowledge of the ventricular arrhythmias, or the physical and intellectual courage to stand there for eight hours trying to make a judgment of what's thin, what's thick – and remember, the heart is lying there as in a butcher shop."[19]

The Toronto Faculty of Medicine has tried to elevate its female pioneers. Here is one they missed.

Chapter Thirteen

Valves

Motto: "The evolution of artificial valves was fraught with both success and failure, and failure often meant that unfortunate patients were the price paid for biomedical and bioengineering errors!"[1]

– Bernie Goldman, 2019

Mechanical Valves

If the mitral valve – or any other valve – isn't functioning properly and can't be repaired, an artificial valve is called for. One constant in the valve story is that sooner or later, virtually all of them fail, unless the patient dies first. Artificial and biological valves competed with each other in the early days. And from the earliest days, ball cage valves were on offer from many manufacturers, none of which were really satisfactory – but all better than the diseased valves. The valve must work under the formidable stress of eighty or so movements up and down, per minute, hour after hour, day after day. And many of the early valves simply didn't hold up. Also, some were too tall, projected into the ventricle, lacerating the opposing wall or blocking the outflow from the ventricle to the aorta.

In 1961 Bigelow asked Ron Baird to begin the first aortic valve replacement program in Canada using the mechanical Kay-Shiley floating disc valve. (It was in 1962 that Albert Starr introduced the subcoronary ball valve.) Bigelow then let Baird do all aortic valve replacements at TGH, "initially with individual 'Kay' valve leaflets and then, in 1962, with the 'Starr Edwards ball valve.'"[2]

Hugh Scully observes of these Starr-Edwards valves, "The initial model had a silastic ball, which occasionally developed a problem with wear-and-tear deterioration over time and the occasional dislodgement or escape of the ball, often with catastrophic consequences. A model with a metal ball was introduced to obviate this problem, but these valves were loud with an audible 'pop'; or 'ping' with each beat, causing great psychological distress in some patients, particularly if two valves had been implanted!"[3] The first 107 Starr-Edwards cases saw only twenty-two deaths in the next four years, an improvement on the grim mortality rate attending earlier aortic operations.

The following year, 1963, saw the first Starr valve replacements for the mitral valve. Scully continued, "Another problem with the Starr-Edwards valves in the mitral position was their high 'vertical' profile from the valve annulus [the dense fibrous ring surrounding the valve]. This could be a real problem in those patients who were having MVR [mitral valve replacement] for rheumatic mitral stenosis not suitable for a 'mitral split' operation. These patients usually had small left ventricular chambers. The implanted Starr valve would present a problem with left ventricular outflow obstruction. As well, though rarely, the high profile cage would erode into the contralateral [opposite] wall of the left ventricle, potentiating catastrophic left ventricular rupture!" For these mitral valves, the mortality was worse than for the aortic valves: seventeen deaths in fifty-two cases operated by 1966.[4]

Understandably, there was great interest in developing lower-profile valves, and in 1968 the Beall floating disc valve was introduced: 101 of these were implanted at TGH. In 1977 it was discovered that the Beall heart valve was subject to premature failure. The valve had been implanted worldwide between 1969 and 1972, and with time it was learned that the five-year death rate was around 25 to 30 per cent. Initially, this news was kept "a tight secret" at the General, as a journalist put it. At the General, ninety-seven patients had received the valve, and by July 1978, when the story broke, forty-five of them had died, although it was unclear whether the valve was directly implicated in their deaths. Leonard Schwartz, a TGH cardiologist, using echo, created a model to predict impending failure of the disc (which could be eroded by the stents). Schwartz and Scully then set up a management protocol for surgical explantation of these "at-risk valves." The General set up a special bed for the investigation of these patients, and while the follow-up proceeded, three of them died. Scully successfully replaced at-risk valves in a number of other patients.[5] It was a front-page story. Thus, said Scully, "The Starr-Edwards valve was still favoured by most surgeons."

There were no valves without problems, and the Starr valves in their turn fell short of expectations. In 1967 Bigelow said, "Our follow up system in the last two or three years has brought to our attention the fact that Starr valves not only produce blood clots, but they can become infected by a rare type infecting organism and we were able to manage this situation once it was discovered and before it was generally known by surgeons doing heart surgery." This is lifesaving in the case of valves. "Such a vigorous follow up is not so necessary in fields of surgery where the operations are standardized and have been carried out for many years and the complications are well known."[6] The surgeons had become entangled in the infections that plagued the unit in these years, and they were unable to locate the source until it was discovered that a window-type air conditioner with bird droppings turned out to be spraying bacteria over the operating field.

Cadaveric Valves (Homografts)

There was an international vogue, beginning in the mid-1960s, for making heart valves out of fascia lata, the strip of fascial tissue running down the thigh. Al Trimble participated in this in Toronto, and was one of a very few surgeons in the world who achieved success with this human-tissue prosthesis.[7] The vogue began in 1966 and was brief because the valves deteriorated quickly; and in 1976 the *British Medical Journal* published a shattering editorial, "Obituary for Fascia Lata Heart Valves," which cited Trimble's work three times.[8] Yet this was merely the beginning of a series of successful, indeed pioneering, Toronto attempts to solve the question of replacement heart valves that either deteriorated, caused clots, or produced annoying clicks.

But how about biological valves from cadavers as preferable to the clunking, defective mechanical kind? The success of the cadaveric valve replacements was like a tidal wave, sweeping all before it. By August 1965 the cardiac surgeons were demanding their own freeze-dying technology, because the patience of the School of Hygiene – with the surgeons using its freeze drier – had run out.[9] "This is really quite an economy for the hospital," Heimbecker told Kergin, "for it is no more expensive than four or five Starr-valves, which would otherwise be the valve used if homograft valves are not available."[10] (Cadaveric valves, of course, were free.)

In 1969 Trimble, who was in charge of the division's finances, said, "We are about to go over from Starr-Edwards Ball Valves (for which we pay well over $60,000 per year) to homograft valves collected in the autopsy room and suitably sterilized and stored."[11]

But where should the aortic valves come from (or, as the phrase went, be "harvested" from)? The city morgue had been quite cooperative, but Ray Heimbecker said in 1965 that demand might soon outrun supply. How about the Department of Pathology, in the basement of the Banting Building? Moreover, "We are willing to consider all age groups and indeed find that a 60 and 70-year-old patient often has large homograft aortic valves which are so often more suitable for clinical implantation."[12] At this point, Toronto was one of the only three North American centres, among them the Mayo Clinic and a hospital in Seattle, doing homograft heart valve transplants instead of the plastic ball valves hitherto in use.[13]

Shiley Valves

From 1973, a number of valves developed by the Shiley company began to be implanted in Toronto. Initially, the valve implanted was the low-profile, tilting, spherical 60-degree model. The valves changed from a spherical disc to a convexo-concave disc, resulting, as Scully said, "in better 'washing' of both surfaces of the disc and therefore less likelihood of thrombus forming across the lesser aperture. An added benefit was an increase in the opening angle from 60 degrees to 70." The "outflow" side had to go face up. For readers who find the valve story complex, it was complex for Bigelow as well. Scully said, "I remember persuading Dr. Bigelow to implant one of these, during a demonstration operation with the overhead visitor observation gallery in 9 POR, but having to quietly 'nudge' him to reverse the initial placement."

Scully continued, "In all of these valves, the inlet struts were integral to the valve ring, and never produced a structural problem." Yet in some of the larger sizes used for mitral valve replacement "there were occasional problems with fracture of the welded outlet struts, resulting in embolization of the disc and severe hemodynamic compromise (cardiogenic shock and embolization of the disc)." Very after these outlet welded strut fractures were reported, the Shiley Valve Company mounted a detailed investigation into the problem and formed an independent international and North American advisory panel of cardiologists, research scientists, and surgeons to study it and give advice. Scully was appointed to the panel, which was very active in Europe and North America.[14]

The problem was confined to a very few production lines of larger diameter sixty-degree and (more frequently) seventy-degree valves usually implanted in the mitral position. Risk profiles, diagnostic guidelines, and recommendations about emergency surgical management were developed and published widely by the panel members.[15]

In the few patients in whom the larger valves had been placed in the aortic position who experienced valve-strut fracture, the outcome was fatal. For mitral-valve fracture patients in the hands of skilled valve surgeons, the successful salvage rate was about 50 per cent if the patient presented for emergency surgery within twelve to twenty-four hours. Scully operated successfully on three such patients who came through the emergency room at TGH, two of whom had been referred from other cardiac centres.

Prophylactic redo surgery was never recommended because the risk of surgery was greater than the prospective risk of fracture in most patients.

The Shiley Valve Company went on to develop the seventy-degree concave/convex tilting disc valve with integration into the valve ring of both the inlet strut and an outlet monostrut with an absolutely clean record of freedom from structural problems. Scully said, "In my view this was perhaps the best mechanical valve ever produced. It proved to have excellent hemodynamics (didn't cause clotting). I have several patients who had had 70° C/C monostrut Shiley valves continuing to function well in the aortic position 30 years after surgery without Coumadin anticoagulation in those patients in regular sinus rhythm." Between 1973 and 1985, 155 of these Björk-Shiley valves were implanted at the General, mainly by Scully.[16] But then the Shiley Valve Company went bankrupt and out of business as a result of an avalanche of prod-uct-liability lawsuits from its earlier line of valves.

After the Shiley valves, the cardiac surgeons went over to the St. Jude bileaflet hinge valve, and that worked well. Yet there was a problem with a particular St. Jude valve that was "silver impregnated." (See "The Valve with the Silver Ring" later in this chapter.)

Butany

The cardiac pathologist at the Peter Munk Cardiac Centre was Jagdish ("Jack") Butany – worldwide the chief specialist in breakdowns of car-diac valves. Butany was born in Karachi in 1944 (which was then in India but is now in Pakistan), and his parents identified completely with India. The family soon moved to the state of Orissa, about two hundred kilometres south of Calcutta, and Butany grew up in Cuttack, attending a mission school. He earned his medical degree in Mysore, south India, in 1971, then trained in general surgery in New Delhi. (But this was not what he really wanted to do; he had wanted to be a fighter pilot, but failed the eye exam.)

Butany came to Canada in 1975, with wife and infant daughter, want-ing to train at the General in surgery. But all the positions were full. A slot, however, was available in pathology.

At the time, the Australian Malcolm Silver was the cardiac specialist in pathology at TGH. Butany told his friends he was going to study with Silver.

"Are you an idiot?" they said.

Butany explained: "Silver could be one cruel – pardon my Hungarian – S.O.B. He had turfed a bunch of residents through the years, and shouted and screamed and really gave them hell. He didn't tolerate idiots very well."

But Butany got on well with him. In those days there were lots of cardiac deaths at operation. Silver and Butany saw many at autopsy. Butany then studied cardiovascular pathology at the National Institutes of Health in Bethesda, at the Heart, Lung and Blood Institute, where for a year he did electron microscopy on "explanted" valves (those that had been removed because they had failed).

Butany thereupon returned to Toronto, initially to Women's College Hospital, then to the General. "Here there were lots of valves going in but also lots coming out. Somebody had to look at them. From that I got my interest in bioprostheses." (A prosthesis is an artificial substitute for a missing body part; "bio" means that it is made of biological material, as opposed to a mechanical valve.) The question of valve failure now arrested his attention.

At this point Scully, who was present at the interview with Butany, intervened. "There were several kinds of tissue valves: pig valves, cow pericardial valves, and then the freestanding valve that Tirone [David] designed." The Division of Cardiac Surgery had a stockpile of valves, and at a meeting the surgeons would decide which they were going to instal. (About 70 per cent of the prosthetic valves were mechanical, so the patient might be on anticoagulants for the rest of his or her life – but this was not invariant.) But the Toronto group favoured either a porcine tissue valve or a bovine pericardial valve. These tissue valves were all mounted on stents. Then creatively Tirone David designed the stentless porcine valves (SPV valve), made by the St. Jude Valve Company in Minneapolis.

The Valve with the Silver Ring

But St. Jude also had a mechanical bileaflet valve that had been highly successful. In the mid-1990s, the St. Jude people decided they would try to improve on this valve, and they sprayed elemental silver on the valve's sewing cuff. (This seemed to make sense; in some countries, when a baby is born, they put a drop of silver nitrate in their eyes to kill off any bacteria from the mother's vagina). St.

Jude's called this the Silver or Silzone Valve, and in 1997 a number were implanted at the General.

But then the mechanical Silzone valve started to fail. Butany said, "I've never seen a mechanical valve, especially a St. Jude, come out in the first month, second month, sixth month or even twelfth month. They don't fail. Once they're in, they're working well. I started seeing one, then I saw two." And Butany went up to Scully and said, "Look, what is this valve? It's different." Yes, the sewing ring was impregnated with silver nitrate. Butany soon had four that had been "explanted" (removed). In all of them, there was an abscess, evidently related to the silver ring. He had never seen this before.

The penny dropped in the surgical suite as well. The valve's silver-coated ring was intended to guard against infection, which is the bug-bear of mechanical devices. Unfortunately, the new valve prevented healing of the remnant valve tissue into the valve's Dacron (silver impregnated) ring. The patients began falling ill. Chris Feindel told Butany, "Something is just not right."

The hospital, of course, stopped implanting the valves, but meanwhile more than 36,000 of the valves had been implanted worldwide. Unlike the prompt response of the Shiley Company to news of occasional outlet strut fractures, the manufacturer's reps reacted poorly to the Toronto news. "Those guys really got after me," said Butany, "and kicked my butt like you wouldn't believe. They didn't want word to get around that Toronto General were not using this valve."

Four more valves came out. He phoned the manufacturer again. "They told me there was nothing wrong with the valve. I said, 'But they've come out.' They said, 'None of these valves have come out in the first eleven months.'"

Butany said, "Why am I seeing them and no one else?" They didn't know.

Butany called Bernie Goldman at Sunnybrook. He was clueless. They had implanted 120 of the valves. Butany called some of the staff in the Sunnybrook clinic.

"Can you tell me what's happening to your 120 patients?"

"More than twenty have died."

"Does Bernie know about it?"

"No."

Goldman was on the case now and took a photo of one of the valves seen at autopsy. St. Jude called a clinical meeting of surgeons from across Canada, to reassure them the valve was all right. Butany was not invited to the meeting, and when Tirone David, head of cardiac surgery, heard this, he blew up.

David said to Butany, "You're coming with me."

At the meeting Goldman "showed the most horrific picture of a heart valve, with a huge abscess around it, and gray, purulent-looking material all around the prosthesis. The prosthesis didn't have to be cut out: it just lifted out. The prosthesis was just rocking in the puddle of necrotic debris. So the discussion was a little bit different now. With Bernie's slide they [St. Jude's] really had no arguments at all."

By this time word was getting around. Butany made a presentation at a meeting in London, England. "The Australians told the company to take it off the market in November of '99. In December of '99, the British said, 'Take if off the market.'"

The company withdrew the valve. Hugh Scully joined Feindel in "explanting," or removing, valves in sixteen of the 147 patients (nineteen valves) who had received them between 1997 and 1999, and Butany found clear evidence of infection and leakage in many of them. But various observers turned on the surgeons at the General, accusing them of not using the proper suture technique. Scully said, "Just a minute. This is our record with other valves, as good or better than anyone in the world. This is the one valve that we're having problems with, and you're trying to tell us that because we're 100 per cent with the others we're screwing up with this one. Get outta here." Scully, Feindel, and Butany wrote a joint article and reported the explantations in the literature.[17] "This was the wrong centre to start accusing people who are doing a lot of valve surgery of not knowing what they're doing," said Scully.

In retrospect, Butany was critical of St. Jude's. "For three years they stonewalled me."[18] Butany and the surgeons became celebrated as the sentinels who had sounded the early alarm.[19]

A Valve from Cow Pericardium

Shiley made another valve from bovine pericardium (the fibrous sac that surrounds the heart and the roots of the great vessels). Scully said, "It worked very well for a while. It was a very good valve but the whole rationale between a mechanical valve and a tissue valve was you could put a tissue valve into somebody in regular rhythm and you might not have to put a patient on lifelong anticoagulants. You had to be much tighter in control [of potential clots] with the mechanical valves. I took out about one hundred of the bovine valves as they tore and replaced them. We picked the Shiley pericardial because we thought it was the better pericardial valve. It turned out none of the pericardial valves had satisfactory durability, Over that time, a vertical shear where the tissue was fixed to the strut would develop, resulting in growing insufficiency and heart failure."

Goldman interjected, "And, yet they had all been tested in a mechanical pulse duplicator. Thousands, upon tens of thousands, of mechanical heart beats, but when you put them in a human body ..." He left the sentence uncompleted.

There is a fine calculus here. Most tissue valves will sooner or later fail. In a younger person, Scully estimated failure after seven to ten years, "because they are more dynamic; there is more stress on the valve." But, "In those days, if you put it in someone over the age of sixty-five the likelihood is the valve would do well for the patient. The rule of thumb was mechanical valve under sixty, sixty is a discussion, and seventy a tissue valve."[20]

Thus, Toronto became known as the centre for valve redos. Scully said, "People like Bernie and me, and Tirone and Chris, got to be very good at redo valve operations, so the first redo mortality was not appreciably different than the first operation. Indeed, Tirone David is he "surgeon's surgeon" for valve redo surgery.[21] For some other centres, that wasn't the case," and Toronto often got redos referred from those centres.

The "Toronto Valve"

Most valves, as noted, fail sooner or later. They start embolizing; they break down; like the Silzone valve, they cause infection. In this endless search for replacement valves, David conceived the idea of using a pig valve, to avoid all the problems – such as a lifetime of anticoagulation – that came with the use of mechanical valves.[22] "[I had to live for years] to be able to develop a pig valve, with no stents," he said. "Take from a pig, put it in a human. I did it in the lab, commercialized it, and then I had to teach all my partners to do it."[23] (The long-term results with this valve were not entirely happy, yet David's work focused the attention of the field on animal valves.[24])

So Tirone David had a go at valve-designing. In 1988, assisted by Jack Butany, he proposed a "stentless" pig valve for the aorta. This valve lacked the surrounding tube, or "stent," in which previous valves sat. It also had no sewing ring (for attaching the valve to the surrounding tissue rim); these innovations should improve the blood flow through the valve, offering fewer obstructions. By the time of the December 1988 report, David had implanted the valve successfully in animals and a few patients.[25] St. Jude's put the valves into production in 1991. It was called the T-SPV: the Toronto Stentless Porcine Valve. Putting it in required surgical expertise that few, except David himself, and Scully, Goldman, and Feindel, possessed.

The valve worked well for seven years or so, and then it began to fail. Calcium started to collect on the valves; they began to tear from the rim. Scully had to undertake redos on them. "A redo on other valves is difficult; these are nightmares. The tissues begin to fuse with the wall of the aorta." Since 1991, the Toronto group had implanted the valve in 270 patients. By 1999, eight of the valves had been "explanted" (removed), three at surgery, five at autopsy.[26]

Yet the valve continued to perform well for another few years, until by 2008 durability problems became apparent that outweighed the safety advantages: 48 per cent of patients younger than age sixty-five experienced valve degeneration at twelve years, and 31 per cent of all patients had redos.[27] The Toronto group were the first to originate the novel stentless valve, and the first to alert the field that there was something wrong with it. David later conceded that the SPV "wasn't as durable as commercially available ones, largely because we humans are imperfect. We cannot implant in a human heart as perfect a valve as nature made for the pig."[28]

Chapter Fourteen

Training

Motto: The cardiac residency was known to be brutal. "We'd operate all day, we'd be up all night saving the patient, who would die, we'd take a shower, have breakfast, and start all over again."[1]

– Bernie Goldman, 2018

Training in surgery does not involve academic courses unless one is in the Surgeon Scientist Program. Surgeons are trained as apprentices, and the history of cardiac training is the history of an apprenticeship, together with intense studies of cardiovascular anatomy, physiology, and pathology. One starts as a junior, opening and closing the chest or harvesting the saphenous vein; one then moves up to first assistant on the other side of the operating table from the surgeon. And finally, as senior resident, one does the operation oneself while the staff surgeon is either the first assistant or variably available to assist as requested. Some of these residents would have started out in training programs in general surgery, others would have directly entered the cardiac program.

In 1936 John Alexander, a thoracic surgeon at the University of Michigan, articulated four "modern-day" concepts of surgical training that apply as well to cardiac surgery. These were later republicized by Toronto's Richard Weisel and colleagues in an effort to distil the essence of superb training as practised in "great institutions," among which Toronto was numbered. They were:

- Firstly, sufficient practice in the OR. Alexander said it was desirable that in a two-year program the resident conduct three hundred to five hundred operations and serve as first assistant in twice again as many.

- Secondly, "broad competencies" in managing the patient from the preoperative exam to the discharge from intensive care.
- Thirdly, exposure to research. Alexander called for familiarity with lab and research methods, plus one published piece of original research.
- Finally, "wellness," by which Alexander meant a constitution sturdy enough to withstand long hours of standing at the operating table, plus "the temperament and personality to succeed in the specialty."[2]

By appending his name to this rigorous program, Weisel implicitly endorsed it as up to snuff for the training program in cardiac surgery in Toronto – and with good cause. Toronto graduates went on to lead many of the cardiac surgery programs in Canada and the world.

After Bigelow's time, there were few interns in cardiac surgery, indeed the junior rotating internship had been abandoned. The trainees were the residents and the fellows, some of them Toronto-bred, others increasingly from abroad. In 1955 Bigelow asked Professor Janes, "Following a meeting of the attending staff of the Third Division, [we request] that the position of resident in cardiovascular surgery be established for an intern who is to live in the hospital. Our present arrangement of having a Fellow who lives out is one that carries with it difficulties when we attempt to give this Fellow surgery of a major nature to perform ... He is unable to take adequate responsibility or follow his cases closely enough while he lives out."[3] In 1958, Bigelow and Bill Mustard organized a course in cardiovascular surgery.[4] This was then the first university program in Canada to train cardiovascular surgeons.

Different Routes

In those days, as Richard Reznick, chairman of surgery at the university from 2002 to 2010, said, "It was five plus two. You had to do general surgery and then another two." That meant four years of surgery following a year internship. He had moved to Toronto from Montreal in 1977 after "some pretty dramatic anti-Anglo sentiment there."[5] He was in the cardiac surgery program but ended up in general surgery. He went on to great prominence in surgical education. He is now the dean of medicine and health science at Queen's University.

Why did Reznick change specialty? He had been a cardiac resident but found it unpromising. "I remember showing a slide of a picture of a corpse being wheeled into the operating theatre, saying 'It's time now to operate.' Cardiac surgery was considered so risky that you didn't want to operate on them, and they had to get so sick that you eventually did operate on them. You folks were being sent very sick patients in the early days for salvage surgery."

A memo in early 1958 outlined "A Two, Three, or Four Year Postgraduate Course in Cardiovascular Surgery at the University of Toronto," to be offered at the General and the Children's Hospital. Training would include one live-out year to work in the experimental animal laboratory of the Banting Institute or the Research Laboratory of HSC. On the clinical side, a two-year live-in residency would be divided between the General and HSC. Finally, there would be a live-out year as a "clinical assistant" at the General. For entry into the program, it was assumed that the major portion of general surgical training would already have been completed. Each hospital would have one "senior resident," preference going to "those who have had previous Assistant Residency positions in the University Fellowship course in surgery."[6]

In 1961 the Royal College of Physicians and Surgeons of Canada recognized both cardiovascular and surgery as a specialty and defined the combined fellowship in cardiovascular and thoracic surgery. The following year, 1962, the General's program for training in cardiovascular and thoracic surgery was accepted by the Royal College. The program was to include a year of pediatric cardiac surgery "to ensure that candidates acquire an adequate experience in surgery of congenital cardiovascular problems."[7] (The thoracic surgery certification was discontinued in 1964.) By this time thirteen Canadian centres had cardiovascular surgery programs. One could do a five-year cardiovascular-thoracic program or become a general surgeon plus two to three additional years of cardiovascular surgery.[8]

In the 1980s, Baird expanded the training program that Bigelow had founded, accepting annually four residents: two American and two Canadian. A form of Medicare, brought in as the Ontario Health Services Insurance Plan in 1969, "had moderated public attitudes about residents operating on private' patients [and] our surgical volume was huge." HSC had become a world-famous children's hospital; at the General, the "sister" program in thoracic surgery was excellent. "During the decade from 1978 to 1987," Baird said, "I was often told we had the best resident training programme in Thoracic and Cardiovascular Surgery in the world. I believe this was true."[9] (Goldman added, "as reflected by the number of Americans who chose to train at TGH."[10]) Indeed, as Scully added further, we became the preferred training centre for fellows from all over the world: China, Japan, Korea, Australia, New Zealand, Europe, and some Soviet Bloc countries.

An important step toward unifying the training program across hospitals occurred in 1987, when Goldman was appointed director of postgraduate education. Teaching was reorganized into citywide programs.[11] In 1988 Sunnybrook Hospital Medical Centre joined the program, under Goldman's leadership.

In 1994 the Royal College split up the exams of the three specialties – thoracic, vascular, and cardiac surgery – and implemented a direct-entry program in cardiac surgery.

These changes welded the training program into a world-class reputation. And Toronto started to become a world destination for trainees. Goldman said, "Superb people flocked to the TGH to augment their cardiac surgical training, especially those returning to university positions in Ivy League hospitals, who became heads of departments, in such places as Boston and Philadelphia" Part of this migration was "the arrival of Tirone David from Cleveland Clinic and Richard Weisel from Milwaukee. Here were two exceptional trainees who were immediately taken on staff for their intellectual and technical skills and clinical innovations."[12] (For more on this, see chapter 20.)

There was also a continual hemorrhage of young cardiac surgeons from the General to centres across Canada. As Neil Watters at the Wellesley Hospital told Bigelow in 1966 on the possibility of getting Heimbecker on staff part-time, "The fact that everyone is raiding your staff at once is simply a tribute to the way that you have trained them. TGH is a tree that flourishes even better after it has been pruned."[13]

How Is Cardiac Different?

How did training in cardiac surgery differ? In surgery in general, you have, as Terry Yau put it, "incremental graded responsibility. Basically, that means what you get to do as the primary surgeon: you're not independent, but with a staff supervision. You start out doing little things like an appendectomy, a closed hysterectomy, and hernias. You work your way up in the increase in responsibility and in the technical aspects of what you are doing."

It's very different in cardiac surgery, Yau continued. "You go from, as a junior resident, learning how to open and close, to the next thing you are going to be doing as a senior resident: valves, cardiac surgery, and anastomosis, where there are consequences of doing things. It is just such a contrast between that and general surgery."[14]

We are not talking about a lot of trainees: In all three hospitals with cardiac surgery programs there were a total of three residents per year. Bigelow explained this to Bill Drucker in 1966: "A trainee can be moved from one hospital to another but he usually takes most of his training in the sponsoring hospital. The Toronto General Hospital now train[s] two, and the Toronto Western Hospital one man per year, which means that the Hospital for Sick Children, in order to rotate all three residents through their hospital, [has] three residents a year."[15]

In 1962 Bigelow beat the bushes for a new senior resident. He explained in a widely broadcast search letter, now that the new cardiovascular area at the TGH is "in full swing," they are very busy. "I must say a service of four staff surgeons operating is rather busy and for that reason we thrust a good deal of responsibility on the shoulders of our senior resident, and they are expected to do a major part of the public ward operating, including open heart procedures on simpler defects with supervision. Our schedule runs about 14 operations a week. These are either heart or artery, and two to four pumps a week."[16] (Assisting at all this work would easily fulfil the Alexander requirements.)

Busy, for sure. Indeed, the senior residents soon found themselves overloaded. (This is probably a universal theme, but it was nonetheless acute at the General.) In 1963 Bigelow told Don Wilson, "The senior resident has too much to do at the present time. With four pumps a week and some of these very sick, requiring his presence in the acute therapy after the patient has left the operating room, you can see that the training of our resident, other than open heart surgery, is a problem."[17]

It is illuminating to see what the residents needed to learn: for example, how to write a discharge note. In 1959 Bigelow instructed Wolf Sapirstein (a fellow from South Africa and among the earliest Jewish trainees in the Department of Surgery): "I wonder if the note could be written with the thought in mind that the referring doctor, living outside the city, is going to use this as his sole guide to understand the treatment that was afforded the patient ... When passing from the paragraph Investigation to Treatment and Prognosis it might be helpful to indicate in a sentence or two why this particular treatment was instituted rather than just go from Physical Examination to a description of the operative procedure." Finally, on treatment, "If the patient is sent out on a low salt diet one should indicate how long he is to remain on it." Ditto for penicillin, or when the patient might "resume their household activities or job."[18] None of this is written in a "Residents' Handbook." It is called learning on the job.[19]

Typical Day

What was a typical day like for assistant residents and junior interns? Here is the schedule for 1964:[20]

6:00 a.m.: Rounds begin. The junior staff meet in the "acute therapy
unit," where acutely ill patients are held just before and after
operations. All the patients here are discussed, and the group
then proceeds to other floors in the hospital "where only the
acutely ill patients will be seen."

7:45 a.m.: "Tuesdays to Fridays, everyone is to report to the operating suite. No one will be allowed in this area without scrub suits
and boots. Double masks will be worn in all pump cases. Everyone is expected to scrub for five minutes."

1:30 p.m. to 3:00 p.m.: Clinics three days a week: "On Monday, the
Medical-Surgical Cardiovascular Clinic will be conducted by Drs.
Bigelow and Heimbecker." There were schedules for the cardiovascular follow-up and the peripheral vascular clinics. "Everyone
is encouraged to attend these clinics." (Don Wilson's formulation
was that in the old two-tiered system of medical care, "the so-
called outpatient clinics were really for charity patients, the rest of
the people who could afford it were seen in private offices."[21])

3:00 p.m. to 5:00 p.m. (or when finished in the operating room):
Ward rounds, accompanied by nurses, social workers, and phys-
iotherapists.

Then all kinds of special events were inserted in the week: combined rounds with the cardiologists on Mondays from 11:00 a.m. to
1:00 p.m.; Fridays 4:00 p.m. to 5:00 p.m., a discussion period with Drs.
Blundell, Trimble, or Firor; "residents' rounds" on Saturdays from
9:00 a.m. to 10:00 a.m. James K-Y ("Jimmy") Yao who, as a senior
resident, composed this schedule, added, "Remember the patients
are human beings and therefore must be treated with care and empathy."[22] Readers, who themselves may have quite different memories
of treatment in other hospitals, may smile at these lines. But the cardiac surgeons at the General were very mindful of the feelings of the
patients and their families.

Quality

The question of the quality of the trainees was very much on the minds
of the chiefs. This is not to say that the residents, many of whom went
on to become leaders in the field in Canada and abroad, were somehow not up to snuff. But cardiac surgery was a demanding field, and
Bigelow and senior colleagues wanted to make sure they got the best
possible candidates. In 1968, Bigelow told Jim Key, on recruiting good

people as residents in cardiovascular surgery that they would have to start beating the bushes, as they do on Wall Street. "It is my observation that successful services start on the outstanding men and make overtures to them rather than having them apply to the service which is the old custom." Bigelow wanted Key to "make a list each year of the top dozen or so of the graduating class and outline their recorded activities, particularly participation in athletics which will probably be an index of their physical co-ordination. As you know this is the routine in business now and a dozen or so of the top banking and financial houses in the United States send representatives to look over the graduating class at Harvard Business School each year, so we might as well get with it."[23] Thus Bigelow was mindful of fulfilling the Alexander criterion of getting "good men" who had the physical stamina the craft required.

Goldman interjects, "Bigelow was big on a past history of athleticism. He loved Bryce Taylor [chief of UHN surgery] who was the U of T quarterback. I disappointed him. I was a high school cheerleader but, nonetheless, the award-winning *best* cheerleading squad in Toronto. I *did* get my athletic letter in med school, so that did help."[24]

Bigelow had a rather cool assessment of the quality of the trainees. Tirone David said, "Dr. Bigelow told me, when I first came here [1975] and he offered me a job, that we train one hundred fellows as heart surgeons. Two or three are superstars. 'Ninety I can make competent, and seven or eight are totally hopeless. I'd tell them to change careers.'"[25]

At a meeting in 1971 of the surgeons-in-chief in the Dean's Office, quality concerns were raised. On opening a cardiac surgery service at Sunnybrook, members were concerned about "obtaining adequate numbers of quality Residents." Owen Gray, who was then surgeon-in-chief at the Toronto Western Hospital, said that "if such a unit is to be opened, then very clearly the supply of Residents and staff members should be worked out before any final agreement is reached." Gray was greatly concerned regarding the paucity and the generally low calibre of current applicants for residency positions in cardiac surgery.[26]

David Naylor, later dean of medicine and president of the University of Toronto, began his career as a resident in cardiac surgery, training with Hugh Scully. One day Naylor was harvesting a saphenous vein, and Scully peered at him, over the top of his half-glasses. Aware of the scrutiny, Naylor (the story goes) skipped a suture. Scully said, "Well, doctor, you might give that one another pass."[27]

Naylor later said, "It was at that moment that I knew I'd never make a cardiac surgeon."

Learning to Deal with Stress

All medicine is, in a certain sense, stressful. You are responsible for people's lives. But the stress in surgery is greater because, unlike internal medicine, things can go wrong under your eyes. And in cardiac surgery the stress is acute because your patients can die in front of you. Ron Baird said, "Cardiac surgery is nothing if not exciting, but the difference in this specialty is that if the patients die, they die in front of your eyes on the table."[28] Thus, the patient dying on the table was a risk that cardiac surgeons had to confront of a daily basis; and in training, residents had to accustom themselves to this reality.

Let's go over a scenario. As Bigelow explained to internist John Oille, who, like Bigelow, also had an office in the Medical Arts Building at the corner of Bloor and St. George streets, there were two circumstances in which the heart failed to maintain "expulsive beats": "(a) ventricular fibrillation, and (b) complete standstill." Now, readers are up to date to this point, as we have discussed these issues extensively. But it got tricky when the abdomen was open, and the patient had no pulse or peripheral blood pressure, yet the heart was still beating. "This can be called cardiac arrest clinically and closed chest massage could very well bring back the blood pressure to normal." That is stressful, but relatively straightforward to master with massage.

But how is this for stressful: The chest is closed and "the heart suddenly stops and ... the blood pressure falls from normal levels to zero in a matter of a few seconds. If a conscious patient, not under anesthesia, develops clinical cardiac arrest, and they proceed to develop dilatation of the pupils, that is excellent evidence, along with unconsciousness, of true cardiac arrest."

So, that is the end of the story, right? Not necessarily. Bigelow continued, "Closed chest massage ... properly applied with a tray, or similar firm object underneath the patient's chest in bed, can be almost, though not quite, as efficient as massage carried out with the chest open. The great danger is in multiple fractured ribs."[29] The scene is pandemonium: the nurse saying she can't get a pulse, the surgeons dumping a tray and shoving it under the patient, then hopping on him and pumping his chest. Or even more challenging: opening the chest on the spot without anesthesia – the patient was already unconscious – and performing direct cardiac massage. In few places in medicine do scenes of such drama occur. The point, however, is that in training you have to learn these responses so that they will be available when you need them.

Thus, there is a certain kind of sangfroid required in cardiac surgery that is not so important in a field like dermatology. It is the ability to keep your head.

Hugh Scully had been visiting a surgeon friend in the cardiac OR in the course of a tour of Vancouver General Hospital. The friend was operating on a young girl with a coarctation of the aorta, but he was feeling quite unwell. "As I went on my way, and was walking down the hall," said Scully, "the charge nurse from the operating room came running out into the hall. 'Dr. Scully could you please come back to the room?' What had happened was the surgeon had fainted and was lying on the floor, the resident had knocked the clamp off the great vessel, and blood was just pouring out onto the floor. So I put on a glove and reached in with my fingers, no clamp, no scrub, nothing, just to stop the bleeding. Got another glove, put the clamp back on, went out and scrubbed, came back in and basically pretty well finished the operation."[30] This is sangfroid, and Scully and Goldman were known for it.

Training Today

Some view the essence of training as mentorship: not just viewing the operating from the other side of the table while the great master does it, but having the great master watch *you* do the operation, so that you learn. Here there is some unease about Toronto. Goldman said of Tirone David, "He was not a mentor. We were all trained by Bruce Tovee, by Griff Pearson, by Bill Bigelow, and by Jim Key, whose methods were mentorship in and out of the operating room. Then I spent a year with Bill Mustard with him as my first assistant, monitoring every single suture. What could be better?"[31] But today, in the division, there are concerns about mentorship. Yet Barry Rubin, head of the Peter Munk Cardiac Centre, is hopeful.

The establishment of the Peter Munk Cardiac Centre, particularly under Barry Rubin's leadership starting in 2011, had a big impact on training. Rubin said in an interview, "When you train at Toronto General, you train in what we call the Peter Munk way. Which is, you train in a team-based approach, so when you go back to Tokyo or Leningrad or Buenos Aires, you say 'Where is my team? This is how I'm used to practicing.' We believe the sum is greater than the parts, and we walk the walk, because I won't fund it if we don't do it that way."[32]

Cardiac surgery itself altered substantially with the migration from open-heart valve replacements to "percutaneous" techniques involving inserting valves at the tip of catheters: no big incision, no opened chest, no prolonged convalescence. Rubin reflected on the change in training in his own allied field of vascular surgery. "I was trained to do this: incision from here to here [sternum to pubic bone]. I was an open surgeon. I loved making big incisions, the bigger the better, the more I could see the greater it was for me. I loved that stuff. And ten years into my practice, somebody comes up with a thing that says, 'You don't have to make that incision, you can just put a needle in the groin and slide a new tube inside the old tube.' Well, what do you think every single patient with an aneurysm wanted? Right. So we had a choice as vascular surgeons: it was either learn how to put in stent grafts or learn how to be a different doctor."[33]

Rubin added that trainees in cardiac surgery were learning this as well. "There's no longer the cardiac surgeon coming with the kind of open surgical expertise. They're just going to be wire guys and girls, just like the interventional cardiologists. So I don't know if we're transitioning to a time somewhere down the road where you won't have cardiac surgeons or interventional cardiologists, you'll have cardiac specialists."[34]

Chapter Fifteen

Research

There were many brilliant surgeons in the division, yet not all were scientists. Bigelow and Baird had both been active on the experimental side, doing dog research in the basement of the Banting Institute. And their residents and fellows had definitely learned that aspect of research. Yet the investigator who anchored the study of basic scientific mechanisms in the division was Richard Weisel.[1]

Richard Weisel

Weisel was born in Alexandria, Louisiana, in 1943 because his father, Wilson Weisel, an assistant professor of surgery at Marquette University School of Medicine in Milwaukee, was in the army medical corps and preparing to go over to Europe for D-Day. In fact, his father was a chest surgeon, and it is no secret why Weisel himself ended up in that field. Weisel grew up in Milwaukee, then earned a BA from Yale University in 1965, where he studied philosophy.

Why philosophy?

"I knew I was going to do medicine. My father and I planned out my career, beginning with philosophy at Yale, because that was my only chance to ever do anything outside of medicine. Since I'd been six years old, I'd been planning to do medicine and heart surgery." His father took him to cardiac meetings, and the greats of cardiac surgery were often at the Weisel dinner table. "My job as a high school student," Weisel later said, "was to go into the Milwaukee Children's Hospital and to carry pails of cold water that I would pour over the oxygenator [part of the pump] to cool kids down. And then when it was time to rewarm, I had to go get warm water and pour it over."

Weisel earned an MD degree from Marquette in 1969, then trained in surgery at the Boston University Medical Center until 1976. At Boston

University, he joined the Surgical Training Program of the National Institutes of Health, which was the first such program in the world. Toronto's Steve Strasberg was also in the program. "Cardiac protection" (see the next section in this chapter) was on the agenda.

Weisel's father had known Bigelow and brought Dick to Toronto in 1969 to look around. Professor Janes said, "This is the place you want to do surgery, you'll get a real large volume." Weisel met Bigelow and told him, "I'll probably come back when I finish."

Weisel began a senior residency in cardiovascular surgery in Toronto in 1976 under Bigelow, Baird, George Trusler, and Griff Pearson. Bigelow retired in 1977, and in the last years of his tenure he was fully supportive of all the research that Weisel as a resident was undertaking. He, Hugh Scully, and Tirone David – all residents – busied themselves at research. Weisel said, "We'd be collecting separate stuff and try to see if what Bigelow was doing was appropriate. Because he would ask the question 'Is this the right way to do it?' And we would say, 'Let's take the next few patients.'"

Cardiac Protection

Then Weisel became a research fellow of the Canadian Heart Foundation at the General and continued to study the problem that would stay with him for much of the rest of his career. It had the opaque name of "cardiac protection."

The story is this: In bypass surgery, the aorta is clamped off just above the point where the ascending aorta leaves the left ventricle. The logic is clear: an unclamped aorta would blow blood back into the open heart. Yet between the clamp and the left ventricle are the two openings (ostia) where the left and right coronary arteries begin. Of course, those arteries are not receiving fresh blood, and the myocardium begins to wilt because it's not being oxygenated. Perfusing these coronary arteries with blood or some other oxygen-rich fluid is "cardiac protection": protecting against anoxia.

Weisel came on staff in the Cardiac Division in 1979 when he passed his Canadian boards and immediately jumped into research. He partnered with Don Mickle in clinical biochemistry; and one of Mickle's students, Ren-Ke Li, whose interest was regenerative medicine, teamed up with Weisel.

For research, surgeons needed PhDs. To better train surgeons to do basic research, this small corps of investigators decided to have academically inclined residents enrol as students in the Institute of Medical Sciences, and with Bernie Langer's support, Weisel and Steve

Strasberg established the Surgeon Scientist Program – which would give surgeons PhDs. (The surgeon-students were assured of funding throughout their enrolment in the program.) This absolutely pioneering venture was widely copied across Canada and elsewhere as the basic motor of surgical research. Weisel later said, "The rigor required to obtain an advanced degree was essential for the clinicians to obtain adequate scientific training."[2] Vivek Rao, who later chaired the hospital division, Terry M. Yau, later chair of the University Division, Steve Fremes, later chief at Sunnybrook, and George Christakis at Sunnybrook were all products of this program.

For the record, Weisel's program in 1978 to get surgical residents into PhD programs funded by the Heart and Stroke Foundation antedated Bernie Langer's 1984 Surgeon Scientist Program (see below). Yet the difference was that Langer arranged for the systematic funding of the surgeon-scientists from a common pool of surgical funds and for the surgeon-scientist program to be extended across the entire Department of Surgery.

To do bypass surgery, it was clear that you had to stop the heart. The Boston surgeons were clear about this. Denton Cooley in Dallas had said "Y'all just have to clamp it and operate fast." When Weisel's father was operating on ASDs, he figured he had four to five minutes before damage to the heart and brain began.

Bernie Goldman, who was present at the Weisel interview, recalled observing Norman Shumway at Stanford, who "believed in clamping [the big veins] and dripping cold water into the heart, which most of us didn't like because you were operating under water all the time."

Nowhere did the surgeons bother to take the temperature of the heart. "Speed was the protection of the heart."

So around 1978 Weisel and company started infusing the coronary arteries with "Bretschneider solution," previously developed in Europe but which gave unsatisfactory results. Then in the early 1980s they started infusing the coronaries with the patient's own blood, into which a bit of potassium had been mixed. They also used "crystalloid," a chilled clear solution with potassium. (For more on this see chapter 18.) These mixtures were infused into the coronaries via the aorta or via the bypass grafts that had just been put in place (and not by cannulas poking directly into the coronaries from the ostia, which would damage those tiny structures).

But how to figure out, during the operation, whether the heart is being damaged? They started measuring "ck" (creatine kinase), an enzyme that is released when cells die. There was much ratiocination about what should be in the perfusate – Weisel ultimately decided that the patient's blood plus potassium was ideal. And this work took a lot of trial and error, but establishing at exactly what temperatures various procedures were to be done had an impact worldwide on cardiac surgery.

Weisel was one of the main surgeon-scientists in the division, and was called "one of the most prolific cardiovascular surgeons in the world."[3] It was mainly Weisel's lab that differentiated Toronto from competing programs in Ottawa and Edmonton. Hugh Scully said, "That was the academic crucible. The people like Viv [Rao] who were brought along through his program are absolutely committed to the academic pursuit of what is going on, and more than any other centre in the country, that's been true here. It wasn't true at that time in Ottawa. Will Keon had a bunch of very good clinical surgeons, but they weren't academic investigators. That's true of Edmonton as well. [What was crucial] was that continued presence and influence of Dick [Weisel] and the Surgeon Scientist Program that was created under Langer, and the fellows that were brought along doing the research."[4]

Surgeon-Scientists

The whole tradition of looking to England as "the Mother Country," and to Ronald Belsey in Bristol as the grand master of chest surgery, began to wither. After thoracic surgery separated from cardiovascular, it was no longer necessary for cardiac residents to travel to Bristol. Bernie Goldman said that residents also stopped going to Bristol because "the research training under Weisel was so superb here that there was no point going anywhere. Although that made us insular, it certainly created a mass research effect, which built on each other because fellows continued carrying the same projects farther and farther. Then that of course attracted outside fellows from all over the world to the PhD program."[5] It was in Weisel's lab that Stephen Fremes received his scientific training, in the context of the Surgeon-Scientist Program, studying techniques of cardioplegia.[6] Fremes then accompanied Goldman to Sunnybrook in November 1989 and later succeeded Goldman as the head of the program there.

Altogether, Weisel trained thirty-four MD/PhD students through the Surgeon-Scientist Program of the Institute of Medical Sciences, as well as sixty PhDs. In 1989 he became associate director of the Centre of Cardiovascular Research at the General, with cardiologist Michael Sole as director. (In 1984 Bernie Langer created the Clinician-Scientist Program for the Department of Surgery as a whole, initially just for the Division of General Surgery; then later, the Surgeon Scientist Program was formally constituted.[7]) In 1990 Weisel began to serve as director of surgical research at the university, and in 1998 became chair of the University Division of Cardiac Surgery, a post he held for ten years. In 2005 he became director of the Research Institute of the General, which he maintained until his retirement from that position in 2011. He continues to be the editor of the prestigious *Journal of Thoracic and Cardiovascular Surgery*, cited many times in these pages. He is also head of Ontario's Innovation Fund Provincial Oversight Committee.[8]

As head of the division, "he emphasized how important it is for young surgeons to 'keep their skis together' by pulling their clinical work towards their research."[9]

Weisel's forte was "bringing the lab to the bedside." He and his fellows would turn up in the OR and, as Goldman recalls, "a few people said 'What the hell are you doing to my patient'? [as] the research fellows shoved in their funny lines to measure things that weren't absolutely part of recovery and survival, but were part of the research effort, and there was a big buy-in from anesthesia and surgery to what he was doing."[10]

All these lines going in and out of the patient permitted Weisel and his fellows to measure things that never before had been measured, such as lactate, as an outcome of the operation. Weisel explained, "We learned retrospectively that when the lactates are up in the coronary sinus [the terminal portion of the great vein that empties into the right atrium], we had injured the heart."

This List Could Be Very Long

Weisel and his fellows achieved a great deal. Weisel did pioneering work on "cardioplegia," as stated, the solution used to nourish the myocardium while the beating of the heart has ceased in bypass surgery. This is known as "cardioprotection."[11] Scully said, "One of Richard's overall greatest contributions was taking the bench to the bedside in terms of cardioprotection. He studied that in the lab and brought it into the operating room where it got great currency and great recognition."[12]

Weisel created one of the first cardiac-surgery databases, with follow-up information on all patients. These databases were very helpful in the creation of the Cardiac Care Network of Ontario (CCNO) in 1988.

Weisel's latest project, working with Ren-Ke Li, now a scientist at St. Michael's Hospital, was using stem cells taken from the bone marrow to recreate the tissue of the damaged heart.[13] At this writing, the latest results from a multicentre trial they organized in 2016 showed that injecting stem cells (CD133+) was safe. Did the left ventricular ejection fraction improve (the crucial measure of the heart getting stronger)? Unfortunately, it improved in both the placebo and active treatment groups, as the trial wasn't powered highly enough to detect subtle changes.[14]

It was under Weisel's aegis that the University Division of Cardiac Surgery became a true jewel in the crown of Canadian medicine. In 2007, Weisel said, "The Division remains the most academically productive unit in the world ... We have greater breadth and depth to our academic programs than any other cardiac surgical unit in the world."[15] Yet, in this vast record, what was really important? We asked, "Of this three decades of excellence and productivity, what would you like to be remembered for: the work on myocardial protection or your work on the hemodynamics of the heart post-op?"

Weisel answered, "The major contribution was the mentoring of these young surgeons, there's no question. That was the output that is most significant."

A Toronto Tradition

So there is a profound Toronto tradition of science. Weisel said there were three pillars in any scientific program in this area: pediatric, thoracic, and cardiac surgery. In a recent review, "we were the only institution in North America that were leaders in all three of those. Each one of them was independently featured in our program. Johns Hopkins had one, UCLA had one, we had all three."

Bernie Goldman asked, "And in terms of the research component alone?"

> WEISEL: I would think we're far ahead of almost all of them, because we do have such extensive research capabilities.
> SHORTER: So you think this is *the* centre for cardiac research?
> WEISEL: It is, absolutely.

PART THREE

The Team

Chapter Sixteen

Cardiologists

At the beginning, the cardiologists were suspicious and unhelpful, and referred patients for surgery only when the illness was far advanced. Anesthetist Sallie Teasdale recalled, "Open heart surgery was still in its infancy and the patients referred for surgery were those that the cardiologists could no longer help. Not infrequently the patients might be outside the OR door in congestive failure or a rapid arrhythmia. As the results of surgery improved the cardiologists agreed to refer their patients at an earlier stage and our results improved further."[1]

The Cardiac Investigation Unit, opened in 1956, represented an inflection point in the history of Canadian cardiology. Here, for the first time, cardiologists and cardiac surgeons became accustomed to working together. Before its formation, as Bigelow noted, "few, if any, cardiologists were ever trained at the Toronto General Hospital." After its establishment, well-trained cardiologists were exported from Toronto to Laval, Dalhousie, McGill, and the University of Turin in Italy.[2] The catheterization unit became, in other words, an important scientific focus as well as an essential prelude to cardiac surgery. In the Cardiovascular Unit in 1970, they catheterized 1,047 patients, with only five deaths.[3] This was a source of pride.

The drama in the cardiology story is the shift from the imaging of "cardiac cath" to the procedures of "percutaneous coronary interventions" (PCI), using a catheter, or "wire," to dilate and stent plugged coronary arteries. The cardiologists learned this from the interventional radiologists, and they went on to make it the core of the specialty.

Heather Ross: "I'm a Surgeon Trapped Inside a Cardiologist's Body"

Heather Ross, head of the Division of Cardiology at the University Health Network, had just completed a very successful term as president of the Canadian Cardiovascular Society, which represents all cardiac specialists in Canada. Ross was a latter-day Bigelow. She had the same ability to inspire research, the same ability to lead, the same confident amicability. But unlike Bigelow, she came from Montreal.[4]

Born in 1962 into the family of a father in business, she spent her early years in Montreal. But following the political crisis of the early 1970s, her parents moved to Orangeville, then to Port Credit in Ontario. She gained a BSc in biology at Queen's in 1984, then an MD degree at the University of British Columbia in 1988. During 1993 and 1994 she passed her boards in internal medicine and cardiology in Canada and the United States. Then from 1994 to 1996 fellowed at Stanford University in cardiac transplantation, studying with Sharon Hunt, "the goddess of transplant cardiology," as Ross later put it.

At Stanford, it was the "incredibly brilliant group" of surgeons who drummed the march in transplant. But when she came to Toronto, Chris Feindel, who led transplant work here, said we do things differently. "When the patients come to the cardiovascular ICU, we should manage the patients together as a team. It shouldn't be the cardiovascular surgeon alone, because they don't have the immunology." But when she came to the General in 1997 as medical director of the cardiac transplant program, there had been no transplant cardiologist. "So it was a remarkable opportunity to come in and make changes. You can desire all you want to make change, but if the people around you aren't engaged in the change process, it won't happen."

Q: But the surgeons were open?
ROSS: Oh my god, yes.

So Ross enlarged the transplant team. "We created a longitudinal heart failure program, and sort of expanding the idea of following the patients, we expanded the team. Now we have fifty people. It's a big change."

Graciously, Ross declined to take the credit for this herself. "This is Chris [Feindel] going, 'Man, this is good,' and getting on board, the recruitment of Viv Rao. Viv and I, we're not allowed to say these things anymore, but we're like a work husband and wife." She said that the concept of the "heart team" had started in a number of transplant centres, because it takes a number of specialized skill sets to get the best outcomes.

Toronto was one of the few centres in which today there is no rivalry between cardiac surgeons and cardiologists. Ross said, "People who come from the outside would always comment on the relationship we

have as a team." Ross said that people considered this spirit of collaboration "unique."

T'was not always so. In Bigelow's days, there was perfect amity with
Heimbecker and Gunton in the investigative unit side by side, and
between Bigelow and Greenwood in the clinical arena. As the cardiologists began doing procedures in the late 1980s, the picture changed.
Goldman said, "It became not only a competition but a confrontation,
because we didn't have first access to the patient. The guy who has the
patient on the angio table has first access. And all the concepts of a heart
team approaching the angio and the patient evaporated as the 'CCs,'
the cardiology cowboys, decided, 'I can fix this' and 'I can fix that.' A
psychiatrist phoned me the other day and said they want to do a third
stent sequentially on him because they thought they saw a little narrowing. Don't go near it!"[5] (All observers were not in agreement with
Goldman's judgment of conflict, and Hugh Scully could not recall a
time when there was anything save complete cooperation between the
cardiologists and the cardiac surgeons.)

Harry Rakowski and the Rise of Percutaneous
Coronary Interventions

Harry Rakowski was born in Stuttgart in 1948; his parents were
Holocaust survivors. The family moved to Toronto in 1951, and
Rakowski attended Bathurst Heights high school, then entered the pre-
med program at the University of Toronto. He earned a medical degree
in 1972.

While Rakowski was interning at Mount Sinai Hospital, the storied
head of medicine at the Sinai, Barney Berris, influenced him to go into
medicine, and Doug Wigle, the head of cardiology, steered him toward
cardiology.

In 1976 Rakowski went to Stanford for a year as a research fellow
in cardiology and learned a new technology, echo cardiography – or
cardiac ultrasound – that a small company near Stanford was just
introducing. "So, I got in on the ground floor," he said later, "with the
first machine that eventually became the first commercially available
machine and brought that technology back to Toronto."[6] The Mayo
Clinic bought "Machine One," and Rakowski brought Machine Seven
back to Toronto. It cost $100,000, a sum that Wigle raised.

Why was cardiac ultrasound valuable? Rakowski said, "There were
invasive cardiologists who with the advent of balloon-tipped catheters
could squish plaques to the side, but those had a high restenosis rate.
With the advent of stents, there was a mechanical way of pushing the

plaques aside and keeping them there and having much better long-term patency rather than restenosis."

"But it was in valvular disease in particular," Rakowski continued, "that cardiac ultrasound was most valuable. Now, in terms of interventions, there's TAVI interventions [transcatheter aortic valve implantation], or being able to replace valves percutaneously either through the tip of the heart, apically, or through an arterial sheath in the femoral [groin]."

What did the surgeons think of that? Rakowski said, "Despite the efforts of some people to say we're going to exclude the surgeons and just do it ourselves, I think the attitude here has been that this is a collaborative process, and it speaks to the long-standing strong relationship that cardiology and cardiac surgery have had over the years. It's not competitive, it is collaborative."

The next technical innovation was using Doppler techniques – an ultrasound method of judging blood flows – to evaluate quantitative degrees of stenosis. Rakowski began publishing on this in 1988.[7] "We could use colour flow imaging to look at jets of regurgitation so we could evaluate valvular disease and whether it was stenotic or regurgitant congenital disease. We could then characterize where the abnormalities were and guide surgeons as to reparability, and now interventionalists as to suitability for using devices such as clips to clip the mitral valve or to guide TAVI insertion." Rakowski led an international team that included Norwegian cardiologist Liv Hadley, "who came up with an equation that allowed you to take a velocity [of blood flow] and convert it into a pressure difference." (Big pressure differences of either side of a valve mean big obstruction of blood flow.)

The disadvantage of transthoracic echocardiology is that the beam had to travel through skin, ribs, fat, and lungs before reaching the heart. A clearer image could be obtained if the probe with the transducer at the end could be planted on the esophagus, right next to the heart. This next step, transesophageal echocardiography (TEE) was pioneered by a German radiologist named Werner Daniel; in 1988 Rakowski took Loretta Daniel, who was his fellow, to Hanover to learn the technique from Werner, and then brought it back to Toronto.

So in the early days, Rakowski, together with David, Feindel, and others, would hold teaching sessions broadcast either to an auditorium or internationally, "where it would show, here's the cardiologist showing the surgeon what the problem was, then the surgeon intervening, showing the surgical technique, then the cardiologist showing the results: whether the results were good enough to finish the operation or whether they needed to go back in and fix something."

Then anesthesia took over TEE from cardiology. The advantage of this was that the anesthetists were already in the operating room (and the anesthetists had a "financial incentive"; the cardiologists were already swimming in work). So Rakowski formed a joint association of anesthetists and cardiologists. "We were the backup for them and we had a video link to the echo labs" so that they could get advice if they ran into trouble. "It was sort of a three-party collaboration. The surgeons needed the information and they got that information from either cardiologists or cardiac anesthesiologists."

At the beginning, the surgeons were clueless about the echo images, "particularly in regurgitant lesions, particularly in the mitral valve," as Goldman pointed out. "It was very important to understand what we were looking at. We weren't expert by any means at all and needed someone to point out, but just as it was essential to go look at an angiogram, it became essential to look at the echo, not just read a report."[8] And here Tirone David's influence made itself felt "in understanding the various mechanisms of mitral valve disease." (And even today, at Friday morning cardiac "triage" rounds at the General, the anesthetists stand at the podium and explain the TEE images, whereas by now the surgeons are competent to interpret the angiograms – which show coronary vessel disease – on their own. Yet the cardiologists in the audience make the decision about whether they can get "a wire" into the plugged vessel or whether bypass is needed.)

So, one day Rakowski and David were together in the OR, David doing some complex aortic valve lesion. The session is being broadcast live around the world. Rakowski tells David, "Tirone, there's a four millimetre hole in the base of the anterior leaflet."

DAVID (LOOKING AT RAKOWSKI): No there's not.
RAKOWSKI: Tirone, you know there's a hole in the leaflet.
DAVID: Oh, you guys with echo, you just see every little red cell that's leaking back. Reverse the patient [meaning end the operation].
RAKOWSKI: Tirone, you know you can't reverse the patient.

Rakowski explains: "And so he trusted me enough that, while grumbling away, 'Oh, okay, fine,' the patient goes back on pump, and you know, this was something that he couldn't easily see, so once I told him where it was, he feels for it and says, 'Oh my god.'"

RAKOWSKI: What's wrong.
DAVID: There's a hole in the base of the anterior leaflet.
RAKOWSKI: What do you think I just told you.

All this on international television.

Percutaneous Coronary Intervention

The first procedures that cardiologists did were actually not "percu-taneous" (via a femoral vessel). In 1974, just as Scully was returning from Harvard with the balloon-pump concept, cardiology got a balloon pump for its Coronary Care Unit, under the direction of Al Adelman.[9] (The pump was for cardiac support, not plaque clearance.) Interest in procedures among cardiologists quickened considerably after Ken Brown, the co-founder of this unit – the first cardiology intensive care unit in the world – himself developed unstable angina. Goldman said, "I put a balloon pump in him, stabilized him and took him to the oper-ating room. He and I had an interesting relationship because his father was a pharmacist and my father was a pharmacist. Brown was very grateful, and it changed my profile in cardiology and surgery here."[10] (But several cardiologists preceded Brown in the use of procedures.) At that time cardiac surgeons were necessary for the procedure because a Dacron graft would be sewn directly onto the femoral artery in the groin and the pump inserted through that. (On the introduction of the balloon catheter on the surgical service at TGH in the early 1970s and Hugh Scully's role in it, see the chapter 9.)

PCI came to mean clearing the coronary artery with a balloon cath-eter and, later, using the catheter to insert a stent. Using the balloon as a ramrod was initiated in Zurich in 1977 by German cardiologist Andreas Grüntzig. In the 1990s stenting began to take the place of balloon angio-plasty, and this started the historic trend toward stenting and away from bypass. Stents to open up plugged coronary arteries are threaded in place by cardiologists; coronary bypass, of course, is the province of cardiac surgeons.

Right up until the foundation of the Peter Munk Cardiac Centre in 1997, cardiac surgeons and cardiologists competed for business, sur-geons offering bypass, cardiologists offering balloon angioplasty and PCI stenting. The cerebral side effects of cardiac surgery – the risk of stroke – started to be discussed because such risks were thought to be greatly lessened with angioplasty. Medical historian David S. Jones writes, "Motivation for this [new attention] came from therapeutic competition. As angioplasty, especially with stents, surged past bypass surgery in the 1990s, one of its selling points was its lower rate of cere-bral complications."[11]

In June 1981 coronary angioplasty commenced in the unit, using a balloon catheter to widen plugged up coronary arteries.[12] (Balloon pro-cedures, in this case the dilation of the pulmonary valve, commenced at the Children's Hospital in 1984.[13])

It was in the early 1980s that percutaneous coronary interventions began in Toronto via the groin. Interventions were either for dilatation or closure of a fetal structure that should have shut down on its own.[14] (When in 1971 surgical resident Lloyd Black and Goldman described the Toronto experience with closing the patent ductus, the intervention was via a postero-lateral thoracotomy. There were substantial adverse effects, and one death in a series of fifty-three patients.[15]) PCI would clearly be the way to go, and this work was led initially by Peter McLaughlin, who graduated in medicine from the University of Toronto in 1970. He was then joined by Leland ("Lee") Benson, who finished his medical studies at the University of Chicago in 1974. In 1988 the intervention team reported inserting with a catheter an occlusive device (an "umbrella") in the patent ductus arteriosus (PDA) of forty adult patients. They went via the "transvenous" route (via a subclavian vessel in the neck), not the groin, and had moderate success: at six months, 21 per cent continued to have some shunting into the pulmonary artery.[16]

In 1996 McLaughlin, Benson, and colleagues reported a percutaneous study of closing the PDA at the Toronto Congenital Centre for Adults.[17] By 2000, the group at the General and the Children's Hospital had moved on to closing atrial septal defects (ASDs) percutaneously.[18] The following year, 2001, they reported efforts going back to 1994 in either stenting or using angioplasty in coarctations (narrowing) of the aorta percutaneously.[19] When one recalls what a major surgical procedure dealing with aortic coarctations once was, the measure of progress here is obvious.

The group reported in 2003 that intracardiac echocardiography gave comparable control in percutaneous closure of ASDs than did TEE (which required general anesthesia).[20]

These contributions were the beginning of a long train of work on PCI; it hallmarks the rising importance of interventional cardiology in the treatment of the heart. In 2002, McLaughlin became medical coordinator of the Peterborough Regional Health Centre (rising to president in 2016), and Eric Horlick, who graduated from McGill in 1996, joined the PCI team at the Toronto General.

Teams

After Feindel and Rubin began presiding over "heart teams" in the Peter Munk Centre for Cardiac Care, collaboration between cardiologists and cardiac surgeons improved further. Rubin told the cardiologists and the cardiac surgeons, "'I don't want to be the one that's driving this decision making, but if you don't sort it out, I'm not supporting the valve program.' So right now, every one of these operations, where there's a valve that goes in without surgery, there's a cardiac surgeon and a cardiologist. Every one." Rubin said, "We did a couple of things that I think are pretty simple. I said, 'If you, the cardiologists, and you, the cardiac surgeons, want me to raise money for new valves or new stents, thou shalt work together. And if thou don't work together, I won't be paying for it.'"[21]

There were other models in Toronto for the team concept. In the Multi-Organ Transplant Program of the University Health Network, there were kidney teams led by urologists and "Kidney transplant docs," a liver team run by liver surgeons and hepatologists, and now the heart transplant team led by surgeons and cardiologists. (Ross did note that Barry Rubin's signal contribution was to have expanded the team concept to the rest of cardiovascular medicine, such as the TAVI team to manage aortic valves, the mitral team, the coronary artery team, and so forth.) Yet under Ross, it was the team concept with a vengeance. She said, "One thing a bit unique about our program is that we have had largely a horizontal hierarchy. By that I mean that when we're at our transplant meetings, the social worker's voice is as important at the table as my voice and the surgeon's voice. At the end of the day the buck stops with us, but in attempting to create a flat reporting style it does make the collegiality and the engagement and investment much higher."

Ross mentioned cardiologist Susan Lenkei at the Western. "Susan Lenkei and Tirone [David] would talk about the plan in a very team-based way, and Susan was one of the pioneers, because she used to come to the CVICU and see the patients." This was unusual for cardiologists (still less usual was cardiologists turning up at operations, which Ross sometimes did, standing at the head of the table).

There was plenty of scope for conflict about the cardiologists' angioplasty dilatation techniques versus the surgeon's coronary bypass. Ross conceded that the transplant team had "had its moments. You get cardiologists, an anesthetist, and a surgeon, and none of us are shrinking violets, put us in a room and you have slight differences in how things might be managed. But we've always tried to come to a consensus. I think it's one of the reasons it's a great place to work, one of the reasons why opportunities [elsewhere] arise but you don't leave."

In 2007, the cardiologists began percutaneous valve implantation, putting a pig or cow valve at the end of a catheter and implanting it. In terms of relations among surgeons, cardiologists, and anesthetists, this was a game changer. Echo-imager Massimiliano Meineri said, "For each of these percutaneous procedures there's a cardiac surgeon assigned to the case. And while in the past we were ready to use a pump to rescue the patient, making the [joint] decision to either use the pump to save the patient or let the patient go, was a big, big important step. When the chest isn't open and you can't see the heart, imaging, particularly the echo, becomes even more important. The percutaneous procedure that they do, clip the mitral valve, they're entirely guided by the echo."[22] (For more on collaboration between cardiologists and surgeons, see chapter 22.)

Ross and Ventricular Assist Devices

Ross's interests turned naturally from transplant to the ventricular assist devices that were just coming in as a way of reducing the waiting-list mortality. "We're the Peter Munk bloody Centre and we didn't have access to it. I think, in truth, it was an absolute quintessential moment of 'Are we going to be what we think we are? Are we going to be *it*?'" So donors were found and funds created to buy the expensive devices.

The team – cardiologist, anesthetist, surgeon – went down to Pitts-burgh to watch the procedure in action. "Once we got our feet completely under us, the cardiologists managed the patients in the VAD [ventricular assist device] clinics and the surgeons come when there's an issue." Rao gives Ross credit for driving the VAD program forward in Toronto.[23]

In scientific terms, Ross has contributed to understanding "patient navigation" in the care of heart-failure and transplant patients.[24] She said that of all her work, what she thought most significant was "patient perspective on treatments. We have done a fair bit of work on what patients feel like to have a treatment. I was told by a senior staff person that I was committing career suicide when I started that project. When you're sitting in front of a patient every day, the thing that matters is how you engage with the patient and that the patient actually feels engaged in the process. We've come a long way toward that in medicine, and away from paternalism."

In 2010 Ross became the Ted Rogers and Family Chair in Heart Function, jointly sponsored by the Children's Hospital, the University Health Network, and the University of Toronto, and situated in the Peter Munk Cardiac Centre. It was here that she and Barry Rubin launched the massive cardiac database, using artificial intelligence, that was designed to pin down the risk factors that would let one predict who would benefit from the transplant and who perhaps not, a matter hitherto for clinical guesswork (but crucial: for every person who received a heart and didn't do well, a heart was wasted). Or who should get angioplasty or a bypass?

Many readers will recall Heather Ross as the cardiologist who founded in 2006 the "Test Your Limits" program, in which she led colleagues and heart-transplant patients on gruelling expeditions to climb mountains or cross Antarctica. In 2013 she and her intrepid band, including heart-transplant patient Dale Shippam, set out to reach the South Pole. These astonishing trips, in which she personally risked her life, raised millions of dollars in donations.[25] This utterly unconventional approach to "patient engagement" gave notice to many readers that there was life after cardiac surgery.

And the impact of her work on Dr. Ross herself? She said, "The legacy I feel is for the patients who died. I don't quite know how to word it, but transplant is the most awesome procedure, and when it goes well, it does so very well. In the right patients, it's getting back to life and having children. When it goes bad, it's an unmitigated disaster, and I have not forgotten the name of any patient I've lost."

Ebb and Flow

There once was competition between cardiac surgeons and cardiologists. There no longer is, partly because the nature of cardiac disease itself has changed. As Mitesh Badiwala said in 2017, "Back in the day, patients did not have acute reopening of coronary arteries and they had myocardial infarction that we treated late; [so] there were other mechanical complications like ventricular and papillary ruptures that we don't see very frequently anymore ... It was far more frequent in the 1980/1990s to have emergency bypass surgery, but it's very rare now because the cardiologists can open blocked arteries with balloons and stents."[26]

Thus, there has been an incessant back and forth between surgery and cardiology. The stents and inserted valves of the cardiologists are less invasive than open heart surgery, but the long-term results are also less certain.

Take, for example, cardiologists inserting a clip to pin the leaves of the mitral valve together in cases of mitral regurgitation (MR). (Surgeons are present in the OR, too.) The leaves are usually not firmly pinned together, and some regurgitation continues. Is that a big deal?

RAO: [The regurgitation] gets from severe [pre-op] to mild but usually moderate. We'd never leave the OR with even more than mild MR, so if you had mild or moderate MR, you [as a surgeon] would say, "I'm not happy with this repair, I'm replacing this valve." As the data comes out from the microclip, mild-to-moderate MR is tolerated, and they're not all hemolyzing and they're not back in heart failure, you might say, "I'm going to leave you in mild-to-moderate MR surgically and not replace your valve, and manage you medically, because the clip data is telling us that this is okay, and it's probably better off for you than putting a pig valve in you that you're going to have to replace every ten years."[27]

Yet the triumphal on march of stenting did not occur without some pushback from the surgeons. In 2007, Goldman deplored "over-reliance on new devices, heavily influenced by industry, with a regrettable tendency to dismiss earlier results [CABG] as 'old technology.' It is essential that the cardiac surgical community promotes the worth of the modern coronary bypass procedure." It is important for the Canadian Society of Cardiac Surgeons (CSCS), which represents all cardiac surgeons in Canada, "to reverse the negativity and pessimism in our field and revitalize the image of cardiac surgery in our hospitals and university residency programs." It was necessary, he said, to "challenge cardiology."[28] (Both Chris Feindel and Viv Rao were elected as presidents of the CSCS and were very effective advocates for this objective.)

Chapter Seventeen

Nurses

Motto: "Rather than the chairmen of boards, the builders of hospitals and the heads of department, these gentle and sympathetic nurses should have their names inscribed on the walls of these great institutions, and on the pages of history."[1]

– Gordon Murray (1960)

What were cardiac nurses good for? Let's ask Gordon Murray. Under Murray's direction, OR nurses might boost the flagging courage of a resident. Murray was mindful of this during a trip to New Zealand in 1951, when demonstrating techniques at a local hospital. The Kiwi resident initially could not summon the resolve to shove his finger into a narrowed mitral valve and open it up. "A slight delay followed, this time not to restore the poise of the heart but rather that of the operator. Under similar circumstances, when this happened to my residents at home, I used to suggest that the head nurse stand behind the faltering resident with an old-fashioned hat pin, then spiritual life could be provided at the given signal, with it being thrust well into the drooping posterior." Alas, there were no hat pins in the operating room in New Zealand, but somehow the resident gathered his resolve anyway. ("He withdrew his finger triumphantly.")[2]

Bigelow Launches Cardiac Nursing

The nursing story takes us from hatpins to the formation of a dedicated corps of professional cardiac nurses. The gathering of this corps was initiated by Bigelow. At first, some surgeons found the nursing side trying. In 1960 an irritated Ray Heimbecker wrote an executive at the Connaught Laboratories, which produced heparin: "We have had another near tragedy in the use of heparin." A patient who should have received 1,000 unit per cc strength was accidentally administered 10,000 unit[s]. "In this day and age when there is such a shortage of nurses and when so many of our nurses are recent immigrants who have language difficulties, I wonder whether further measures might be taken," such as plastering red warnings on the label.[3]

These are grunts of exasperation from this privileged male elite against recent immigrant women struggling to acquire the new language. But from the get-go, nurses have been integral to cardiac care. As he was organizing care in the little ward for blue babies at the General, Murray praised the nurses, "who, either by native endowments or as a result of their work and associations, developed spiritual qualities which set them above the mundane routine and inspired the dedication of their lives." He mentioned supervisor Marjorie Ferrie and the "tender care" of Betty McFarlane.[4]

Working alongside Murray on Ward C, Bigelow realized that a specialized corps of dedicated cardiac nurses was necessary and did everything he could to encourage its formation. Cardiac nursing as a specialty dates back to a surgery in the early 1950s on a patient named Gordon Graham. He was made aware of the existence of private patients, who received "special" nursing care, and public ward patients who received the "shared care" of busy nurses. A female patient down the hall was receiving non-special care, and Graham, in Bigelow's words, "immediately requested that [the patient] be assigned 'specials' for each shift at his expenses." As Graham was discharged from hospital, Bigelow continued, "He gave me a generous donation each year (the Graham Fund) that was provided anonymously to ensure that all cases we operated on henceforth would 'have the same full nursing care I received.'"[5] (Graham couldn't see into the future, but on the later Cardiovascular Division, there was no separate public-private care, and ironically, in the hospital as a whole it was the public patients who received the better care because these wards were thick with trainee nurses, medical students, interns, and residents.[6])

This notion of specialized nursing care was dear to Bigelow. In September 1957, outlining plans for the future cardiac surgery service, he emphasized that operations such as those lasting five to ten hours on the aorta, "require post-operative management beyond the scope of special nurses chosen by the Central [Nursing] Registry. The concept of a recovery room with *specialized nursing care* must be extended in these cases to become an 'intensive therapy unit' with specialized nursing care for one to five days."[7] It was Bigelow's diligence that ensured that in cardiac nursing there would be three patients to one nurse; in general medical nursing (on Ward H), twelve.[8]

Bigelow took a role in nurse training. He had a budget to send the nurses on road trips to visit other centres. Around 1958, as the service was being set up, he asked several head nurses to "take a tour of two or three surgical centers in the United States to enable them to organize our units more efficiently." Then in the fall of 1961 he proposed sending several others on such a tour. He told "Miss" Jean Dodds, the hospital's superintendent of nurses, "Our techniques in the operating room are changing continually and with the added complications of open heart surgery, I think it is important not only to the efficiency of the operating room but the welfare of the patients that Miss [Patricia] Holder see something of other units. The same situation applies to the acute therapy where Mrs. [Christine] Jeffries has pretty well set up her routines and methods of nursing care from her own experiences."[9] (Patricia Holder later became Bigelow's secretary.) Never, ever, did Bigelow disparage the nurses or suggest that their views and skills were inferior to those of the staff surgeons. Well might he have refrained, because the eighth floor was chronically short of nurses,[10] even though many nurses sought out cardiac experience for their skill set.

In 1965 Bigelow told Jean Dodds, the director of nurses at TGH, how pleased he was with the appointment of Judy Wass "as our nursing supervisor. She is absolutely first class and has taken on a very intelligent and dynamic manner. She is young, full of energy and ideas and also quite diplomatic in the way she is going about things, We are all very pleased and we feel that this was a very astute appointment on your part."[11]

In 1972 Joan Breakey replaced Judy Wass as nursing coordinator. A photo of her and her team survives. Sometime thereafter, Doreen Craig replaced Breakey, and managed the ICU until 1996. Goldman writes, "I remember Doreen well as calm, caring and compassionate equally to her nurses, the patients, the families and the exhausted surgeons. She was exceptionally so when my father lay dying in the CVICU."[12]

So a head nurse would have to be properly accommodated, in her own office, as planning for the eighth floor was conducted. "At the present time, on the 6th floor, the nurses must go into the bathroom to read their report to the incoming group of nurses because the hubbub and confusion around the nursing station is too great to allow this to be carried out. The nursing office would thus not only be the private office of the nurse, but would be a quiet place in which the report could be read. In this regard, I believe we shall have to sacrifice one of the doctor's offices and make this a nursing office." As for nursing instruction, sharing a classroom with the medical students simply did not work.

"There would be almost daily conflict in timetable. [The nurses] have found that they need one room, specially for their nursing teaching."[13]

Distinctive Contributions

Cardiac nursing may occur under intense pressure. Scully said, "What happens in a cardiac intensive care unit is that you sometimes have to open the chest in the bed. We all did that more times than we were comfortable with. It wasn't infrequent twenty years ago. And that puts immense pressure on the nursing staff."[14]

The distinctive contribution of the nurses to cardiac care is often not appreciated. With junior surgeons, they become tutors. Scully was pretty junior when he started at the General. Claudia Koropecki, the head nurse, "would come along and say, 'Dr. Scully, there is a way of approaching this, and I suggest that you do this.'"

Nurses are teachers. Scully said, "What I would do with the young surgeons and residents is say, 'Pay attention to the nurses. You'll learn a lot more from them than you will from me in the operating room.' And that was a fundamental lesson. A lot of what I learned in the operating room was from ladies like these [gesturing to Heidi Duringer and Leda Parente]."

What other special skills set cardiac nursing apart? Said Heidi Duringer, "Cardiac is one of the only services where you're talking to a patient when they're going to sleep, and it may be the last time somebody speaks to that patient. Things can go seriously wrong in cardiac. People don't die in the other ORs the way cardiac patients can."[15] If something is urgently needed, like more blood, the circulating nurse is "the runner," sprinting down the corridor.

What Makes Cardiac Nurses Special?

What specialized care might these nurses provide? Closed chest massage in the event of heart failure, for one thing. Bigelow said of nurses, "The challenge of sick patients, the necessary acquisition of highly specialized knowledge, the skill to perform immediate (closed-chest) cardiac massage and not wait for a doctor ... the need to be alert, involved, and tireless attracted a superb group of talented and dedicated young women." Bigelow noted they were often so tired that "their social life suffered."[16]

Leda Parente, who entered nursing in 1976, began on the wards in ear, nose, and throat (ENT), "We used to take our patients from the ENT floor right down to the operating room, so I would peek into the windows and went kind of 'hmm, this looks good,' so off I went. I started in the cardiac OR in 1978."

Cardiac OR was seen as a plum posting. Heidi Duringer started in nursing at the Western in 1980 on a surgical-geriatric floor. Like Leda Parente, they would have to wheel their patients to the OR, and she would look in and want to be in the OR, "because I didn't like the floor [ward nursing]." She'd regularly ask the head cardiac nurse, "'Is there an opening?' and I'd ask because back then you just begged for your position." She continued, "At the Western, you had to do everything, neuro, orthopedic, everything. Then when you were 'allowed' – you had to show that you were capable – they let you into cardiac. Anyone who wasn't capable could not step through the doors because it was the highest pressure place." Goldman commented, "Nurses like Leda understood the flow of the operation and created a rhythm of correct instruments and sutures to the surgeon as the operation evolved."[17]

Going on pump, was one example. There were only so many nurses who could do it. Leda Parente said, "That's a particular skill. Without a cardiac nurse you can't go on pump. You can't take somebody from ENT and get her to go on pump."

So, that is literally what you do, get the lines ready for the pump. Leda Parente said, "While the surgeons were putting their sutures onto the aorta to prepare for cannulation, I was getting the lines ready [which she got from the perfusionist]. Then they would have to use a number eleven blade, go in with the cannula, take my line, connect the line, arterial to arterial, and then do the same with venous to venous. That was my job."

Scully put in, "On a couple occasions in the middle of the night there were no cardiac nurses, and it's a nightmare working with people not trained. It demands that the surgeon understands what the different lines are, and what you do with them. So I would do what Leda describes when she gets the lines ready. The skill set is extremely important to an effective and efficient operation."[18] This is indeed important: the surgeon needs to stay calm, focused, and gently carry things along so as to create a flow, not chaos.

How about psychological qualities? Heidi Duringer gave an example: "I have the 21 [OR] rooms, I'm walking around. They have one room in oncology, they do mastectomies and they reconstruct. That room, very quiet, very peaceful. People are having reconstructive surgery, the music is on, it's very calm, people are sitting under microscopes, quiet. It's very peaceful, it's very Zen in there. So those type of nurses like it calm, there's one case in a day, they're set up for that case; it's eight to ten hours, it's going to be finished and it's nice."

And in cardiac surgery?

> DURINGER: There's a pace. There's movement. You're constantly moving, you're constantly watching, things change every minute.

But then something goes wrong.

> SCULLY: I would say, "Hey, folks, we have a situation. Nobody talks, and turn off the music." And then, "Okay, here's what we need to do."
> DURINGER: When things get tight, the music always goes down. Don't get erratic. Because that anxiety, that angst, that tension runs with everybody, and then everybody else starts to get like *this* [gestures catatonically] and people start to drop things, they start to fumble because they're getting shrieked at.

The nurses considered themselves part of a team. Heidi Duringer said, "You have to be able to listen to [what's happening with the surgeons], that's part of it. Every surgeon had their own coping mechanisms. Some people shut down, some become very quiet. Some become louder, some, their accents are accentuated, and nobody knows what they're saying [laughter]. Some stress, some people shake."

Leda Parente recalled the comradeship of the team. "To me, my most pleasurable time in cardiac ORs was upstairs [ninth floor], and for one major reason, and that is the camaraderie we had within the team. The camaraderie was unbelievable, we ate with them [the doctors], we had coffee with them." They congregated in the lounge on the ninth floor. Parente said, "There was the only one place to congregate. We knew about his family, he knew about mine. We always socialized together, and it was always nurses and doctors." They would all go to a restaurant together to send off a departee. Linda Mickleborough would have everybody out to her farm for a barbecue.

Bigelow, it must be said, did not share in all this camaraderie with the nurses. And it started to dissolve when cardiac surgery moved to the second floor of the Norman Urquhart building, where they lost their special lounge. And then in 2003 they moved again to the second floor of the Peter Munk Building, and the camaraderie steadily gave way to new behavioural codes and bureaucratic realities. At Friday morning rounds today, the nurses are helpful when asked for information but otherwise are silent and do not join in with the raillery among the surgeons.

Crashing on Pump, and Other Emergencies

The cardiac nurses did not see themselves in any sense as rivals to the surgeons but as their *protectors*. Heidi Duringer said, "We like to embrace our surgeons. We want to take care of them because we *like* them. So we take care of them." Some of the now-older nurses were inclined to be indulgent with the surgeons in moments of tension. Said one, "Tirone [David] in his younger days was rough on the girls. 'I cannot cope!' 'You're killing my patients!' 'Hurry up!' 'Give me my suture!' 'Oh, my God.'" (Some of this changed when the hospital brought in a code of conduct.)

How to protect the surgeons? Leda Parente said, "In an emergency, if he needs something, I want to make sure I have that something to give him. So I would go through certain scenarios in my head [as she lay in bed at night]. Certainly crashing on pump was something that was scary, extremely scary."

Q: Crashing on pump means what?

PARENTE: It means you have three minutes to put that patient on the heart-lung machine because he's arrested.

SCULLY: It doesn't happen often, but the patient may be unstable coming into the room, and gray, then has a cardiac arrest. Now you've got to resuscitate the patient and get the airway going. You've got to get the patient on the heart-lung machine if you're going to salvage the situation, and that's where having a skilled integrated team makes a huge difference.

PARENTE: Sterility at that point goes out the window, because you are to the point where you are saving a life.

She has a pack lying ready for her on the table. "Inside the packs are your drapes. You open the pack, quickly. I've got to get myself gowned first. Then I open everything out. I'm dependent on my circulator [the circulating nurse] to flip all the sutures I'm going to need, so I expect her to know that the only sutures I want her to give me are the cannulation sutures, which are the sutures I need immediately."

She gets her instruments on the table as fast as possible. Often I don't have time to *unstring* my instruments. I have to get them [the surgeons] dressed, put gloves on right away. One of them is doing compressions, and the other one hopefully is throwing prep on the patient, and we are draping as much as we can. Once that is done, the saw is in use, crack the chest open, and they do open massage to the heart."

Scully said, "A patient came off the elevator, blue as a boot. I was in my street clothes, moved the stretcher into the operating room, I opened a prep tray, tore off his clothes, prepped the chest. No anesthetist, but the guy's out of it. I opened his chest and I reached in and put my finger in the hole. He had a stab wound in the heart. So the bleeding stops. 'Somebody get an anesthetist and let's get a setup here.' It was a straight thoracotomy [chest incision] set. At this stage the guy wakes up."

Scully continued, "He was a professional wrestler. These great hands come up. 'Jesus Christ, doc! What the fuck do you think you're doing?'"

Scully said to him, "I think you better let me go." He continued, "He collapses back again. No anesthetic, no anesthetist, but the guy was out of it. He had a stab wound in the heart. Then I got a pair of gloves on and I actually fixed the hole before we did anything else. Knife wound to the heart is usually fatal. The guy walked out of the hospital against advice two days later."

Pride

The cardiac nurses had a real sense of pride. Linda Jussaume said, "At one point in time the rest of the hospital and the other ICU's felt that CVICU nurses thought they were that little bit cut above ... We were a very cohesive group, very avant-garde, very leading edge, and proud and motivated."[19]

Doctors used to ask Bev McParland, head nurse of the cardiological intensive care unit in the mid-1980s, why she didn't go to medical school, as she seemed so knowledgeable about medicine. "Medicine's over there," she would declare, indicating with a sweep of her arm the giant hospital. "Do you know what we do? We are *there*. We do the people part. We look at you as a person, as someone who relates to *us* as a person, who lives in a family and has a job, and a past and a future. We are there – twenty-four hours a day, seven days a week. That's our strong point. Everybody else looks at you as a piece."[20]

Leda Parente said, "I was a little reluctant to go to cardiac, because I knew those girls were going to be tough on me. Because those are the standards up there. You've got to know what you're doing, otherwise you're told, for sure. They were tough nurses, they were really, really tough."

Heidi Duringer added, "You came into the OR, *they* accepted you. They'd have their pow-wow, 'She can come, she has to go, she can stay.' You were selected. Your initiation is 'You stand there and don't move.'"

Danna Blakley, on leaving the cardiovascular service in 1966, wrote to Bigelow to express her appreciation. As well, "I am happy to report that, slowly but steadily, more senior [nursing] students are requesting clinical experience in the cardiovascular department. I have endeavoured to show the students how care of the cardiovascular patient can be interesting and a challenge for their nursing care."[21]

How was cardiac OR nursing different from floor nursing? There were obvious differences: on the ward you are responsible for changing dressings and giving meds to thirty patients. In the closed space of the OR you may have just one patient. You've got to learn the instrumentation. But the big difference is that on the floor you aren't really a team. Heidi Duringer said, "The doctors walk in, and you're sort of ... They give you orders, and then they walk away."

Q: There's no team there?
HEIDI DURINGER: No.

It did happen that a surgeon might enlist nurses of such loyalty that they stayed at his side for much of his career. Tirone David had a loyalist, a nurse-assistant named Joanne Bos, who became a kind of queen bee, to the irritation of the other nurses, when she moved with him from the Western to the General. Clare Baker at St. Michael's had, according to one source, "his favourite nurse in the operating room and she operated with him all the time. And he sometimes let her close the patient, including closing the chest."[22] The Nursing Office at St. Mike's would not have been thrilled about this, but the point is that senior nurses were often vested with extraordinary trust.

ICU Nursing

Cardiac ICU nursing was something special; such nurses were an elite among nurses, an elite among ICUs. The surgeons acknowledged this. In June 1973, following the recovery of an Iraqi patient from a difficult operation, Heimbecker told journalist Joan Hollobon, "It is the specialized nursing in the General's intensive care unit that is the most important factor in the recovery of a patient like Najat. For five days highly trained nurses constantly monitored Najat's heart rate, noted the heart rhythm, took her blood pressure, took blood samples to measure the levels of the blood gases ... and watched the tube to her heart to measure central venous pressure." Under these conditions, Najat, though unable to speak English, "just sailed through."[23]

Linda Jussaume, who started cardiac nursing at the Western in 1984, said in an interview, "You had to prove yourself for a year or more before you went into the cardiac ICU room. It's like a specialized ICU room, you need more skills, you need experience. So the people who weren't performing as well would not go into cardiac. You had to be at least a year, two years into the MedSurg ICU before you went into cardiac. And it was very intensive because of all the machines, and the pressure, and the temperature." Linda Harris supplemented her thought: "In cardiac surgery it really has to be a calling, because of the hours that it takes and the length of time you're in the OR in the middle of the night, and the number of patients you have to take back [to the OR] because of bleeding."[24]

Nurses as Members of the Team

Cursing at the nurses? Does that happen? Wayne Johnston recalled being on the search committee that hired Betty Watt to come from Montreal as head nurse in the operating room. Bernie Goldman was on the committee. "Bernie turned to her and said, 'Mrs. Watt, cardiac surgeons sometimes face a lot of stress and sometimes they behave badly in the operating room because of this stress. And sometimes they use bad words. And how would you deal with a cardiac surgeon like that?' She looked straight at Bernie and she said, 'I have three teenage children. What's your question?'"[25]

Only in the movies and maybe Montreal do doctors bark orders at nurses. Linda Jussaume said, "When I arrived in Toronto, it was better than when I was in Montreal for my first job. I was talked down to, 'You do this, you do that, you're the nurse.' In Toronto, in CVICU I always felt that I was part of a team. I never felt that I was talked down to."

She continued, speaking of Toronto: "I remember somebody was yelling at a nurse, and he was spoken to very sternly afterwards. 'You do not do this on this unit. I don't care where you come from, you do not.'"

At the General in cardiac surgery, the nurses were indeed members of the team, and the surgeons were keen to bring them along. Leda Parente said, "When I was a young nurse, you always saw me at the head of the [operating] table. Because that was my time to watch him." She didn't learn much as a scrub nurse because she couldn't see into the open chest. "So the way I learned, as a circulator, my role was to go to the head of the table, peer over at what he was doing. Then I would watch him use whatever the scrub nurse would give him. That's how I learned. *That's* how he uses that." Surgeons Scully or Goldman might say, "'Come and feel this valve, the calcification of a valve, come and feel it.' He would take my finger and feel around a valve. Or the arteries that were clogged, 'Come and feel the plaque.'"

Doreen Craig said, "I always felt that we were part of the team with Dr. Bigelow, really."

Q: Did he solicit your opinion?
CRAIG: Yes, yes he would.
Q: How was cardiac surgery nursing different from urology?

Linda Jussaume said of this, "We were a partnership. I remember a surgeon asking 'What do you think?' In urology I don't think they would do that."[26]

When Richard Reznick was a resident in cardiac, one evening he assisted Lynda Mickleborough in an operation. "We brought back the patient at seven or eight at night and there was a lot of blood coming out of the chest tube. Cheryl [McKay] was in charge [of the ICU] at the time; she looked at me, looked at the situation, and said 'You had better get back to the operating room.' I think she might have said something a little bit more strongly."

Now, this story has a sequel, aside from making the point about the sovereign judgment of the cardiac ICU nurses. Reznick continued, "As I was wheeling the bed back myself, I looked over my shoulder at this pretty young nurse and decided to go and chat her up at the end of the reopening. We flirted for the next two or three months and starting dating at the cardiac ICU Christmas party at Casa Loma. We continued dating, living together, and then got married." And stayed married. Thus, at the cardiac ICU there were happy endings for the staff as well as for the patients.[27]

These nurses developed a kind of Spidey-sense that something might be going wrong. Linda Harris was "milking the chest tube" and not getting the usual results, "and was really worried," nurse Linda Jussaume explained. "Chris Feindel [a surgeon] comes in, and Harris says, 'This is not good,' and Feindel says, 'What do you think?' and she says 'I think he should go back to the OR.' The patient was on the way to the OR and arrested."[28] Good call.

The ultimate sign of respect for a nurse is a staff physician's willingness to jump out of bed in the middle of the night because a nurse, not a resident, has called. Jussaume said, "[You need] a good, trained, experienced ICU nurse who picks up right away, because it's always the subtle things, and this is what makes the team." She said, "Chris Feindel told me, when some of the experienced nurses called him saying, 'I don't like what I'm seeing, I'm really worried,' they would drive down whether it's 2 a.m. or 3 a.m. to go in. Now that is real trust between us and them."

So the cardiac nurses spoke right up! Scully said, "Tirone [David] and I were making rounds together in ICU, and the nurse came up and said, 'Dr. Mickleborough's patient is in real trouble.' So we went in, and the patient arrested. Between the two of us, he intubated, I massaged, we got things organized, the drugs reorganized, and the patient's fine."

She thanked them for "helping her out."

Chapter Eighteen

Perfusionists

You can't do bypass surgery without a perfusionist. The story goes that a drummer with the Jimmy Dorsey Band was among the earliest perfusionists. Dick Weisel, cardiac surgeon at TGH, said that his father, an academic cardiac surgeon named Wilson Weisel in Milwaukee, used to play trumpet in the 1930s with some of the big bands of the era. He would come down from Milwaukee to Chicago to jam with them. "After they were finished on Saturday, he would bring the drummer up to Milwaukee, because the guy was good with his hands. He ran the pump, and he became a founding member of the American Academy of Perfusion. His name was Ace Adams."[1] Indeed, Ace Adams became the director in the early 1970s of the St. Luke's School of Perfusion in Milwaukee.

Perfusion had an even earlier beginning in Toronto. At TGH on 10 January 1958, Bigelow, Key, and Heimbecker "performed the first successful open-heart surgery in Toronto when they closed an ASD on a twenty-five-year-old female utilizing the commercially available Travenol bubble oxygenator."[2] Daniel Stanford, a young technologist-engineer, was the first perfusionist at the TGH. Bigelow disliked Stanford and dismissed him.

Life in the early days of perfusion was not the simplest. Barrie Fairley, who was administering the anesthetic, recalled of one operation, "Bigelow was standing with the heart cannulated and the pump behind him primed and ready to go. When he told the technician to start, [the technician] delayed taking off the arterial line clamp and one of the latex hoses split and came apart. Blood was spraying at several litres a minute up and down Bigelow's back, then his front when he turned, shouting at the technician, 'Danny, what are you doing?' The technician coolly picked up an unsterile piece of tubing that was there by chance, stopped the pump, switched the tubing and restarted – all in a very brief period of time. The operation was completed successfully," without infection.[3]

In open-heart surgery, there has always been a perfusionist. The names of the earliest perfusionists have been lost in the mists of time ("Gerald and Mike"), Englishmen who also, of course, were trained on the job – but in England. The earliest reference we have seen is 1969, when Heimbecker's homemade pump met a rather ignominious end. Al Trimble told the manager of the operating rooms, "Dr. Heimbecker along with the Engineering Department and our perfusionists devised and constructed a portable pump oxygenator for managing emergency pulmonary emboli and heart failure on the wards. It is a makeshift apparatus, and the perfusionists are open to electrical shocks from it and it is, of course, not dependable." We therefore require one of the commercial models that is now on the market.[4]

Jennifer McDonough was one of the last perfusionists to be trained on the job.[5] She had been a nurse at the West Middlesex Hospital in London, England, then came to Canada in 1968 and started working as a nurse at TGH, then slowly moved into perfusion around 1973 after starting in the cardiac OR. She recalls the early days on the job as "nerve-wracking." She had to hook up the oxygenator, the heat exchanger, and the filters, and then attach them to a pump. "When we went off bypass and they had pressure in them, suddenly they go psssst! psssst! so you have to tighten it like this [screwing motion]. There were a lot of things that could potentially go wrong. And we didn't have any way to measure the amount of heparin on board a patient, so we gave a loading dose. Every hour we gave a half-dose again, and just hoped for the best ... The cases went on quite long. I remember if you ever left the room and came back in, you had that horrible hot blood smell, you know, like a butcher's shop."

Being a Perfusionist

The perfusionists were responsible for the several pumps that infused the entire body and the coronary arteries. The perfusionists were also responsible for the suction. "I was working with Dr. Bigelow," said Jennifer McDonough, and he got really mad at me because the suction wasn't working. Already told him that I was cranking the pump. I had one hand doing the main thing, but I couldn't suction with the other. There were a lot of things like that. You didn't know what the day was going to bring."

The surgeons themselves were under great stress because the perfusion of the coronary arteries was not continuous. It had to stop if an artery were open, then resume. The perfusionists were counting off the minutes of anoxia. "It's been ten minutes since she was given cardioplegia [meaning here crystalloid, a fluid with electrolytes] it's now fifteen minutes, it's now twenty minutes." "So you're trying to concentrate and you've got this nagging situation going on because the heart hasn't had any replenishment in that time."

"OK," the perfusionist says, "It's been twenty minutes, we have to do something." (The heart muscle begins to die after twenty minutes without oxygen.) This was very tense-making and led to surgeons and perfusionists snapping at each other.

Two areas are being perfused: the entire body with blood from the bypass, delivered via the aorta, and the coronary arteries themselves – because the aorta is clamped further down and blood from it can't get into the coronaries, which originate at the root, or base, of the aorta; the bypass feeds into the aorta beyond the clamp.

How does this work? Remember that if nothing is done, the entire myocardium is anoxic during the bypass procedure; the heart is stilled and bloodless. Nancy Pretty said, "If you're doing coronaries, you've put a needle into the root, which is separated [from the rest of the aorta] by a cross-clamp, and that needle is delivering down both coronaries." The anoxia was intermittent, depending on whether the surgeon had a coronary or a heart chamber open to air.

When the surgeon opens a coronary artery, the perfusion to both of the coronary arteries (left main and right) stops. You can't just perfuse the coronary artery you're working on? No, Pretty said, the perfusate goes to all the coronary arteries because they're interconnected. So while you've got one artery open, the perfusion to the rest stops. "It has to, because if it goes to the other vessels that you're not working on, you get retrograde flow; it floods the field, and you can't see. So this group is under a lot of pressure, and the surgeons are aware of time; they're under pressure of time all of the time, and some handle it better than others."

Perfusion of the coronary arteries began in the early 1970s with aortic-valve surgery. Scully recalled, "We would perfuse the coronaries with blood at intervals to get some oxygen into the tissues."[6] McDonough illustrated some of the agonies about getting the perfusate smoothly into the coronaries. "Originally we perfused it by pump bag, put in a litre of fluid that would hopefully go into the coronaries. We had these glass cylinders that we put together with a seal and screwed up tightly [to keep out air], filled them half full with a manometer [pressure gauge] on top. After we primed it and they were ready to go, it would say there was no flow, [the line] was kinked or the vessel was very small, the pressure on the manometer would go up. So we would say, 'We can't perfuse the right but the left is okay.' You're running the pump whilst you're looking at that, and it was 'no flow, yes flow, no flow, no flow' – terrible. I don't know how the heart survived."

Scully said, "One of the problems was you often had a lot of calcification around that area [called the ostia, meaning the entrances to the two coronary arteries]. You always worried about knocking out a chip of calcium either into the coronaries or into the aorta, where it would go north [into the brain] at some stage later." (Chips of calcium and air are the great enemies of the cardiac team: sending either "north" can cause a stroke.)

Here, the readiness of the perfusionists was crucial. Scully said, "We were absolutely dependent on the training and professionalism of the perfusion group to do their best to protect the heart, because otherwise we wouldn't get through."

By the time Nancy Pretty, a nurse-perfusionist, came on board in 1988, they had started to use a perfusion pump rather than just a bag to perfuse the coronaries. With the motorized "roller" pump they could deliver from 100 millilitres to 300 millilitres a minute to the table. The chilled solution was still in a bag, but it was no longer pressurized, and the pump let them gauge exactly how the flow was going.

What was the solution made of? Nancy Pretty said, "It was called crystalloid, mainly high potassium, but usually a bit of magnesium, maybe a little bit of lidocaine [an anesthetic]. The chemicals were suspended in Ringer's solution, a fluid electrolyte replacement. Each centre made its own solution." Or rather, the hospital pharmacy made it up (and then in the mid-1990s the cardiac team started buying commercial preparations after the pharmacy grew tired of all the sterile precautions involved in making the crystalloid). The crystalloid, or potassium cocktail, hangs in a bag at the perfusionist's work station. The concentration can be adjusted with the coronary artery pump. The crystalloid solution is mixed with blood and delivered into the aortic root via a dedicated line. From time to time, the perfusionist may also add a solution called "plasmalyte" to restore the volume of blood lost through surgery, and this solution goes into the aorta, not into the coronaries.

The perfusionists delivered it at about 13°C, in line with the general objective of cooling the body. (Today, some perfusionists use a single pump head that Toronto surgeon Richard Weisel [see chapter 15] designed; it infuses the patient's own blood with a bit of potassium trickled in. It is marketed by the Quest company.)

The Michener Institute, the technical training college for the hospitals, began in 1958 with a lab technician pilot training program; it introduced in 1979 the Post Diploma Program in Cardiovascular Perfusion. Therewith, perfusionists continued to learn on the job but also with the aid of a program of instruction. (The Institute became independent in 1967 when it was incorporated as the Toronto Institute of Medical Technology and in 1990 was renamed in honour of the governor general.[7]) The program is very demanding. Nancy Pretty said of the eighteen-month program that nurses were accepted, likewise physicians from other countries who didn't have an Ontario medical licence, and medical technicians. For admission, you had to have three to five years, minimum, of clinical experience. "I remember Jen [McDonough] telling me, 'You'd better get yourself organized, because you're not even going to be able to do Christmas shopping.' You felt guilty taking an hour off for dinner, it was that intense. They look at it that they're pushing you to the limit because if you couldn't handle the stress you certainly couldn't handle the stress inside the operating room when you're now by yourself." Half of the class dropped out.

Relations with some of the surgeons might be snappish. "I know, I know, it's fifteen minutes, leave me alone!" But the perfusionists knew their mission. Nancy Pretty said, "You're there to protect the heart, you're there because it's part of our job to let them know that this heart has been anoxic for fifteen, twenty, thirty minutes, but they're working in a very difficult situation. They're trying to get things done, and they really don't need somebody basically giving them an ultimatum."

And then crisis! The perfusionist says, "I've got no venous return." The bypass pump won't work if there's no venous blood flowing into it. This might happen because the surgeon lifts up the heart and blocks the venous cava (two of them) that return the de-oxygenated blood to the heart.

So, the surgeon says, "It's not my problem."

Pretty says of this situation, "Meanwhile you're giving cardioplegia [crystalloid], meanwhile you're doing the sucker, meanwhile you're making sure you're doing blood gases, and everything else to make sure the patient is staying stable and safe. You're giving the anesthetic drugs because the anesthetist is out of the room, you might be giving vapour. You're doing all of this and all of a sudden you see *whoosh* everything disappears [meaning, the venous return stops]."

Then the surgeon lowers the heart, and it's "Aaah, I've got all this volume back. I can put my flow up."

The term "cardioplegia" is used in two senses; in one, it means the cold potassium solution that stops the heart; in the other "plege" means the electrolyte solution that nourishes the heart at intervals when the coronary arteries are not open.

Teamwork is essential, despite the irritability. The perfusionist is off to the side and has no view of the operative field. Nancy Pretty recalls, "I would hear a 4–0 Proline suture, which could be an emergency suture, and I'm thinking 'That's not what it's supposed to be,' because I know what's going on up there. I know the sequence of events. The next thing I know, I'm paying attention up there and now here, I'm watching very diligently for air in the venous line because there could be a hole someplace. Your antennae are up, and the next thing is you're aware that they may need another sucker line up there. Because you're part of the team – and everybody else is up there and able to see what's going on – you're back here outside of the sterile area."

Do we cool the patients today? Not as relentlessly in the past, given that studies showed that cold-heart surgery was not superior to warm-heart surgery. At the General, Nancy Pretty said, "we don't really cool them, we let them drift down unless we're doing really big cases like [aortic] arches or [aortic] dissections or whatever."

Drift down? Pretty: "You've got an open chest, you've got a big huge room." And meanwhile, cold "cardioplegia" is being delivered to the heart itself to give it nourishment. Cold versus warm is still being debated.[8] The last chapter in this story has not yet been written.

Emotions

Q: How do you deal with patients dying on the table. Some of the surgeons are pretty cool about that. Are the perfusionists cool about it too?

Jennifer McDonough said that when she was at Sick Kids, she would leave the OR as the patient was being brought in, "when they were awake. So I didn't know their character. I'd come back in when they're asleep."

She did it to create psychological distance. At Sick Kids, "I remember one little girl once, I could remember so clearly, and when I went home they were still working. I phoned to find out what happened and I burst into tears. My husband said, 'It's not your fault.' 'I know, I know,' but you can't help it, you have that empathy."

At the General, McDonough once sat up all night with a patient whose heart had not started beating after coming off bypass and was now on long-term circulatory support (called ECMO – extracorporeal membrane oxygenation). "I remember his family coming in and I thought, 'Oh my goodness these children and this wife are going to have no father now.' Or the other thing we see is somebody's only child, and they died. That's probably why I like the operating room, because I'm not dealing with [family contact] day to day. It sounds like an awful thing to say, but I always liked Emerg, ICU, and the OR because they're sort of not nursing the sick." (What the "floor" nurses do, of course, is nurse the sick – and interact psychologically with them constantly.)

Nancy Pretty tried to avoid working in the cardiac ICU because "you're in very close contact with the family. The worst ones are the younger people. There was a sixteen-year-old that had been misdiagnosed, came in. I spent about four days with her. They decided they weren't going to keep her on [alive] anymore, and all of her classmates started to come in, and her family came in. I left, I went out in the hallway and cried and cried and tried to contain myself. I came back in and the pastor's arrived, and they're doing a service and singing and it was like, 'Oh my God.' It's horrible."

Later, she tried to distance herself as well. "I would come in and it would be 'Hi, how are you,' and that would be the only connection. It used to be 'Where are you from?'"

When the nurse-supervisors of the cardiac ICU – several of them over the years – heard these stories, they shrugged. "You've got to be tough to do cardiac surgery," they said.

Chapter Nineteen

Anesthetists

Motto: Nobody comes to hospital for an anesthetic, but good luck having cardiac surgery without one. The goal is not that the patient comes for surgery but leaves intact after surgery, which is a team effort."[1]

– Gerald O'Leary, cardiac anesthetist, 2018

Stephen Evelyn, a medical graduate of the University of Toronto in 1919 and member of the Toronto General Hospital's Department of Anesthesia, was Murray's favourite anesthetist. A paper that he wrote with Iain MacKay, presented at a meeting in October 1953 – and published the following year – laid down some of the basic principles of cardiac anesthesia. Anesthesia might be light, to preserve the body's natural control over blood pressure, respiration, and heart rate ("vasomotor control"); it was essential to keep the lungs fully oxygenated (via intubation); and depressing drugs must be used sparingly, "if at all." The authors concluded, with a touch of wounded pride, "The anesthetist ... must not be relegated to the position of a piece of standard operating equipment, with mainly nuisance value. He is part of a therapeutic team and harmonious teamwork among surgeon, anesthetist and operating room nursing staff is absolutely essential for the proper care of the patient."[2] Interestingly, it was the anesthetists and perfusionists who led this emphasis on teamwork – vis-à-vis the surgeons. (This pioneering paper remained widely uncited.)

Later in the 1950s, H. Barrie Fairley, an English medical graduate (1949), was Bigelow's favourite anesthetist, and it was Fairley who brought to the cardiac OR the scientific perspectives of anesthesiology. Why was the early death rate so high? Fairley writes, "One of the major problems was acidosis [decrease in blood pH] in the rewarming period." Unable to measure at that point the concentration of oxygen or carbon dioxide in the blood, "we attributed the pallor and the shivering to the patient being cold, not fully recognizing that we were probably also dealing with significant hypovolemia [low fluid volume] in many cases." They thought they had discovered a unique acidosis of rewarming and were humbled to discover later that, in fact, they had not.[3] In any event Fairley did propose in 1957 for hypothermic cardiac surgery a "lytic cocktail" that had just been developed in France as a means of anesthesia: The cocktail was a mixture of two phenothiazines (then coming into use as antipsychotics) – chlorpromazine and promethazine – plus the sedative-anesthetic meperidine. It was designed to prevent shivering and during cooling and rewarming to keep the body's acid-base level constant.[4]

It was Fairley who initiated the team of specialized cardiac anesthetists, including Tom Hanley (who went to Oxford for a year) and Ray Matthews (to London, at Westminster Hospital), and John Nunn (at the Royal College). It was Fairley and his team of anesthetists who helped establish the Cardiac Surgery Post-operative Unit on the ninth floor, later on the eighth.[5]

After Fairley's departure in 1969, it was Sallie Teasdale who led cardiac anesthesia.

George Boddington (Toronto MD, 1937) also figured prominently. Scully recalled, "George was actually one of my father's boyhood friends, and when we visited Toronto we would go there, and George would tell me stories about the early days of Bigelow in the operating room; and some of the stories would just curl your hair. The courage Bigelow had to continue what he was doing when the mortality rate was 50 per cent was just unbelievable."

Scully continued, "One of the things that really blew up in Bigelow's face at one stage is that a patient did die, and he – to the family – blamed anesthesia. It never went to the College [of Physicians and Surgeons of Ontario], but it created quite a blowup, as you might imagine."

  Q: Was Bigelow just shuffling the blame, or was it really the fault of
  anesthesia?
  SCULLY: There is a principle of leadership, which I've always followed. If
  there's a problem and I'm the leader, it's my problem. I've had patients
  who have died because other people made mistakes. I have always
  acknowledged that that happened, and when I'm asked for the name
  I don't give it. I say, "I'm responsible." Anyway, Bigelow had a lot
  of trouble with anesthesia for a few years after that, and ultimately
  apologized.
  Q: Oh, did he? There's no trace of this in the letters I've seen.
  SCULLY: There wouldn't be.[6]

The Growth of Anesthetics

The anesthetists, previously the handmaidens of the surgeons in the OR, now began flexing their muscles. In 1957, as mentioned, Fairley laid out a whole program of anesthesia in cardiac surgery.[7] In 1962 Fairley decreed that surgical residents had to stop adjusting respirators, because they didn't know what they're doing. "Previously, their enthusiastic but untutored efforts were responsible for mortalities on more than one occasion ... Only when it became routine for the anaesthetists to be consulted over each change did the overall picture improve."[8]

Gerry O'Leary and Anesthetic Imperialism

Gerald O'Leary, a Dublin medical graduate in 1980, did his internship and residency in Ireland, then came to Canada in 1986 as a fellow in intensive care at the Hospital for Sick Children. In 1987 he moved over to the General as a research fellow in anesthesia and trained further there until joining the staff of anesthesia in 1993.[9] He was in fact the first cardiothoracic fellow in anesthesia. An Irishman, O'Leary was not impressed with what he found in anesthesia in Canada. "A lot of the drugs we used were about five to ten years behind Europe. Everyone thinks Canada's way ahead. No, no, it's five to ten behind." Colonial oppression of the Irish and the Canadians? "There were three English-trained anesthesiologists, and they weren't mean to me, but they certainly felt free to put me in my place."

Nor was he any happier with the pace of work. "I came over and saw the OR list and said, 'Okay, that's the morning. What do we do in the afternoon?' Because there was this obsession with spending time at work, rather than actually getting work done. People were incredibly slow. We could easily do twice the volume of cases in Ireland."

And the tediousness of cardiac surgery, where O'Leary was a whirlwind: "I would come to work at five to eight. I would find the patient, set up the room, bring the patient in, because that's what you would do. I would put in the intravenous, I would apply the monitors, I would put in the arterial line, I would give the drugs, I would intubate, I would put them on the ventilator, I would pre-op them, I would put in the catheter. I'd be finished in sixteen minutes. Sixteen past eight, and I'm done. I look at the other rooms around me, people have been setting up since seven or seven-thirty and they're still not finished."

On O'Leary's watch, new drugs came into cardiac anesthesia. In Stephen Evelyn's day, he and Murray had used ether, which O'Leary had now abandoned entirely. Then there was cyclopropane (invented in

Toronto): "I really like cyclopropane," he said. "Cyclopropane was one of those really fantastic gases, came in a lovely orange cylinder. You give it to somebody, they'd be asleep in ten seconds."

Why don't we still use it?

"The problem with cyclopropane, if you don't pay attention and get a leak, it explodes. If something happens to that cylinder, you will blow up the OR. Literally. It would demolish the operating room and everybody in it."

The anesthetist is often the imager in a cardiac operation, and they now rely heavily on an imaging technique, transesophageal echocardiography (TEE), a form of echo imaging. O'Leary said, "It stemmed from being able to miniaturize an echocardiographic probe and putting it at the top of a gastroscope, so you could put it down the esophagus and then look at the heart from behind. You are right next to the heart, and the quality of the images is very good." Also, the probe could be rotated, giving a series of standard cuts of the heart. Add colour to that and you can "look at the flow through the valves and measure the velocity of blood flow."

It was, as we know, the cardiologists who first started doing echoes in the OR. Then Tirone David pushed to have TEE available when he was doing mitral and aortic valves – so as to know if the new valve had been properly positioned. The anesthetists were already in the operating room and, said O'Leary, started to become interested in using this new technology themselves. "The cardiologists weren't that interested in having someone in the operating room all the time, so that became an opportunity to collaborate and train the first group of [anesthetists]." The first Canadian guidelines for TEE in the cardiac operating room were issued in 2006.[10]

Why would the anesthetists have so avidly seized control of an imaging technique from the cardiologists? They just give anesthesia, don't they?

Wrong there, said O'Leary. "Anything to do with the whole patient is what we're interested in. If we want to know what the heart is doing, what the lungs are doing, any of the information that helps us get the patient off the table, get well, and go home." So this articulates a highly ambitious vision of anesthesia as responsible for the whole patient from the moment he or she is wheeled into the OR until the patient leaves the ICU.

O'Leary maintained that the anesthetists were in charge of the cardiac surgery ICU, a view that several surgeons disputed, emphasizing that the two specialties managed the unit *together*. Were there rivalries between the two disciplines? Anesthetist Massimiliano (Max) Meineri made an interesting point: "The Department of Critical Care and the intensivists in the general ICU over the years have tried multiple times to take over our cardiac ICU, and apparently those who were on our side and wanted us to manage their patients were the cardiac surgeons."[11]

Goldman's take: "Nearly everywhere where the med-surg ICU has taken over the cardiac ICU, it is to the detriment of the cardiac patient, because the patients have not been in the cardiac OR and you cannot treat a cardiac patient like a peritonitis or pneumonia or trauma patient."[12]

O'Leary's is a vision that downplays the role of the cardiac surgeon. "The surgeon does the surgery, that's it. We're the people who actually adjust the medication to make the heart function better or not." This idea confronts cardiology's role. "We're the people who decide the course for the whole patient. Surgeons think they're in charge of the patient, but as chief of anesthesia, I'm telling you, I'm in charge of the patient."

Q: Is the surgeon the captain of the team, or is he just a player?
O'LEARY: They can be the captain of the ship, if they want to be, but I'm the Admiral of the Fleet.

The cardiac surgeons, it must be said, have a slightly different view of this. They conceive the management of ICU patients as a partnership. Bernie Goldman said, "In fact the cardiac surgery ICU is still owned, that is, bed-controlled, by us. [Surgery] determines throughput. Nobody discharges an ICU patient, ain't nobody coming from the OR [without the assent of the surgeons]." Goldman said the cardiac ICU at the General was the only one where the intensivists or anesthetists were not in charge, and even at Sunnybrook the surgeons had lost control. There, where Goldman was chief of cardiac surgery, "we [would] have guys who say, 'I see you have an empty cardiac bed, and we have a trauma coming in.' At the General if anything like that would happen you'd just stamp your foot and say, 'That ain't gonna happen.'"

Goldman remembered coming back from his rotation in England at Ronald Belsey's chest unit in Bristol, "thinking I could bronchoscope anyone, forgetting that in England at that time they didn't have any teeth, that's why it was so easy. So anesthesia [which inserted respirator tubes] was our partner, but we as residents were boss. We stayed up in that damned ICU on the ninth floor all night long and all weekend long." They had a sleeping room there.[13]

Looking back, Sallie Teasdale, who was chief of cardiac anesthesia at the General from 1975 to 1991, summarized the changes over those

years: "In the twenty-seven years that I was involved, the surgical techniques progressed through cold hearts, warm hearts, beating hearts,
arrested hearts, unperfused hearts, and finally transplanted hearts.
In parallel, anaesthetic technique progressed through nitrous oxide/
oxygen, halothane, fentanyl, succinylcholine, curare to sedation and
mechanical ventilation in the recovery room (sometimes for days), to
being awake and extubated [going off respirator] in the OR."[14]

There are different worlds of training here. One is the training of
intensivists. The other is the joint training of cardiac surgeons and
anesthetists. What's the difference? Linda Harris, who manages the
twenty-one ORs in the Munk Centre, said, "If you want to really, truly
bring excellence to the ICU setting, you need to be able to bring a sick
patient, and get that patient through the operation, and get that patient
through the ICU, and I see today a difference between people that are
intensivist-trained versus cardiac surgery-anesthesia trained."

Q: What's the difference?
LINDA HARRIS: They have to have the ability to do a bedside echo [TEE].
   That's the gold standard in ICU care today, and you have to have that
   ability. If you're looking at a patient and can't [put the] puzzle together,
   go and get the echo machine, do that echo within ten minutes. It saves
   lives. And that's what's kept me in the ICU. It's having the excellent
   surgeon and the excellent anesthetist and the complex patient and the
   nurse. That whole four pieces, that's what's kept me there, really.[15]

Thus, the members of the team marched through this odyssey, more or
less, hand in hand.

PART FOUR

Today

Chapter Twenty

Tirone David

Motto: "As residents, Dr. David would say to us that if this patient came in the door carrying a briefcase and he left in a pine box, the only thing that happened between Point A and Point B was you."[1]

– Terrence Yau, 2010

Tirone David was born in 1944 in the city of Ribeirao Claro in Brazil, a small town in the province of Paraná, one of six children. His father was Jewish, an immigrant from Syria who had become a successful businessman and mayor of the town; his mother was Italian, a Roman Catholic, and the children, all of whom were named after movie stars, were raised as Catholics. Tirone owed his name to the dashing leading man Tyrone Power (but it was written as Tirone, there being no "y" in Portuguese). His middle name was Esperidiao, which means "he who hopes in God."[2]

His father wanted him to be a doctor, and there was much talk of medicine at home. David's own interest in medicine kindled in high school when he did a project on the missionary-doctor Albert Schweitzer in Africa. "After completing his research on Schweitzer, David wanted to go to Africa, too," said one journalist. "'What a great man,' he thought, 'what a giving soul!' He, too, Tirone David would become a priest and go to Africa to heal the sick."[3] Well, David, who liked women, at least carried through with the medical part of the plan.

Tirone David graduated from the Universidade Federal de Paraná in Curitiba, Brazil, in 1968, where his mentor was Giacondo Artigas, known as a brilliant technical surgeon. Artigas required him to learn English and rewrite in English a paper on bile duct strictures that he had written in Portuguese.

David interned at the State University of New York in Brooklyn in 1970. "It was a great year," he later said. "New York was wonderful for a young foreign doctor. Very cosmopolitan and one never feels a 'foreigner.'"[4] He then trained in general surgery and vascular surgery for four years at the Cleveland Clinic Hospital, under George Crile, Jr. Said Toronto surgeon Martin McKneally, in a brief biographical summary, "Caldwell Ecklestein, Crile's son-in-law, took a strong interest in the gifted young Brazilian surgeon and served as his mentor. Crile, a very conceptual surgeon, taught Tirone to 'follow nature's rule: form follows function.'"[5]

David then decided to become a heart surgeon and in 1975 came to the University of Toronto to train with Bigelow. Why the choice of Toronto? "Bigelow was a visiting professor at Cleveland Clinic when I was a resident," said David later. "The resident took care of the professor. So I'd pick him up at the airport, take him to the hotel, watch him operate." David's boss, the famous heart surgeon Donald Effler, told Bigelow that David wanted to become a heart surgeon, and immediately Bigelow was interested. Thus, David came to Toronto for training.[6]

But stay in Toronto? "I thought I would go back to Brazil to practise cardiac surgery," he said. "But by the time I finished eight years of training I was overtrained and could not practise there anymore." He joined the staff of TGH in 1977.

Have things gone well in Canada? Despite his thrill at interning in New York, he said, "I felt a foreigner in the USA. I never felt that I belonged. This feeling never existed here. From the moment I arrived to the present, I have never felt a foreigner. Canadians made me feel part of them."

But Canada in those days was over-doctored. It was difficult to get permission to immigrate. No problem. "Dr. Bigelow and Dean Holmes went to see the late Pierre Trudeau in Ottawa. Mr. Trudeau solved the problem by sending a letter to the Department of Immigration and Manpower stating the reason for my entering the country as 'national interest' and the next day I became a landed immigrant."[7]

David's initial tenure as a staffer at TGH was brief. Bigelow recruited him in July 1977. Then a problem surfaced at the Western: Susan Lenkei, the director of cardiac investigation at the Western, had demanded that the surgery unit there be closed "due to poor outcomes."[8] So they needed someone to take over the unit, and it was in December 1977 that "Ron Baird 'forced me' to go to TWH to reopen the cardiac unit that had been closed in August 1977 because of 'unacceptable clinical outcomes.' I recall that you [Hugh Scully], Bernie, and John Gunstensen (who soon moved to Hamilton) all said 'no' to Ron Baird, and as the lowest man in the pole I had no choice but moved to TWH. I was not happy going there because the main reason I stayed in Canada was to work at TGH." [9] David said he had received a job offer from the Cleveland Clinic.

Baird said diplomatically of David's move to the Western, "In the fall of 1978 [sic] I persuaded Tirone to work at Toronto Western Hospital two days a week, and in 1979 he agreed to move over as Head of that division. Although not very enthused at the beginning, he soon realized he had inherited a unique opportunity."[10]

All did not go well for David at the beginning. Cardiologist Harry Rakowski recalls that his colleague Susan Lenkei, who was known as something of a "bulldog," wanted to check on David's results. "She just said, 'Okay, I am going to take a hundred consecutive bypass patients that you are going to do and I am going to re-cath them.' No research ethics assessment, just going to do it. And after the hundred, she sat Tirone in her office like a little boy and said, 'Your results are shit. You know, here are the results of failed grafts at six months or a year.' And he was horrified that they were so high, and he learned from it and improved."[11]

So the story of Tirone David at the Western has a happy end. It was a training ground for David to become a great surgeon. In David's own view, "Within 6 months I realized how lucky I was. It was the best thing that happened to me professionally because instead of doing surgery one day a week at TGH, after 2 months at TWH I was given an extra OR and I began to operate 5 days a week. In no time I was doing 450 cases a year and that was when I matured as a clinical surgeon." David then introduced many innovative operative procedures.[12]

This might be the place to give credit to Irving Lipton, who, as Goldman puts it "was David's colleague at TWH and quietly supported the flamboyant David. Tirone ultimately performed multiple CABGs on Lipton."[13] Lipton began a residency under Bigelow in 1968, accompanied fellow trainee Claude Labrosse to a staff job at Sherbrooke University, then returned to Toronto, this time to the Toronto Western Hospital.

Tirone David's Innovations

In the history of the General, David will probably be also remembered as a tremendous fundraiser. Stephanie Brister said, "He brought huge resources in, that paid for most of our fellows. And so we could train fellows from all over the world because of the money that Tirone brought in." Scully added, "Tirone has been the most prolific, productive fundraiser of any surgeon in the history of this hospital."[14]

Q: More than Barry Rubin?

BRISTER: Oh, yeah.

In the history of cardiac surgery, David will be remembered as an innovator *sans pareil*.

In an echo of the praise of Gordon Murray a half-century previously, David's operating style was routinely characterized as "brilliant." Though the other great surgical centres of North America, such as Mayo, the Cleveland Clinic, and the University of Minnesota, doubtless have had many gifted operators, extraordinary virtuosity seems somehow to flourish in Toronto as well. Or perhaps it was merely a matter of luck: Bigelow and Baird were not brilliant operators, though Bigelow embodied the Pasteurian principle, "Chance favours the prepared mind." Murray and David were, by all accounts, brilliant. The term is not out of place here.

"Innovation" also characterized David, and with David, innovation was not so much a matter of being first to try new concepts in the dog lab, as Bigelow and Baird had done, but the sudden flash of insight. Cardiologist Harry Rakowski was often present with David in the OR: "I would look down at what he was doing and say, 'You know, Tirone, I haven't seen you do that before.' And he said, 'Yeah, I just thought of it.'"[15]

David learned from others, and in Oxford he saw surgeons extubating patients in the operating room (rather than waiting for hours) and not sedating them heavily, to avoid intensive care. "I saw that and I was blown away. So I came back home, took five or six people back here, intensivists and anesthetists, shipped them off to Oxford, and they learned, and the next day we started doing the same thing here. Of course, very cautiously, because we had some concerns. They always ask the surgeon, 'Is it safe to wake him up?' and the surgeons say, 'Well, there's no technical problem, no bleeding, the heart functions well, wake him up!' In North America this was a major breakthrough."[16] The morning after an operation, "the patient is sitting up in bed eating breakfast instead of unconscious and on a ventilator," said Toronto Hospital president Alan Hudson. David said, he "believes the most dramatic results are in the quicker recovery after a heart operation. Because people wake up alert and in control."[17] In Toronto, the custom established itself of not keeping patients in the ICU for more than a day.

When the Peter Munk Cardiac Centre opened in 1997 (see chapter 22), the practice of carting the patients around the hospital from service to service came to an end. It was all under one roof. "Why move the patient? Move the nurses!" said David. "Again, another revolutionary change in patient care."[18]

Other ideas came to David on the fly. One was an operation he and Chris Feindel originated in 1992, which was named after him – the David Procedure[19] (sometimes the David-Feindel operation[20]) – and which is for eliminating an aneurysm around the aortic valve, something that occurs in children with Marfan Syndrome, in addition to other circumstances. (David did operate on children, but the David Procedure is used on adults as well.) "The first was [a young] girl. The parents did not want her to have a mechanical valve. 'Use a human valve for her, so at least she can get pregnant and have babies.'" She was sixteen.

"So I opened the patient up: entirely normal valve, but there was an aneurysm. So I had to come up with an operation that preserved the valve but took the aneurysm out."

Q: So you just saw spontaneously that there was an aneurysm around the valve, and you just fixed it like that?

DAVID: Absolutely. And this is called a great achievement. But you don't become great if you don't know the aortic valve well, how the pulmonary valve looks, what an aneurysm looks like. That's why I say it was stepwise. I could never develop it in 1980. I had to live seven or eight years, doing what I did [to hit on the idea of this particular procedure].[21]

Why was this procedure important? "This resulted in young patients being able to resume full activity on no medication after surgery."[22]

David innovated across a wide variety of cardiac fronts. In 1978 he established a cardiovascular surgical database to track outcomes for each procedure. In the judgment of one surgeon, "Much of the academic productivity of the unit is directly attributable to the formation of this clinical database."[23]

He was probably best known for his innovative surgery on aortic and mitral valves. Beginning in 1983, he authored a series of articles that reoriented the approach of the field to the valve.[24] In Goldman's view, "His contributions to the field ... have made TGH almost as important as Broussais Hospital in Paris, where Alain Carpentier is considered the father of reparative surgery on the mitral valve."[25] "David evaluated mitral annuloplasty with fixed versus flexible rings, chordal preservation, the David I and David II aortic root sparing reconstructions. [He] developed the subcoronary stentless porcine valve."[26] This was the SPV, an aortic valve manufactured by St. Jude Medical of St. Paul, which David first described in 1988. For details on this, see chapter 13.)

David originated in 1989 a new procedure for replacing the chordae tendineae – the tendinous cords that connect each cusp of the mitral valve to the papillary muscle in the left ventricle – with Dacron sutures in reconstructing the valve.[27] David also pioneered operations for endocarditis, mitral regurgitation, and aortic dissection.[28]

In 1998 David proposed a novel method of handling ruptures of the septum between left and right sides of the heart, the patients in cardiac shock, and blood being pumped back from the left side to the right (causing low cardiac output and death). These were grave complications, and the mortality in cardiogenic shock in various centres ranged from 20 to 88 per cent. The previous strategy had been infarctectomy, cutting away the dead cardiac muscle (originally proposed by Gordon Murray). David argued for stitching on the left side a big piece of bovine pericardium to the healthy tissue around the infarct. Further manipulation of the right ventricle, he said, would only worsen the patient. His results were impressive: of nineteen patients operated on, there was only one death.[29]

But perhaps the procedure for which he became best known – aside from the aortic aneurysm operation – was replacing the patient's aortic valve with the patient's own pulmonary valve, then implanting a cadaveric pulmonary valve in place of the one just removed. This was known as the Ross Procedure, first described in 1967, and it required a great deal of manual dexterity, so much in fact that it was going out of use because surgeons found it too challenging. But it had the advantage over a mechanical valve of freeing the patient from a lifetime of taking the anticoagulant drug warfarin. The disadvantage was a nontrivial failure rate. David began aortic valve replacement with a pulmonary autograft in 1990.[30] What he added were instructions for doing the Ross Procedure safely, minimizing mortality and reinterventions. David followed his patients carefully, and at twenty years (or less; median follow-up was 13.8 years) the results for the 212 patients on whom he performed the Ross Procedure from 1990 to 2004 were that 82 per cent were free of reoperation on the new aortic valve; 93 per cent free from operation on the cadaveric pulmonary valve. Free from reoperation of any kind were 80 per cent. David remarked, "These outcomes are much better than those obtained after aortic valve replacement with bioprosthetic (pig etc.) aortic valves or aortic valve homografts (cadaveric aortic valves) in patients of similar age." It was a good operation for young people and those who are physically active. Mortality from the operation was comparable to that of the general population of the same age – so it was a safe operation. But it was not every surgeon's cup of tea. David said rather puckishly, "The Ross procedure is a complex operation that transforms aortic valve disease into combined aortic and pulmonary valve disease."[31] You had to perform about thirty of them before feeling even vaguely competent.[32]

After such a record, David was held literally in awe by his surgical colleagues – and by much of the field. When in 2008 he gave a talk on "creativity in medicine" at citywide surgical rounds, it was to a "rapt" audience.[33] In an interview, John Wedge, who headed the University Department of Surgery from 1992 to 2002, said, "If I had to list the five most distinguished academic surgeons in the entire 250 surgeon cohort of the University of Toronto, Tirone David would be up there as number one, two, or three. He has brand recognition everywhere."[34]

It was on David's watch that the government's first efforts to regulate a medical specialty began. In 1988 Hugh Scully became a founding member of the Cardiac Care Network of Ontario (CCNO), established by the Ministry of Health to coordinate the provision of cardiac services across the province. Heart surgery was thus far in the lead of other specialties in establishing a database that would allow systematic comparisons of results across centres and across procedures. Bryce Taylor later said, "People are getting used to having the statistical analyses now because they are part of a North American network, and that's coming gradually division by division. But cardiac was basically twenty years ahead of everyone else."[35]

While the CCNO increased the resources available to heart surgery, it had also the effect of making many surgeons risk averse. As Scully later said, "You didn't necessarily want to take on high-risk patients, because your mortality was being compared. So various surgeons stopped doing high-risk operations."[36] It was in this high-risk pool that David dazzled.

What Makes for Success?

David was such a success in cardiac surgery for several reasons. One, he is very fast – which counts for a lot when a patient's heart is open.

David had a big reputation for his technical virtuosity and speed. According to one journalist in 1985, while David was still at the Western, "The 41-year-old cardiovascular surgeon believes the less time a patient spends on a heart-lung machine the better his chances of recovery. So David works quickly." Said Carl Cardella, director of transplantation at the Western, "He's fast, confident, precise. If I had to have a heart operation, he would do it. I trust him."[37]

Two, he is technically very inventive, able to devise new solutions on the spot, which then enter the literature. One journalist said, "On more than one occasion, David has leaped off the beaten path, so to speak, in mid operation, devising an ad hoc solution to a unique puzzle in a patient's wounded flesh – spontaneously inventing a technique that his peers around the world will soon be copying."[38]

Three, he is better able than many to see the heart in three dimensions. A colleague said, "This man has a 3-dimensional mind, he always sees things in three dimensions, that's why he can do the things he can do in the operating room."[39] David said, "Remember, we operate on a still heart, but then we have to imagine, this is how it is in three dimensions, but it's going to be moving ... The David operation [procedure] is much more geometrically defined, because once you put the valve inside of a [Dacron] tube it doesn't move anymore." Scully added, "It demands of the surgeon a very detailed, intimate knowledge of the anatomy, and how the anatomy can vary in a pathological way, and how that structure functions when it isn't just sitting quiet on the table. You have to translate that into the three-dimensional concept, and that's what Tirone did better than anyone I've ever met."[40]

There was one more skill David had that wasn't necessarily generalizable:

> DAVID: Yesterday I was helping a partner do a mitral valve repair, and I kept talking. Everything that came into my head I kept telling him. He just couldn't do it, what went through my brain.
> Q: Is that right?
> DAVID: So there must be something else that is innate.
> Q: But you aren't able to put your finger on what this other thing is?
> DAVID: I think it's innate. It's the only thing.[41]

Merger: David Begins Three Terms as Chief of Cardiac Surgery at the General

In Toronto by the mid-1960s, there was a terrific shortage of patient beds, and the costs of the publicly financed system were soaring. In March 1965, the Ontario Hospital Services Commission formed a Metro Toronto hospital council to achieve efficiencies by, among other things, merging expensive specialty services. Among them was heart surgery.[42] But this did not happen right away.

In October 1986 the Provincial Legislature passed the enabling Toronto Hospital Act. But, said Baird, "the merger process was not complete until the end of 1992."[43] The merger created a single superpower in cardiac surgery. David was unabashed about preferring the principle of excellence over accessibility. He said in 2017, "I am against unrestricted competitive medical practice ... Concentration of Centres of Excellence requires that patients have to travel, but that is a worthwhile price to pay for higher quality of care ... Perhaps we could consolidate three hospitals into one in Toronto [as at the Cleveland Clinic] to achieve this goal."[44]

The merger is recalled as a very trying experience. Said Bernie Langer, who at the time was head of general surgery at TGH, "The hospitals were competitors ... completely independent institutions, and they competed fiercely with one another. The Toronto General was in a way the cement that held everything together, because all the rest of them could agree that they hated the General. And there was probably good reason for that."[45]

But who was to head the newly merged General Hospital division? Baird apparently threw his hat in the ring but was rebuffed. The search was to have been, supposedly, "open." But Goldman said, "I knew from Tirone that the deal was done at the level of the board and Tirone would come over and be the chief ... It was a good deal. Tirone was the ascending star, we all knew it and we all benefited from it, all of our skills improved because of him."[46]

David, who had led cardiac surgery at the Western from 1980 to 1988, became head at the General in that year. In 1989 he moved his office from the Western to the General. The merger was arduous for cardiac surgery. During the transition to a single service at the TGH, Hugh Scully, as deputy head of cardiac surgeon and deputy surgeon-in-chief, operated at both the General and the Western. He found it very stressful, always being reminded that "Tirone does not do it that way." The nurses and perfusionists hated not knowing where they were going to be working. Nancy Pretty and other perfusionists were at the Western: "All of a sudden this very professional but almost cottage, friendly, small-town hospital was being eaten by this big corporate hospital, and we resented it." The General ended up with two ICUs, because the ICUs refused to merge. Pretty said, "We had the Western ICU and the TGH ICU because the paperwork was different, and 'we're not going onto your paperwork.' They were both on the same floor of the General, the TGH ICU with something like twelve beds, the Western with ten." David retained an office at the Western for a year but started operating at the General from the get-go. It was Scully who went back and forth. "It was one of the most uncomfortable transitions of my life, trying to deal with that."[47] The whole thing was consolidated around 1990.

David told Scully, "We became the largest cardiac surgical unit in Canada and, braggadocio aside, one of the best open-heart units in the world. Our annual courses on 'Innovative Approaches to Heart

Surgery' became legendary and our auditorium was always filled with Americans, Europeans, and even Asians, and soon after we began to broadcast live-surgery internationally to European, Japanese and South American cardiac surgical meetings. We had a long list of operative procedures that surgeons want to learn."[48] There have been some big success stories in this book, but even by those standards, this is extraordinary. One can understand why David was chosen to serve three terms as head of cardiac surgery at the General. He laid down the headship in 2011.

For the first time, the hospital chiefship at the General was held separately from the university chair. Tom Salerno at St. Michael's Hospital, not David, was the university chair. Salerno was first to use the title "Professor of Cardiovascular Surgery." The previous heads had called themselves "Chairman of the Inter-Hospital Coordinating Committee for Cardiovascular Surgery."[49]

David in Action

Toronto started to become a Mecca for the training of cardiac surgeons. David said, "We averaged 200 visitors a year in our operating rooms. 200! And this went on for a good ten years. We had two or three guys [residents], we nicknamed them tour guides."[50]

Hugh Scully, who was listening to this interview, added, "In the late 1980s and the 90s, it was his leadership and innovation and creativity that generated the reputation and the attraction, because he would challenge us all to think differently. He has always thought differently."

David added, "Why? I believe that perfection is impossible, no human being is perfect. But if you seek perfection, I guarantee to you, you'll obtain excellence. And this was our motto."

In an interview in 2017, David talked about mentors who had influenced him: "Bill Bigelow was my principal mentor here. He guided me to seek a niche in cardiac surgery and excel in it."[51] But David also remembered, while he was a resident at the Cleveland Clinic, a talk by hematologist Maxwell Wintrobe. "[He] said that just about any coagulopathy could be corrected by the transfusion of fresh whole blood. I never forgot that coming from Dr. Wintrobe. This led me to donating my own blood to an exsanguinating patient after an extensive open-heart procedure soon after I started practicing." (There are stories of nurses doing this on the spot too.) On another occasion, "Midway through a heart valve operation, David decided that the bleeding was so profuse that he could not wait for whole blood to arrive from the hospital blood bank and called for donations there and then from the operating team."

We are not surprised to learn that the volunteer donors included the surgeon himself, and the procedure saved about 20 minutes."[52] "Too bad we can't do this any longer," said David.[53]

The appeal of cardiac surgery for David? "Heart surgery is mechanical, simple, and gratifying," David said in 2010. "Its problems are highly technical. But with heart surgery I can more easily transform a patient's life. I can save someone who's about to die."[54] David's concern for his patients very much belies the image of the Very Important Man. Bigelow on one occasion told a journalist that he was struck "by the sensitivity [David] displayed around patients. He never forgot that these were human beings, that's what impressed me."[55] Once, David was operating on a woman whose heart had been badly damaged by earlier radiation therapy for a chest tumour. David said, "The consequence of the radiation was that everything turned and twisted in her heart, and arteries closed with scarring from being burned and one lung was destroyed ... Parts of her heart were so scarred and calcified that they shattered like eggshells." What he found as he opened her up was even worse than he anticipated. At one point he was said, as a journalist put it, to have "looked up around the operating table and said he wasn't sure he should continue." Then he said, "This woman has three children to go home to."

Here is what he did: "I cut her leg, took the vein, cut the main artery, replaced the aortic valve, the main pipe, as well. It was not conventional surgery. It was something creative that I do sporadically and only out of desperation." At nine that evening he came out of the OR to speak to the family. He told them she had survived the surgery. "But he was sombre. When her sister cheered, he admonished her, 'Don't cheer yet. I'm not sure she'll make it through the night or the week.'" But the patient did make it, and after a long convalescence, returned gladly to her family.[56]

Like many Brazilians (and non-Brazilians) David liked to take the occasional glass of red wine. One Friday evening he was invited to a stag, and given that he had no patients scheduled the next day and that his current patients were all stable, he accepted, and drank "half a bottle of wine." At eleven p.m. his pager went off. A twenty-eight-year-old man with a history of five cardiac operations was now just on the brink.

"Is he stable?" David asked the nurse.

Yes.

"Can it wait until tomorrow?"

Yes.

So David went home and lay down to sleep. But he couldn't sleep. "At one o'clock in the morning, I'm fully awake, same thing at two o'clock. How could I sleep? The kid had had cardiac arrest and been resuscitated. So finally I thought, to hell with that, and got in the car and came here. The kid had been crying, because the surgeon on call told him he couldn't do the operation; it was too complicated. So at three, they wheeled him into the OR, and I operated for the next five or six hours. I finished about nine a.m., had some coffee and went home. And slept."[57]

David was known, not always in an admiring way, for his sardonic wit. Residents trembled to hear the phrase "It's my fault," as in "It is my fault for thinking you could tie that knot." Or, in the absence of his trusted assistant Joanne Bos, a former nurse from the Western who had assisted him for more than thirty-three years, "It is my fault for doing this operation without Joanne." He trusted her to do procedures: "If you cannot do, Joanne can do."[58] This would be humiliating for a resident or fellow. (David was the only surgeon who had a permanent assistant.) Anesthetist Gerry O'Leary remembers once in the OR, David said to a *staff surgeon* who was helping, "No, no, it's okay, Joanne, you do it. You're an idiot. It's my fault, I didn't teach you right, you just don't know what you're doing."[59]

"You're killing my patient," David would say, if the patient were on bypass and there were delays. Just what one wants to hear: You're killing my patient. For all his technical brilliance, David was known for having a bit of a rough edge in human relations. One senior faculty member, who wished not to be quoted, said "I've had numerous people over the years tell me that when they come out of meetings [with David] they are thinking of looking elsewhere and they just can't stand it any longer."

The Waiting-List Crisis

By 1995 the chronic waiting-list crisis had become acute. Patients on the list were classed according to "emergency" (treatment that day), "urgent" (within 14 days), "semi-urgent" (wait up to six weeks), and "elective" (wait up to three months). Elective makes it sound like kind of a voluntary thing, but septal defects and valve replacements were typically labelled "elective." For patients on the elective list at Sunnybrook, the average waiting time in the spring of 1995 was 132 days; at the Toronto Hospital, 108 days; and at St. Michael's, 62 days.

"We are doing rationing," David told the *Toronto Star* in 1995 with typical bluntness. "Old folks can have an operation all right, but they cost the system immensely more because 10 percent of patients over 80 suffer stroke. If they suffer stroke, you can imagine what it costs the hospital. They can no longer go home so they block a bed permanently." And, Dr. David, what happens to those patients who don't get operated on? "They go home and die, block up a medical bed or have a heart attack."

But David said, "We don't tell them that we don't operate on them because we don't have the money, we tell them we don't think an operation is going to help. But it could potentially."[60] (Nonetheless, the mortality of bypass operations in the elderly was dropping dramatically – and there was actually no clinical reason why they shouldn't get bypass.[61])

David said he felt "'awful' having to make these decisions, saying, 'My gosh, do I ever feel bad. You're playing God, aren't you? We have to play God sometimes, that's decision-making.'"[62] This kind of conversation, of course, would scare the pants off a seventy-six-year-old with a bit of angina and led to renewed pressure to pour resources into cardiac surgery. It was in 1997 that the Institute for Clinical Evaluative Sciences, headed by David Naylor, brought out its report, "Waits and Rates." Under its influence, cardiac surgery expanded and waiting lists shortened. Waiting list deaths for coronary bypass declined from 0.6 per cent in 1996 to 0.3 per cent in 2000.[63]

The needs of cardiac surgery were now desperate. Funding was short, and waiting lists grew. Goldman, chair in 1997 of the Association of Cardiac Surgeons of Toronto, said, "The waiting lists in Ontario are now unacceptable, both in the number of patients (more than 1,000 patients) and the average waiting time (up to six months or more). There is an increase in the number of patients who have died while awaiting surgery." He said that "there are first-rate cardiac teams around this province capable of world-class results." But what was needed was long-term funding.[64] This arrived with the founding in 1997 of the Peter Munk Cardiac Centre (see chapter 22).

Worldwide Reach

David's fame gave him a worldwide reach, as indeed Bigelow had possessed, but magnified this time with technology. In 1991 David began televising operations on closed-circuit television for an international medical audience that would assemble in a lecture hall at the General. An overhead camera would broadcast the operation to the breathless audience, with a running commentary, provided on this particular occasion in June 1991 by Delos Cosgrove who had come up from the Cleveland Clinic. A live audio link between the operating room and Cosgrove on the podium permitted a back-and-forth banter.

"Tirone, it's beautiful," said Cosgrove. "We've got a great view."

This "teleconference" was the first ever staged in Canada, and gave the audience a view of such immediacy that, as reported, "when blood squirted, it looked like a geyser. Some sitting in the front row automatically ducked." That day, David did four different operations, moving from OR to OR. On a following day, further operations were planned.[65] By 1996, David's highly successful biannual interactive live video conferences were attracting more than 250 practising cardiac surgeons internationally.[66]

One peg higher on the international-reach scale was David travelling, often to exotic places, to demonstrate something such as his pigvalve operation, while Goldman commented, "describing each and every step as moderator."[67]

But not only did David do videoconferences and travel; sometimes, patients travelled to David himself! "From every country they come," exulted a journalist. "Kings and queens, princes and potentates, Vatican monsignors and chief rabbis, the most exalted and most humble ... all make the pilgrimage to his surgical theatre. From every country they come, not only for quintuple bypasses and valve replacements, operations that have become almost routine, but for the most complicated, most intricate – the riskiest procedures, consigning their hearts, their very lives, to his remarkable hands."[68] One would wince at such gush, were it not true.

Scully ranked David "among the top five in the world. I consider myself to be a very good heart surgeon, but Tirone's in a league of his own." Said Michael Baker, head of the University Health Network of which the Toronto General Hospital is a part, "We have many brilliant doctors here ... But there are very few where the world literally beats a path the way they do with Tirone. And they're coming from some of the most skilled medical centres in the world. I consider Tirone a genius."[69] (Interestingly, insiders considered Scully a superior bypass surgeon to David; anesthetist Gerry O'Leary said, in an interview, "Hugh Scully's successful bypass rate is very good. I do know that Hugh isn't recognized for how good a bypass surgeon he is, or was. He was good at valves but he was better than Tirone at bypass, and also very good at bypass surgery."[70])

"I used to work longer hours," David confessed in 2001. "There was a time when I lived at the hospital. I came to work on Monday and went home – we lived in Willowdale then – on Saturday. My record was 11 consecutive operations without sleep. Once, I came home, and my daughter Adriane was two and a half, and I drove up and she was looking out the window and I stood up on the car to wave at her, and she ran to tell her mother, 'Mommy, there's a strange man waving at me outside.' It's sad, isn't it? But that was my life."[71]

Yet all this work paid off. As Richard Jonas, vice president of the American Association for Thoracic Surgery, told the audience in 2005 – as David became president – it was well known in Canada that "Wayne Gretzky is the Tirone David of hockey."[72] An observer estimated that David had operated on around 7,500 patients over a twenty-five-year period. "If each of his 7,500 patients has gained, say, an average of 12 years, that's 90,000 bonus years – 90,000 extra birthdays, anniversaries, grandchildren's kisses, walks in the park."[73] This is worth something.

At the time of this writing in 2019, David has no plans for retiring. But when he retires, there may be consequences. Vivek Rao, who succeeded him as head of the Division said, "I think we're going to lose a big area that we may or may not be able to capture, and I think it's a group of patients that no one else wants to do, and those are the multiple-time redos with extensive calcification that need an extensive reconstruction of their heart. He's got a unique capability in getting those patients through the operation. Most of us can't."[74]

Shadow Side of Brilliance?

For all the worldwide wonder that David's virtuosity provoked, there were shadow sides to his often one-person show. In training, for example, some of his residents felt they were not receiving sufficient hands-on instruction; the places at the operating table they should have had were now occupied by the nurses that David brought from the Western and the international fellows who crowded about. The phrase "You guys are now the tour guides" was sardonically repeated.

As well, several staffers deplored the loss of a sense of community the division had once enjoyed under Bigelow and Baird. Bigelow in particular had invited people to his home and encouraged teamwork. David, by contrast, often humiliated in public errant staffers. One female resident was said to have fled the program demoralized and tearful.

Lynda Mickleborough, full of praise for David's technical brilliance as a surgeon, said, "He is not like Ron Baird. He does not have the capability of seeing the division as a whole and nurturing the division as a whole and encouraging people. Now, he never *dis*couraged me, he was always very supportive, but on the other hand he was never really aware of what I was doing, not hands-on, not 'Lynda, what do you need, what might you need.'"[75]

What was the basic problem here – lack of empathy? No, not really. David came from a very hierarchical Brazilian system, where you were compliant with highers-up and often unbridled in criticism of those below you. This is not really the way things were done at the General, and there was probably some cultural dissonance.

Stephanie Brister defended David on the empathy question. "I felt very strongly that we had to treat our fellows fairly, we had to pay them fairly, and I have gone to him on a one-to-one basis: 'We accepted this person, they don't have enough funding, they are here with $15,000, they can't make it, we need money.' And he would come up with the money. There would be no discussion of, no, we need to talk to the other surgeons; he just came up with the money. So if you went to him, you had to make him empathic. You had to give him a reason to care. But, he did."[76]

Chapter Twenty-One

Vivek Rao

Each head of the division has left a distinctive imprint. Murray was too problematic as a personality to have headed anything but he founded cardiac surgery. Under Bigelow it was hypothermia and the pacemaker. Under Baird it was vascular surgery and cardiac transplants. Under the three terms of Tirone David it was new approaches to aneurysms and valves. And under Vivek Rao, who became head in 2011, it was heart failure.

"There are a million people in Canada with heart failure right now," said Barry Rubin in 2017, medical director of the Peter Munk Centre for Cardiac Care at the General. "And this number is going to increase by 25 percent in the next 25 years, so we need to have new approaches ... to deal with that, or else hospitals will be full of people with heart failure."[1]

The larger tableau here is the plateauing of open heart and bypass surgery in the new millennium, to the advantage of new cardiac drugs, stenting, and other "percutaneous" (through the skin) procedures involving catheters. Vivek Rao said, "In the 1990s, a group of anti-cholesterol drugs called statins significantly lowered the progression of disease, while percutaneous or minimally-invasive therapies, such as [balloon] angioplasty and stenting, provided alternatives to opening up the chest ... Today, many patients opt for angioplasty and stenting."[2] These latter techniques were done by cardiologists, not cardiac surgeons. These techniques had the advantage of democratizing cardiac care to the vastly expanding aging demographic. They had the disadvantage of sometimes requiring redos.

Early Years

Born in India, Rao came to Canada as a small child, and, as he puts it, "I've basically lived in Toronto for most of my life since then, so Toronto born and bred."[3]

His father was a nuclear engineer, his mother a forensic pathologist. In arriving in Canada, the family was a bit uncertain about what educational arrangements to make for their children. So to give their son a leg up, the family put Viv in Upper Canada College on a scholarship; UCC is an elite private school where Rao boarded. (The family lived in Burlington.) UCC is a very sports-minded place, and Rao played cricket the entire five years he was there, and captained the basketball and volleyball teams as well.

Was the UCC background helpful to him? "Very few UCC graduates go into medicine," he said. "They're mostly all shunted into business or finance – but in a lot of circles I travel in now, where we're fundraising, being a UCC grad had been a little bit helpful to me because you go into a room and I've never met you, but 'Oh, you went to UCC, what year were you?' and there's automatically a connection point."

Why cardiac surgery? "My family has a long history of physicians on both sides. My mother's first cousin is a pediatric heart surgeon in India, so I had some exposure to cardiac surgery through him. In my early years I had some difficulty deciding between neurosurgery and cardiac surgery. I knew I wanted to be a surgeon. I just couldn't figure out which organ. I figured that with neurosurgery you'd have no idea if it worked for months or years, whereas cardiac surgery had that immediate gratification."

Rao studied medicine at Toronto, graduating in 1996, then trained in cardiovascular sciences under Bernie Goldman at Sunnybrook. He also enrolled in the Surgeon Scientist Program under Richard Weisel. As a PhD student, he led a study of the outcomes of combined lung cancer surgery and heart surgery. The view had been that simultaneous cardiac procedures lessened the prognosis of the cancer patients. But after examining the records of thirty patients who'd had the combined procedure at the General between 1982 and 1995, the investigators found the five-year survival of the combined patients was 73 per cent, versus the actuarial survival of patients with malignant disease of 64 per cent at five years.[4]

Rao's interest in heart failure started to percolate under Christopher Feindel. In 1997 on the transplant side, as a research fellow at the General during his PhD program, Rao helped Feindel, surgical director of the heart-transplant program, improve a vastly vexing problem in procuring donor hearts: With previous techniques, the heart would last up to four hours only in transit, which ruled out using donors in the Maritimes for heart patients in Vancouver. The investigators found that perfusing the heart in a sack with the donor's own blood doubled the permitted transit time to eight hours.[5]

A year at Columbia from 2000 to 2001 under Mehmet Oz followed, where Rao became interested in the mechanical assistance of patients in heart failure who were waiting for cardiac transplants. It was this expertise that he then brought back to Toronto. The choice of heart failure was, as Rao later put it, "a little bit opportunistic. I looked around and I saw that going forward at TGH specifically they could use someone who had a dedicated focus in transplantation because although Chris [Feindel] was doing it, he was doing it because no one else wanted it at the time. He said to me, 'As soon as you're finished [at Columbia] I want you to take over the transplant program, because I've been doing it for ten years and I don't want to do it anymore.'"

Then, as Rao was getting set to return to Toronto from Columbia, Tirone David said, "'One of the things we want for a transplant program is a VAD program,' because at the time – around 2000 – it was part and parcel of the concept."[6] (VAD stands for ventricular assist device, and it is an artificial heart, in a sense: patients can be kept alive with a VAD until they can have a transplant. On the US origins of these devices, see Shelley McKellar's excellent study, *Artificial Hearts*.[7])

The era of sending recent trainees to Bristol or to US centres had, on the whole, now passed. "In cardiac no one went anywhere because Tirone thought this was the centre of the universe, so why should we go anywhere else to learn heart surgery?"

But transplant and VAD were different. Rao told David, "The one thing you guys don't do here was VADs." David said Rao had a choice between Stanford and New York, and Rao chose New York "as a matter of convenience, to be honest with you, because New York was an easier commute than Stanford." Some ground laying for the LVAD program was necessary, and in 1999 to 2001 Chris Feindel spent two years at Harvard earning a MSc in healthcare management. As part of the program he had to organize a special project at his home institution, and he laid the basis for the arrival of the LVAD at Toronto, under Rao. (The "L" means left, assisting the left heart.[8])

This story is actually a little more complicated. When Rao was still a resident at Sunnybrook, Goldman offered him a job, and copied the letter to David, then head of the hospital division. "That got Tirone all flustered and he dragged me into his office," Rao said.

DAVID: What is *this*!
RAO: What is it! I got a letter from Dr. Goldman saying he wants me on staff at Sunnybrook.
DAVID: I thought you wanted to do transplant?
RAO: I do, but you haven't given me a job offer, so I have to consider what's on my plate.

"And so," Rao continued, "very soon after that – like, literally twenty-four hours – he drafted an offer letter saying, 'Sign on the dotted line. I'm sending you to New York, and you can come back and work for me.' Okay."

When Rao joined the Division of Cardiac Surgery in 2001 it was as their youngest recruit ever. He had an awe-inspiring figure, Tirone David, looking over his shoulder, because if you count David's chiefship at the Western and then three terms at TGH, he had been in office for twenty years. "I thought we did stagnate a little bit," said Rao, "because the last ten or fifteen years it totally became about what was best for the valve program. I think he just got into a rut, and it was just this [valves] is what we're doing. Our volumes were falling so we weren't recruiting new people; we didn't have any new blood. Whereas the first thing I did when I became chief was to hire Maral [Ouzounian] and hire Mitesh [Badiwala]."

At the time of Rao's arrival, heart transplantation was out of the hands of the cardiac surgeons (David had little interest in it), and being run by a nephrologist at the Western, Carl Cardella. Then the program transited to cardiologist Paul Daly, "but again," said Rao, "Paul was an interventional cardiologist, and, very much like Chris [Feindel], he did it because he was told to, and didn't have a huge interest in it."

The VAD, and Other Life-Saving Devices

Then the Division of Cardiology hired Heather Ross, who was fully trained in transplant. Rao said, "She came here and she just basically rewrote the book on how we manage patients, how we select them and how we treat them post-op. She was the first one to say, 'We need a VAD program here.'" The VAD was used in three different situations: for acute support in heart failure following major heart attacks or after cardiac surgery; in transplantation support to bridge the patient until a new heart becomes available; and in destination therapy, where the patients are not candidates for transplantation but can be maintained indefinitely on a VAD.

On arrival, in 2001 Rao introduced Canada's first HeartMate artificial heart program with Thoratec's assist device HeartMate I, which became the largest ventricular-assist-device program in the country. (On a predecessor of this assist device that surgeons Hugh Scully and Robert Kormos introduced in 1983, see "A Very Early Assist Device" in chapter 11.) The LVAD itself reached Canada around November 2001 in the person of Rao's patient Mike Schmidt of Kitchener, who was within hours of death before Rao implanted the device. Schmidt, forty-seven, who had been so short of breath that he couldn't even brush his teeth, said two weeks after the operation, "So far, it's great. I haven't been able to breathe like this in years. I can't wait to play golf."[9]

In March 2002, the *Globe and Mail* featured a beaming Leona Parsons, who, with little hope of survival from her myocarditis, had received in December 2001 a HeartMate I; three months later, her heart recovered sufficiently, and she was able to have it removed. Rao said, "This is an exciting development in heart failure surgery," and the journalist added, "The unusual move raises the prospect that ... a failing heart can fully recover if it is given time to rest and repair itself." (At that point, only a third of assist-device patients survived the explant; a third died, and a third received heart transplants.)[10]

In 2006 the second HeartMate edition was introduced, the first continuous flow VAD in Canada.[11] The Munk Centre was the first site in North America for the launch of this device, the HeartMate II Pocket Controller,[12] and Rao at TGH participated in the trials. The following year, 2007, the Levacor VAD (from World Heart Corp) arrived in Toronto. The year 2010 saw the arrival of the HeartWare HVAD, and in 2014 the CE Mark HeartMate3 underwent its first Canadian trials at the General.

On 31 October 2014, Rao implanted in Robert Power the HeartMate III.[13] Rao said, "Robert's options were rapidly running out and given the increasingly weak state of his health, a transplant was simply not an option. Having this type of assist device available to support the pumping of blood from Robert's heart was really his only lifeline." After the operation, Robert's wife, Gail, said, "There really wasn't much of anything that Robert could do anymore. I've seen a big change in him in such a short time. And he smiles a lot more now."[14]

Rao was thus among the leading international trialists of these devices that allowed a weary heart to restore its energies and made it possible for patients to avoid a transplant.[15] Canadian VAD centres grew from five in 2001 to eleven in 2019, implanting at total of 125 VADs a year. At the General, survival in patients with previously shattering conditions had started to look up: by around 2017, survival in cardiogenic shock was 35 per cent; and myocarditis, 66 per cent – both previously high-mortality conditions. The goal was, as Rao put it, "to unload the heart for rest and recovery."

It was only in 2010 that Ministry of Health funding of these expensive devices began, which previously at the Munk Centre had been paid for by private charity.

Rao presided over the introduction of several other leading-edge therapies for patients who otherwise would have died. Post-cardiotomy, some patients went into shock and died of cardiogenic shock. Fewer than 25 per cent were ever discharged. Under Rao, extracorporeal membrane oxygenation was instigated for these patients. It involved a complicated apparatus on a pushcart that patients, now freed of intubation, could push around the ward. Extracorporeal life support (ECLS) meant a variety of devices, one of which (Novalung), the innovative chest surgeon, and professor of surgery Shaf Keshavjee had pioneered for blowing off carbon dioxide. If patients at other hospitals needed to be transferred (via helicopter) to the General for ECLS, the Big Hospital would send a "ECLS retrieval team," with an ICU physician, an ECLS surgeon, and a perfusion fellow – all of whom would remove the tubes (cannulation) the patient had received locally and transfer him or her to the Medical Surgical Intensive Care Unit (MSICU) at the General.

Rao himself in 2002 became surgical director of cardiac transplantation, in 2007 the De Gasperis Chair in Heart Failure Surgery, and in 2011 chief of the Division of Cardiac Surgery.

The VADs cost $100,000 apiece. They were definitely not in anybody's budget. The Ontario Heart Foundation wouldn't fund them, and Tirone David told Viv Rao, "This is your program so you need to go out and meet the donors and beg for the money." Rao recalls his response: "Fine. So I went to cocktail parties and shook hands and tried to get $100,000 per device." Rao succeeded. The Toronto VAD program became the largest in Canada. In 2010 Ministry of Health, as mentioned, stepped up to the plate, and in 2012, the ministry began funding the bridging concept. So Rao went "back out on the cocktail circuit, saying, 'These other people aren't getting transplants and need devices, and we want to offer this to our patients because it's being offered in America.'" In 2018 the ministry began funding VADs for non-transplant patients.

For Rao's work on the VAD and for his aura of general dynamism, he became one of Canada's "Top 40 Under 40," a program for identifying future Canadian leaders. Thoracic surgeon Shaf Keshavjee and pediatric neurosurgeon Peter Dirks preceded him on this list.

In these proceedings, it became apparent that there was another aspect to Rao's life apart from cardiac surgery: He sponsored an Olympic athlete, Joe Montgomery, who was a member of the Canadian bobsled team. It was reported that "[Rao] was disturbed by learning how poorly Canadian Olympic athletes are supported and resolved to replace their Wal-Mart jobs with personal support so they could devote adequate time to preparing for their events."[16]

The force driving the adoption of the LVAD in Canada was a US study, in which Rao had taken part, assessing the LVAD in end-stage heart failure patients who were ineligible for a transplant. Sixty-eight

LVAD patients were compared to sixty-one patients on "optimal medical management." The results were stunning. The LVAD group had a 48 per cent reduction in the risk of death from any cause. The survival at one year was 52 per cent in the device group versus 25 per cent in the medical-therapy group.[17]

With the LVADs making it possible to wait peacefully for the ideal donor heart to come along, the General's cardiac transplant program achieved a 90 per cent five-year survival rate, as opposed to 75 to 80 per cent for the rest of Canada, "Once an advanced heart failure patient comes to PMCC," said Rao, "they're here for life." They selected their patients carefully, treated them with multidisciplinary teams, and gave long-term follow-up care.[18]

Krystina Henneker of Hamilton, Ontario, became one of Viv Rao's patients at twenty-four. Her heart was four sizes too big for her. At fourteen, she had seen her mother, age twenty-nine, die of cardiomyopathy: an enlarged heart, the same condition that Krystina had.

In the spring of 2010, Krystina "felt extremely tired, for days on end. It went on for a couple of weeks," reported a journalist. "She could hardly make it up the stairs." She was diagnosed locally with "a rapid heart rate," then transferred to the General in Toronto, "where they discovered the enlarged heart."

What to do? Wait for a new heart while on the transplant list? Rao said that "one in 10 will die waiting for a heart. So most likely she would have died within 10 weeks had we not intervened." They decided to implant an LVAD, and on 11 June 2010 Rao's team inserted the device.

Krystina became "the only person in Hamilton with an LVAD." She went to the closest EMS station to let them know, should she need to call for help. There were backup plans in the event of a prolonged power outage. (The device has to be recharged daily.)

"At first Krystina was uneasy with it all, this machine keeping her heart going, and having to go out in public with the wires and battery pack front and centre. 'I was wondering if people were staring at me, at my fanny pack holding the batteries.'"

"It's tough knowing someone has to die to save my daughter," said her stepmother. "Emotionally, that's a difficult thing to deal with. We will rejoice when she gets a heart, but a family will suffer."

Rao said it was not uncommon for a patient to opt for continuing to wear the LVAD rather than get a new heart. He said, "There are 50 patients out there who have worn an LVAD for more than five years."[19]

Mitesh Badiwala completed his residency in cardiac surgery at Toronto in 2012. Working in Rao's lab in the Surgeon Scientist Program, he went on to earn a PhD in 2013. He also became the go-to guy in harvesting donors' hearts. With a Detweiler Travelling Fellowship, he fellowed for a further year at Northwestern University learning valve repair under Patrick McCarthy. He joined the cardiac surgery staff at the General in 2014, and the following year became director of the cardiac transplant program. Thus, Badiwala was in on the ground floor with the LVAD.

The VAD was transformative. If you needed a heart, and one wasn't available, there were not many options. Badiwala recalled from around 2007, "a young man in his 20s landing on [my] operating table." Badiwala said, "His skin was dry, he was really sick. We couldn't get a heart for him. Because he was too sick to wait, we put a [LVAD] pump into him. And that in and of itself transformed him." He was able "to walk around with a backpack controlling the loud pump ... Seeing him get better with the pump was an eye-opener for me – a guy who was almost dead being kept alive with a pump."[20]

That was a first-generation pump. Then successive generations of pumps began to shrink in size, migrating from a backpack to a cartridge that can fit in the same sack as the heart (the pericardium).

In April 2005 after her exams, an exhausted Sally Fung became terribly tired. She told her boyfriend she couldn't breathe. It was 1 a.m. He insisted they go to the hospital. At the Markham Stouffville Hospital there were almost no doctors, and her only real symptom was plunging blood pressure. "They didn't want to admit me," she remembers.

But her boyfriend persisted. "She doesn't look right. You need to examine her."

They admitted her to the ICU, where she was given an ultrasound of her stomach. The doctor told her, "Since we're here, I'll ultrasound your heart, too."

The decision saved her life. Her heart was swollen. "I've never ever seen such a big heart," he said.

Now things started happening. At 3 a.m. technicians were called in to perform a CT scan, and her records were put together for the one-hour ambulance trip to the Munk Centre. "It's not that I feel they saved my life," she later said. "I *know* that they saved my life."

Said Vivek Rao, "When she arrived, I was worried she wouldn't make it to the operating room in time." They put her at once on the LVAD. Both of her ventricles had stopped working, and the LVAD was "doing all the work." Many such patients would have received a transplant, but Fung's own heart recovered and took over in less than two weeks. She stayed at the Munk Centre for six weeks, then went home well. "Life is normal now," she said a decade later.[21]

Destination Therapy

Rao was on the cusp of the ever-improving mechanical heart wave. As the devices got steadily better, they started increasingly to seem as alternatives to a heart transplant, not just stopgaps. Rao said in 2007, that mechanical hearts are rapidly becoming a "destination therapy" rather than a mere bridge. A heart transplant would have a normal life expectancy of about ten years, a LVAD device about the same length.[22]

In 2016 Rao, as part of a cross-Canada team, reported on the results of an LVAD manufactured under the HeartWare label called HeartWare HVAD. This was one of a variety of LVADs on the market. From its introduction in 2010 until 2016, 137 patients had been implanted with an HVAD device, with the idea of bridging to transplant (at that point 65 were transplanted with new hearts). Of the 137, 29 had died on support, with an average survival of 231 days. The others were either still on HVAD support or had had the devices removed for one reason or another. The authors concluded that "the HVAD constitutes an important tool in the management of end-stage heart failure patients that are awaiting transplant."[23]

The mortality statistics remain considerable. Yet virtually all of these patients would have died in the days before transplant and assist devices.

In heart failure, Rao did not limit himself to VADs. After Lynda Mickleborough retired in 2003, he inherited all the left ventricular aneurysms and bad ventricles. In 2017 Rao concluded that in patients who had already sustained significant damage – with enlarged hearts and low ejection fractions – bypass surgery could be life saving, and that surgical "remodelling" of the left ventricle might also contribute a benefit, though this was less certain.[24] But in the management of heart failure, as opposed to acute heart attacks, it was all a new departure.

Tirone David was a support, and sometimes a hindrance, for the new head. "All the functional MRs [mitral regurgitation] with bad ventricles that Tirone didn't want to repair, he sent over to me," said Rao. But David was set against microsurgery. Rao said, "When the biggest valve surgeon in your institution doesn't believe in minimally invasive valve surgery, it's very hard for a junior surgeon to come and launch that."

What does Rao see as his own legacy? "I reinvigorated the heart failure program here, took over from what Lynda [Mickleborough] did, expanded into artificial hearts and transplants. I'm happy to say that Mitesh Badiwala took the baton from me and moved the programs even farther ahead, and we're doing some stuff that has never been done before. I'd like to say that I established UHN-PMCC as a heart failure centre of excellence, building on the reputation that Tirone had on valve surgery, and Baird had in vascular surgery, and Bigelow had in heart surgery generally."

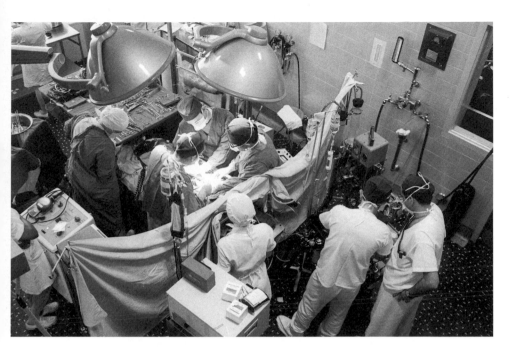

Plate 1 Cardiac surgeon Wilfred G. Bigelow (dark cap and glasses at right) and team operating in one of the twin Pavilion Operating Rooms (PORs) on the ninth floor of the University Wing (Private Patients Pavilion) at TGH, 14 March 1972. Photograph by Robert Lansdale. (UTARMS, LAN72071–079, Robert Lansdale Photography fonds)

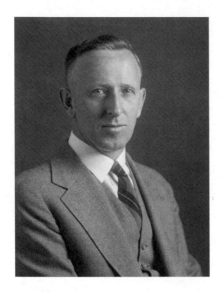

Plate 2 Gordon Murray, 1930s. Following extensive surgical training in North America and the UK, Gordon Murray became a staff surgeon at the Toronto General Hospital in 1929. He quickly established a reputation for technical brilliance, setting the stage for cardiovascular surgery by pioneering the development and clinical use of the anticoagulant heparin. (UTARMS, 2011–26-IMS)

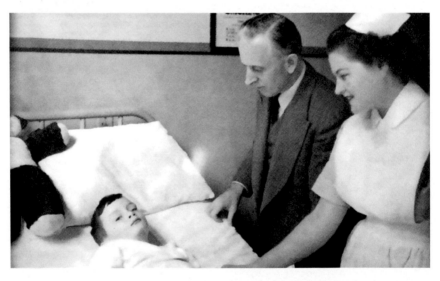

Plate 3 Gordon Murray, the "blue baby" surgeon. Unlike subsequent generations of cardiovascular and cardiac specialists, Murray remained a general surgeon throughout his career. Yet by introducing the new "blue baby" operation at TGH in the years after the Second World War, he paved the way for the new field of cardiac surgery in Toronto. (Gordon Murray, *Medicine in the Making* [1965])

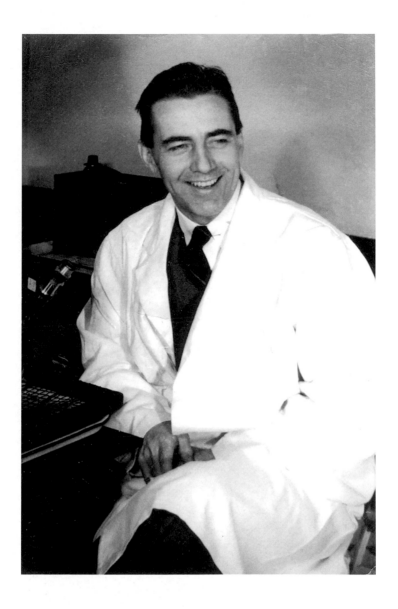

Plate 4 Wilfred G. "Uncle Bill" Bigelow. Following Gordon Murray's resignation in November 1953, Bigelow became the chief of Ward C. Under his leadership the golden age of cardiac surgery as a team effort was launched with his pioneering use of hypothermia. (Bigelow fonds)

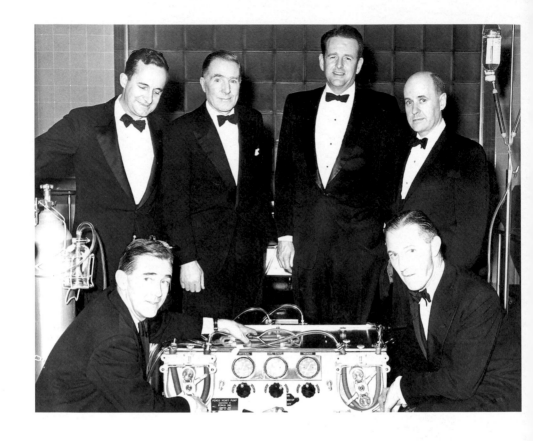

Plate 5 The new CV Unit opens, 1962; commercial heart-lung pumps are
introduced. Bill Bigelow and Jim Key kneel beside the new Pemco heart-lung
pump at the official opening of TGH's expanded Cardiovascular Surgical Unit
in January 1962. Joining them in the celebration are TGH heart surgeon Ray
Heimbecker, Frederick Kergin, head of the Department of Surgery, and two
special guests: pioneer heart surgeons Henry Swan from Denver and Edouard
Gagnon from Montreal. (Photograph by Bill Cole; originally published in W.G.
Bigelow, *Cold Hearts: The Story of Hypothermia and the Pacemaker in Heart Surgery*
[Toronto: McClelland and Stewart, 1984], fig. 9, p.127)

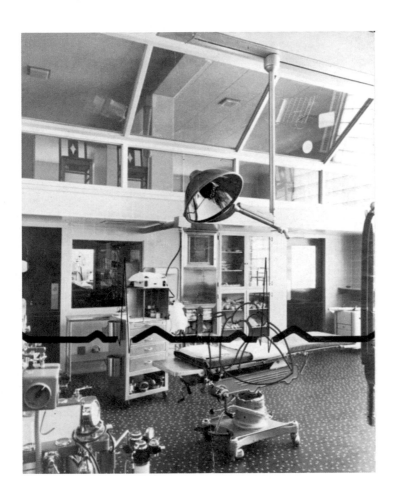

Plate 6 One of the two new PORs on the ninth floor of the Private Patients
Pavilion, 1962, featuring its advanced equipment and observation gallery.
(Photograph by Andrew Smith, PANDA, from the "Souvenir Programme,
Official Opening of the Cardiovascular Surgical Unit of the Toronto General
Hospital, January 19th, 1962," ed. James A. Key; Hugh Scully collection)

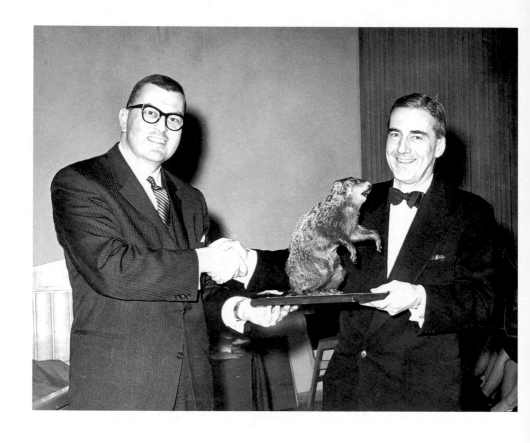

Plate 7 The "Hibernin" fiasco. John McBirnie, the first of numerous fellows assigned to the hibernation project, later presented Bigelow with a stuffed groundhog in tribute to the failed experiments. (Photograph by Bill Cole; Bigelow fonds)

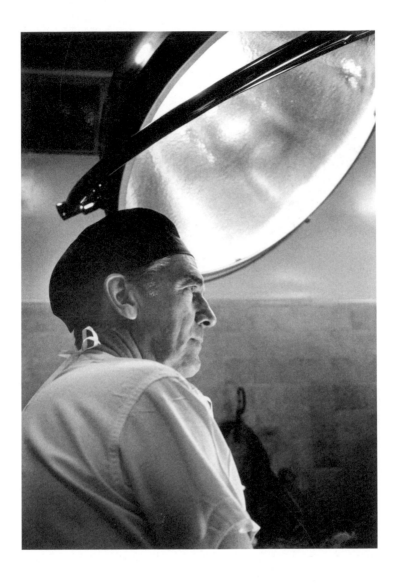

Plate 8 Bigelow as the mature master surgeon, 1972. He stepped down in 1977, and during his retirement wrote important histories of his experiences with hypothermia and the pacemaker (*Cold Hearts*, 1984) and the development of heparin (*Mysterious Heparin*, 1990). (Photograph by Robert Lansdale, UTARMS, 2014–37-SMS)

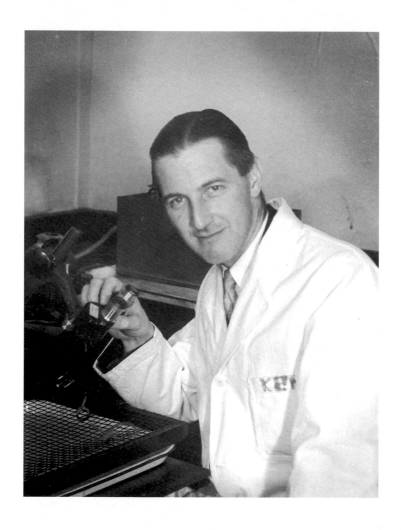

Plate 9 James A. Key, "Gentleman Jim." Scottish-born Jim Key joined the
new cardiovascular team at TGH in 1953, becoming Bigelow's close personal
friend as well as his first colleague on the service. In addition to being a skilled
surgeon and a gifted clinical teacher, Key was an accomplished concert-level
pianist. (Bigelow fonds)

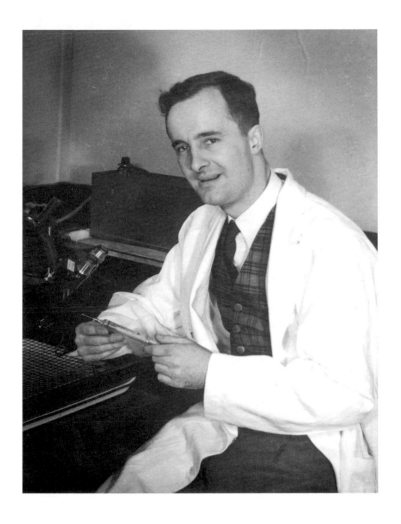

Plate 10 Raymond O. Heimbecker. Heimbecker was added to the team in 1955 and became Bigelow's closest early collaborator. In 1974 he went on to head the cardiac service at Western University, where he performed Canada's first heart transplant with the immunosuppressant cyclosporine. (Bigelow fonds)

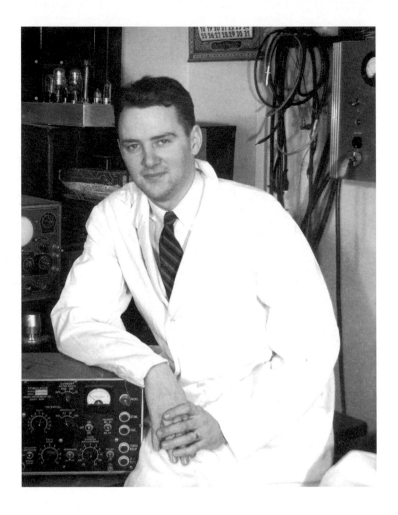

Plate 11 John C. Callaghan. Surgical resident John Callaghan entered
Bigelow's research lab reluctantly, yet ended up taking charge of the project
that resulted in the first cardiac pacemaker in 1950.Seen here with the team's
Grass stimulator, which could re-start a stopped heart but was not a pacemaker.
Following his training, Callaghan became a founding member of the Division
of Cardiac and Thoracic Surgery at the University of Alberta, performing
Canada's first on-pump heart operation in 1956. (Bigelow fonds)

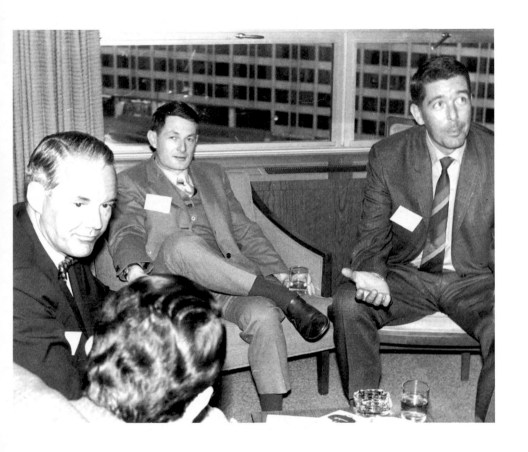

Plate 12 George Trusler, Will Keon, and Al Trimble, 1970. Three of Bigelow's
trainees, seen at a meeting in Washington, DC, April 1970. George Trusler
(left), a student of both Murray and Bigelow, became a distinguished pediatric
cardiac surgeon at Toronto's Hospital for Sick Children. Wilbert Keon (centre)
founded the University of Ottawa Heart Institute. Alan Trimble (right) was
noted for his surgical brilliance and research innovations as a member of the
Cardiovascular Service in the 1960s and 1970s. (Bigelow fonds)

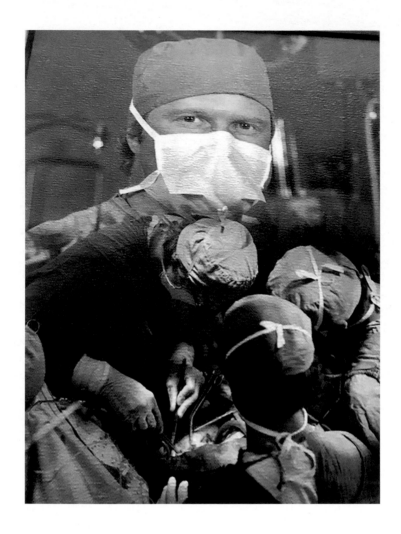

Plate 13 Photo montage of Hugh Scully by motorsport and Olympic
photographer Allan de la Plante, 1970s. This shot was taken from the
observation gallery above the cardiac PORs on the ninth floor of the former
University Wing/Private Patients Pavilion. (Photograph by Allan de la Plante;
Courtesy of Hugh Scully)

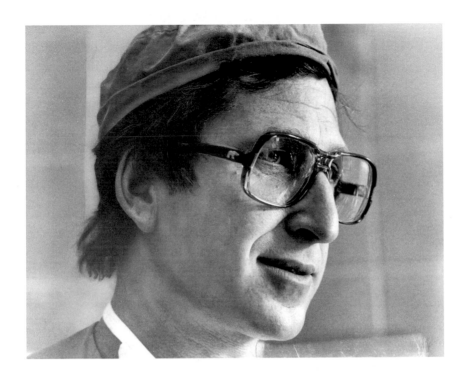

Plate 14 Bernie Goldman, 1980. Bernie Goldman became a staff surgeon
at TGH on 1 July 1968, after returning from Boston and Bristol, England,
on a McLaughlin Surgical Fellowship. He is seen here in November 1980
after performing one of the last heart operations on the ninth floor of the
University Wing (a valve implantation) before the division's move to the newly
constructed Eaton Wing. (Photograph by Dick Loek / *Toronto Star* via Getty
Images)

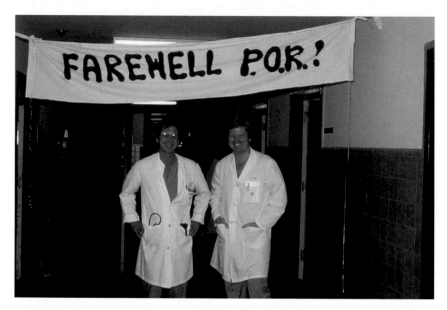

PLATE 15 "Farewell POR!" Goldman and Scully pose outside the ninth floor Pavilion Operating Rooms after completing the two final heart procedures done there before the facility was decommissioned in November 1980. (Courtesy of Hugh Scully)

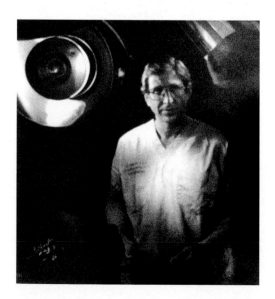

Plate 16 Goldman in the Eaton Wing OR, 1980s. In 1989 Goldman left TGH to become the inaugural head of the cardiac surgery unit at Sunnybrook Health Science Centre. The new unit was created to help relieve long wait times for treatment. (Courtesy of Bernard Goldman)

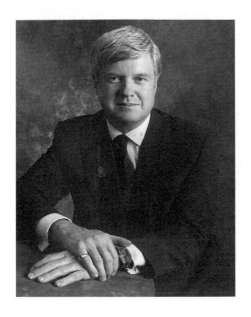

Plate 17 Hugh Scully, 1988. Unlike most academic surgeons, Hugh Scully has had a long parallel career in medical leadership and activism. In July 1987 he was elected president of the Ontario Medical Association during a fierce battle over "extra billing," and effectively terminated a strike when some physicians advocated limiting hospital emergency services. (Photograph by David Street, Toronto)

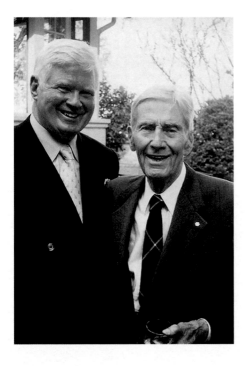

Plate 18 Scully presents Bigelow with the Canadian Medical Association's Starr medal, its top honour, in 1992. Scully: "For me this is a very poignant picture … for the last seven to eight years of his life, I would pick Bill Bigelow up, stay by his side at social functions, and get him home early and safely. He was becoming more frail, but for this event he was engaged and energetic!!!" (Courtesy of Hugh Scully)

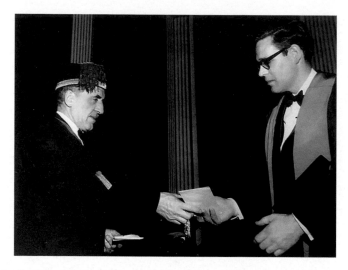

Plate 19 Bigelow (left) presents his colleague Ron Baird with the Royal College's Medal in Surgery, its highest award, at its 1969 meeting in Vancouver. (Courtesy of Hugh Scully)

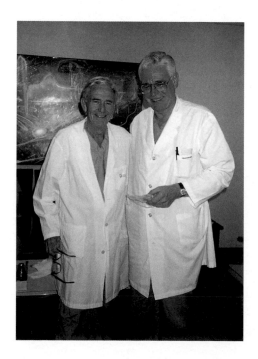

Plate 20 Ron Baird (right) succeeded Bigelow as head of cardiovascular surgery at TGH in 1977. He became known as an innovative vascular surgeon and a leader in valvular surgery and heart transplantation. (Courtesy of Hugh Scully)

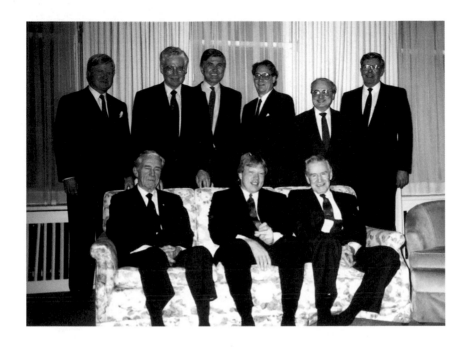

Plate 21 A historic moment: the Division of Cardiovascular Surgery gathers at the Faculty Club, 1988. Standing: Hugh Scully, Ronald Baird, Tirone David, Richard Weisel, Irving Lipton, Alan Trimble. Seated: W.G. Bigelow, Xavier Mousset (senior fellow), Donald Wilson (former university chair of surgery). Bigelow and Wilson were retired, and Baird was completing his term as chief. (Courtesy of Hugh Scully)

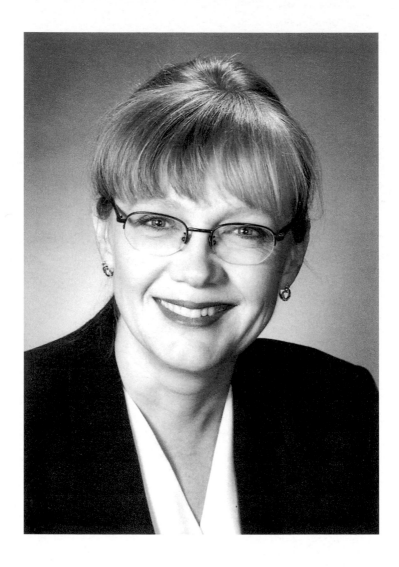

Plate 22 Lynda Mickleborough. A star of the McGill training program, Lynda
Mickleborough came to Toronto in 1980 as a fellow. She went on to became a
pioneer of left ventricular reconstruction in patients with chronic heart failure.
(Courtesy of Lynda Mickleborough)

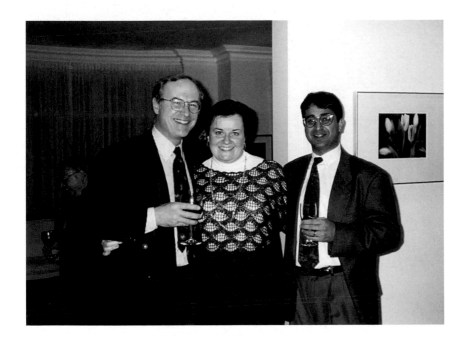

Plate 23 Christopher Feindel (left) became a master of reconstructing heart damage so severe that the cases were dubbed UFOs. With him and nurse Vicki Morley is thoracic surgeon Shaf Keshavjee, now surgeon-in-chief at UHN and creator of its world-famous lung transplantation program. (Courtesy of Hugh Scully)

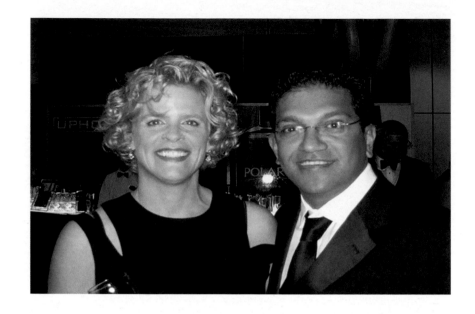

Plate 24 Two leaders of the present Peter Munk Cardiac Centre: Heather
Ross, head of the Division of Cardiology and leader of its Ted Rogers Centre of
Excellence in Heart Function, and Vivek Rao, head of the Division of Cardiac
Surgery. (Courtesy of Heather Ross)

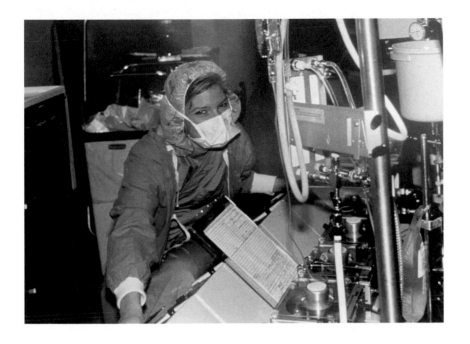

Plate 25 Open-heart surgery has always required the special skills of a perfusionist. Here, TGH perfusionist Kathy Deemar is running the heart bypass pump in the OR. (Courtesy of Michael Aubin, Michener Institute of Education at UHN)

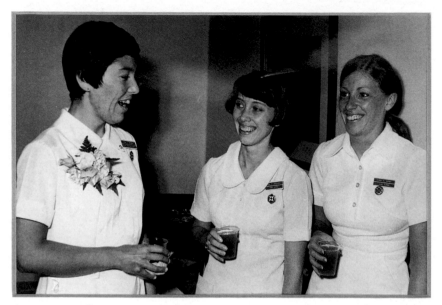

Joan Breakey   *Karen Abourbih*   *Carol Moran*

"*The First Team – 1976*"

Plate 26 Nurses as traffic wardens. In 1972 Joan Breakey became head nurse
for the cardiovascular service. She warned the surgeons that TGH lacked the
bed space to take on a heavier patient load (a recurring problem). This photo
was taken at a birthday celebration in her honour. (Bigelow fonds)

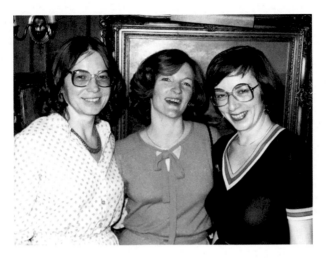

Plate 27 Nurses as teachers. Three successive head nurses: Claudia Koropecki (L), Pat Turner (R), and Jessie McMillan. Scully recalls that as a junior surgeon Koropecki would quietly take him aside and say "Dr. Scully, there is a way of approaching this, and I suggest you do this." (Courtesy of Hugh Scully)

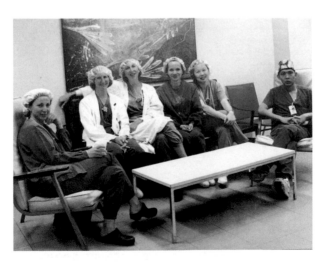

Plate 28 Nurses taking a break. Leda Parente, Joanne Bos, Heidi Duringer, Mercedes Koh, Ester Ko, and Ferdu Datu. (Courtesy of Hugh Scully)

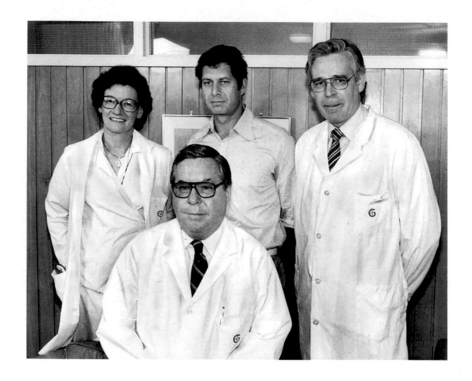

Plate 29 Cardiac anesthetist Sallie Teasdale was on the team that successfully
performed a simultaneous open heart operation and Caesarian delivery in
1981. Teasdale described the case as requiring subtle use of anesthesia to avoid
harming the baby. With Teasdale are pediatrician Hartley Garfield, Ronald
Baird, chief of cardiovascular surgery, and (front) John Harkins, chief of
obstetrics and gynaecology. (Photograph by Ron Bull / *Toronto Star* via Getty
Images)

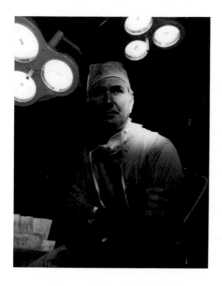

Plate 30 Tirone David in the OR, 1995. Tirone David headed the division for an unprecedented three terms, becoming world-renowned for his technical brilliance and innovative approach to heart surgery. (Photograph by Boris Spremo / *Toronto Star* via Getty Images)

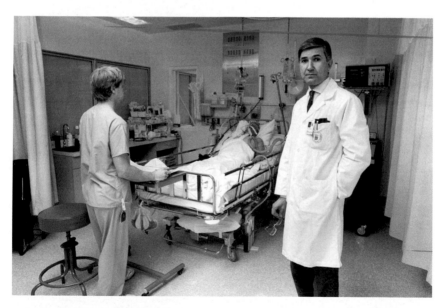

Plate 31 The waiting list crisis, 1988. Long waiting lists for cardiac surgery have been a recurring problem, dating back to the Bigelow era of the late 1950s and early 1960s. In 1988 division chief Tirone David spoke out in the *Toronto Star* about patients dying or suffering strokes while awaiting surgery. (Photograph by Mike Slaughter / *Toronto Star* via Getty Images)

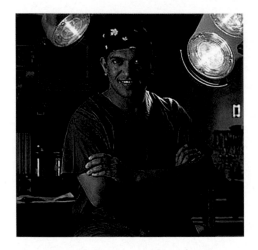

Plate 32 Vivek Rao, a specialist in cardiac transplantation and mechanical circulatory support in heart failure, has been head of the division since 2011. (Courtesy of Vivek Rao)

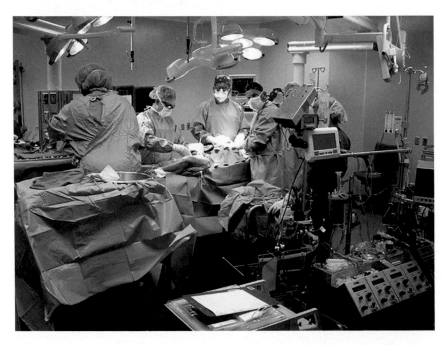

Plate 33 Cardiac surgery today, showing the position of the heart-lung pump (foreground). Rao is in the centre (red cap), accompanied by Wojciech Kaflinski-(blue cap), turned toward the photographer, and Yong Sung (regular OR cap). (Courtesy of Vivek Rao)

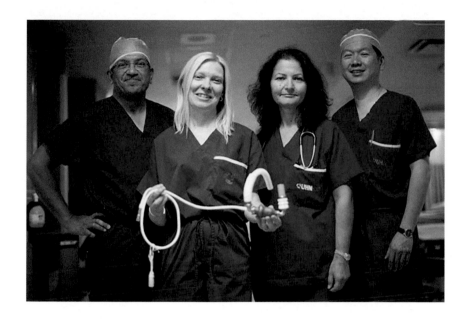

Plate 34 The LVAD program. Rao introduced LVAD (left ventricular assist device) technology to UHN as a bridge to transplantation or for ongoing use in patients ineligible for transplant. Here he is joined by nurse-practitioners Marnie (holding the device) and Phyllis, and cardiac surgeon Terrence Yau. (Courtesy of Vivek Rao)

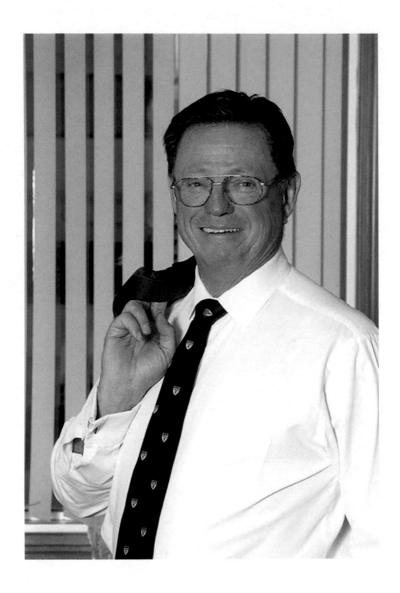

Plate 35 Alan Hudson, President and CEO of UHN, 1991–2000. It was at Hudson's home that philanthropist Peter Munk met Tirone David for the first time. Munk was so impressed by the surgeon returning to the hospital to care for a patient that he began supporting the heart centre that came to bear his name. (Courtesy of Alan Hudson)

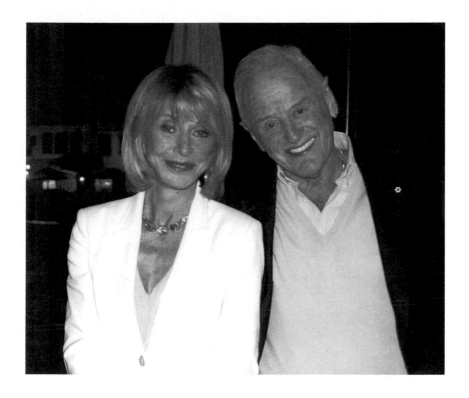

Plate 36 Peter and Melanie Munk. In May 1997 the new Peter Munk Cardiac Centre opened in the Gerrard Wing of TGH. The couple donated $6 million of the $25 million cost, and its grand lobby was created by Melanie's favourite interior designer, Robert Noakes of Toronto. (Melanie Munk)

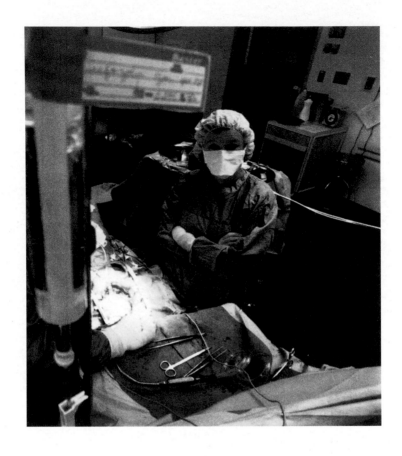

Plate 37 Stephanie Brister spent her surgical and research career at the Munk Centre, where she also played a major role in training fellows and residents. Like her colleagues Goldman and Scully, Brister was known for keeping a cool head during emergencies. (Courtesy Stephanie Brister)

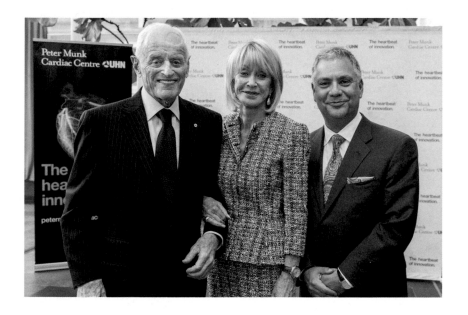

Plate 38 Munk donates $100 million to PMCC. In 2017, UHN announced
a landmark gift of $100 million from Peter Munk, bringing the family's
donations to a total of $175 million. Here, Peter and Melanie Munk make
the announcement along with Barry Rubin, head of the Peter Munk Cardiac
Centre. (Courtesy of Barry Rubin)

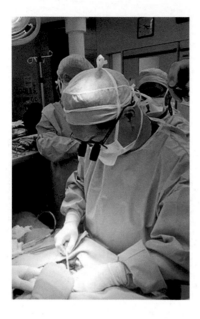

Plate 39 Terrence Yau carrying out a stem cell infusion at UHN, a major advance. He performed Ontario's first stem cell cardiac procedure in 2012. Yau is the current university chair of cardiac surgery. (Courtesy of Vivek Rao)

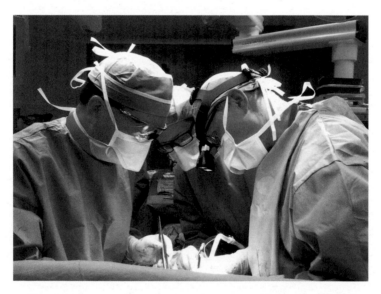

Plate 40 R.J. Cusimano and Yau performing heart surgery. Like several of his colleagues, Cusimano developed a reputation for finding innovative surgical solutions for difficult cases. (Courtesy of Hugh Scully)

Chapter Twenty-Two

The Peter Munk Cardiac Centre

Alan Hudson

This story begins with hard-driving Alan Hudson, formerly chief of neurosurgery at St. Michael's Hospital and chair of the University Department of Neurosurgery, who became surgeon-in-chief at the Toronto Hospital in 1989 and president and CEO in 1991.[1] Hudson, who graduated in medicine in Cape Town in 1960, interned with surgeon Christiaan Barnard – who of course did the world's first heart transplant – and at Barnard's urging he almost went into cardiac surgery himself. But fate intervened. After training in general surgery in London – and writing his fellowship in Edinburgh – Hudson fell in love in London with a Toronto woman. They decided to relocate to Toronto, and he got a post at the Children's Hospital. He worked for six months with Bruce Hendrick, head of neurosurgery, "and what he did was that he intercepted my application, crossed out general surgery, and wrote in neurosurgery." So that was the end of cardiac for Hudson. He spent the next twenty-five years at St. Mike's, where "goddamn General Hospital was one word."

We're in the late 80s. The merger of the Toronto General and Western was in progress, creating the "Toronto Hospital." Not surprisingly, that name aroused political tensions with the other teaching hospitals in Toronto. These hospitals were justifiably proud of their good reputations as teaching hospitals and resented the perceived arrogance of the claim to be "The" Toronto Hospital.

After an open international search, Alan Hudson, who had been head of neurosurgery at St. Michael's Hospital, was chosen as surgeon-in-chief.

He was the first James Wallace McCutcheon Chair of Surgery, which was created to support the surgeon-in-chief at TTH/TGH. This was

generously funded by James (Jim) McCutcheon, a personal friend of
Hugh Scully and a long-time board member of TGH with a particular interest in the Department of Surgery. The project was facilitated
with the Jim McCutcheon Foundation by Hugh Scully, Griff Pearson
(whom Alan Hudson was succeeding as surgeon-in-chief), and Bill
Bigelow.

He quickly took charge.

To improve and assure quality and accountability in all surgical services, the "on call" requirement for all staff surgeons became that they
must be physically present on site during any emergency operation carried out under their name (not just available by telephone).

Neither hospital could be all things to all people. Neurosurgery, ophthalmology, and orthopedic surgery were based at the Western, and
cardiovascular, thoracic, and transplantation surgery were based at the
General.

General surgery was present in each site, although predominantly at
the General, focusing on cancer surgery. Ear, nose, and throat surgery,
plastic surgery, and urology were also based at the General.

These selected programs needed space to grow, which meant
"shedding" other programs. Level one trauma centres for the city
of Toronto were created at St. Mike's and Sunnybrook. While emergency rooms were maintained at both hospitals, the orientation was
focused on the specialty services located at each; for example, a limb
fracture to the Western, not to the General, or a chest injury to the
General, not to the Western.

Obstetrics moved to Mount Sinai. The now combined cardiac unit
moved into the space vacated by obstetrics.

Hudson began contacting philanthropist Peter Munk as a prospective
donor to the hospital. Plan A didn't fly. "Met him about a month later at
the Toronto Club," Hudson said, "and tried something else. This went
on and on. Peter was trying to size me up, I was trying to size Peter up."

"I then had Peter and Melanie, and Jackie [David] and Tirone David
at our house for supper. And here was the exact key moment. Peter met
Tirone for the first time. At my house, at our supper table. And they fell
in love with each other. Tirone kept telling Peter how important he was,
Peter kept telling Tirone how important he was. It was one of those
magical moments [laughter]."

So they reached dessert. "Tirone had done a case that day. The phone
rang, and there was a problem. Tirone said, 'Excuse me, I'm going back
to the hospital.' And Peter's mouth fell open. He was so impressed that
Tirone was actually going to go back and look after a patient. So that
was how this started."

Munk focused his charity like a laser: Israel, cardiac surgery, and the School of International Affairs at Trinity College of the University of Toronto. "He encouraged other people to give money," Hudson continued. "Big event at Peter's house, and Ted Rogers was there, so Ted Rogers got in right at the start."

Hudson retired as CEO in 2000, and his involvement in the story ends almost there, but not quite. "We would see the Munks three or four times a year, then we sort of drifted apart. But in the last two or three years of his life, Peter and Melanie invited Bob Bell [who became the next CEO but one] and me over to his house, and he said when I'm gone would Bob and I please support and advise Melanie on the whole Peter Munk Centre. So that's what Bob and I now do."

The cardiac field has had many generous donors in Toronto. The De Gasperis family are fondly remembered as early benefactors. The Rogers family made the largest single donation in the history of the hospital. (See "The Donor World," later in this chapter, for more on both De Gasperis and Rogers.) Yet cardiac surgery in Toronto in ineffably associated with the name Peter Munk.

Peter Munk

It is 1989. Tirone David and Peter Munk are having lunch at Munk's office on Hazelton Avenue. "He and I clicked for multiple reasons," said David in an interview. "So he came back to Vickery Stoughton CEO of the General, and Fred Eaton" – chair of the TGH board – "and he said 'If I'm going to support, I want to support heart surgery.'"

Munk's father had a pacemaker, which Bigelow had implanted. And Munk himself had had several pacemakers. He also had a new cardiac valve installed with a catheter in 2014. There was a big family history of cardiac disease. "I don't want you to worry about money," Munk told David. "Just go to work."[2]

The Faculty of Medicine has departments. The University Health Network has programs. Alan Hudson created the cardiac program. Because Peter Munk had shown such a lively interest in supporting work on heart disease, the program became named after him. (It was, in fact, a condition of his support.) Tom Closson, who became CEO of the University Health Network in 2000, said that cardiac was one of the seven lead programs of the merged hospitals.[3] The cardiac program became the Centre for Cardiac Care.

It was Tennys Hanson, CEO of the Toronto General and Western Hospital Foundation, who did the actual negotiations with Munk. Closson explained how it worked: "Munk was donating to the foundation, he wasn't donating to the hospital. The hospital was giving up a space where a name would go, but the way I looked at it, Tennys had an incentive not to give away too much. You know why? Because if she gave it away to him she couldn't give it away to somebody else. There are only so many things to name so she wanted to give away as little as possible for naming rights."

Each one of the programs, Closson said, was given a "strategic plan." And Peter and Melanie Munk paid close attention to the reports from the cardiac program. "They wanted the hospital to be accountable for their donations. So they wanted regular reports back about what was being accomplished. If it was a research chair, it would be the chair themselves. If it was the program, it would be Chris Feindel [one of the leaders of the program] who would report back and meet with them."

Closson agreed with several other observers that philanthropic considerations played the principal role in the Munk donation. "I believe, based on my interaction with him, that the reason he did it was because he really wanted to create a heart centre that was world class here. So that people could get served well by the Canadian healthcare system in the heart realm." But, continued Closson, even if Munk had been uninterested in seeing his name in lights, "the foundation would've encouraged it. Because if John Smith who also has a lot of money sees that Peter Munk made a big donation, every time he goes down University Avenue he sees Peter Munk's name. That might make John Smith more interested in making a big donation."

The Peter Munk Cardiac Centre

In December 1993 the Toronto Hospital announced a new fundraising campaign for a cardiac centre, with a target of $25 million. Co-chairs were Peter A. Crossgrove, a member of the Toronto Hospital Board of Directors, and Peter Munk, who was also a member of the board and, at the time, CEO of a large mine, the American Barrick Resources Corporation. Munk himself was donating $5 million; the hospital was kicking in $6 million of the $25 million needed.[4]

In May 1997 the new centre opened in the Gerrard Wing of the hospital. It was called the Peter Munk Cardiac Centre (PMCC), "a marvel of beauty, efficiency and state-of-the-art everything," in the words of one journalist, with four operating rooms, a central ultrasound lab, and an intensive care unit with up to twenty-five beds. Cardiologist Michael Sole was the head,[5] his colleague Harry Rakowski the deputy head. Rakowski recalls that at the beginning, the logic for the collaboration was more "an administrative thing" concerning budgets and resources.

But the opening was splendid. "It is here," noted the *Globe and Mail* at the opening, "that Dr. David and his seven fellow heart surgeons ... will perform 2,500 open-heart operations a year, 20 percent more than a year ago." Cardiac care, noted hospital CEO Alan Hudson, consumed a quarter of the hospital's entire budget. Peter and Melanie Munk had now increased their donation to $6 million, and an academic chair in the Melanie Munk Chair of Cardiac Surgery was created. There were many donations from private individuals; said one hospital executive, "95 percent of Peter's friends gave." The decor of the centre was fashioned by Melanie Munk's favourite designer, Robert Noakes of Toronto, who said that in the hands of the centre's previous designers, the lobby was well on its way to becoming "a third-rate Holiday Inn in Las Vegas."[6] "The Baby Boom is coming through," Sole said. "There's no way that even a centre as large as this, which is one of the great centres of the world, can keep up with the boomers moving into the coronary artery [disease] group."[7]

The centre actually never left its original home in the Gerrard Wing but expanded steadily to the surrounding wings. "The idea," said Tennys Hanson, "was pulling together all the cardiac services into one building, and that was the Peter Munk Cardiac Centre. The building was not named after Munk but inside the building was the centre."[8] Then, quite separately, the "Munk Building" was erected, and the inpatient units and imaging are on two floors of it. The clinics and offices of the centre are in the Norman Urquhart building.

In 2003 Chris Feindel became director of the cardiac and circulation program. (For more on Feindel, see "Chris Feindel" later in this chapter.) He had known Hudson, and, of course, neurosurgeon Hudson knew Feindel's father, who had been director of the Montreal Neurological Institute. Hudson was caught up in controversies. Feindel later said, "Hudson's a very strong individual and certainly had opinions." Chris Feindel himself never had any problems with Hudson. "He knew my father pretty well. So I could skirt around all this stuff just by saying, 'Dad said to say hello.' So that would always put me in good stead. But I knew if people had opinions that he didn't agree with there would be sparks."[9]

Barry Rubin Takes Command

There were then other directors and finally another new one was needed. Vascular surgeon Barry Rubin said, "There was to be a presentation to the board of trustees in three weeks, and the CEO at the time, Dr. [Bob] Bell, came to a meeting and said to the assembled group,

'Who's going to give the quality presentation to the board?' I put up my hand. I said 'I'll do it.'"

Bell was happy with the presentation, and a week later he called Rubin into his office and said, "Do you want to be the head of PMCC?"

At this point, Rubin met Peter Munk. "I remember vividly being in Bob's office, and the elegant Peter and the stunning Melanie walked in, they were holding hands. He sits down, he's eighty-three or eighty-four at the time. Melanie sits on his lap [laughter]. They're calling each other 'Lover' and 'Darling,' and I never saw anything like this. It was remarkable."

Rubin got to know Peter and Melanie well and was often in their home. As well, as Peter became ill with heart disease, "I coordinated his care, and there was not one time that Peter Munk came to this hospital, if I knew he was coming, that I wasn't standing – I get emotional about this [tearing up] – I wasn't standing at the front entrance of the Munk Building, waiting for him. Not one time."[10]

At PMCC, Rubin had a distinctive philosophy. He said of the many international fellows training at the centre (ninety-three by 2018), "While at the PMCC, fellows learn the 'PMCC Way.' It is a philosophy that is the cornerstone of the institution and includes three pillars: a mandate to work in multidisciplinary teams, a commitment to using the best equipment in the world, and an unremitting focus on innovation."[11] Rubin said, "After I started, there was more of a transition to running the enterprise as a program as opposed to different areas that were loosely affiliated. I established core operating principles for the program."[12] It was Rubin's job to coordinate cardiology, cardiac surgery, vascular surgery, and interventional radiology into a functioning unit. (Anesthesia had its own autonomous hospital department.) Shaf Keshavjee, as the surgeon-in-chief, organized actual operations in cooperation with Heidi Duringer, the nurse-coordinator of the twenty-one operating rooms.

Peter Munk's Donations

Does all this program building require money? Yes, said Rubin. "I remember vividly discussing this with Peter, who just loved it. If you're going to be a place that does first-in-the-world type things, you take some risks. If you want to be the place that's always trying new things, there has to be some mechanism to fund those initiatives. I wanted to create an environment where everybody was aware that innovation was encouraged. So we solicited some capital, one to two million dollars a year."[13]

Having already funded the cardiac centre, in 2006 the Munks donated another $37 million to help buy new diagnostic equipment for the PMCC; it was at the time the largest single gift ever to a Canadian hospital.[14] The pricey devices would go into the PMCC's new home in the TGH's Clinical Sciences Building and Ambulatory Centre, where it moved in 2003 and help cardiologists in particular do procedures such as implanting heart valves via catheters. Operating Room 21, for example, contained a CT scanner right next to the operating table so that the patient could be instantly assessed. Said Bryce Taylor, chief of UHN Surgery, in November 2009 as OR 21 was opening, "I think the marriage of imaging and intervention is where everybody's going, no question about it. I'll bet you most major academic centres in North America are at least thinking about this, if they haven't already got one." At $5 million a pop.[15]

In addition, Peter Munk connected the centre with other donors. Anesthetist Massimiliano (Max) Meineri, an echocardiogram specialist, recalled that Peter Munk brought him "in touch with a donor [Arnold Irwin] who was interested in funding something for the hospital." Meineri needed a three-dimensional imaging lab. So Meineri and Cardiology jointly proposed "an imaging lab where we would archive and manage and three-dimensionally study images that we would have acquired in the operating room."[16]

In 2011 Munk donated yet another $18 million, this time to fund people rather than equipment. There were to be four centres of excellence within the PMCC – in valve disease, clinical trials, molecular medicine, and aortic diseases – each led by a significant figure. The valve-disease centre would be led by Tirone David, who had retired as chief of the division in 2011 and would devote himself to mitral valve issues. The entire concept was really an effort to keep David from being lured away by an American centre – as many other Toronto specialists had been – by salaries in the millions.[17] (David later said that he was indifferent to these staggering offers because one could only spend so much money.)[18] The imaging equipment itself purchased with the grant greatly increased the ability of cardiologists to do procedures.

Munk said in December 2010, just before the donation was announced, "I realized that heart disease, which is endemic in my family, also happens to be the number one killer in Canada." (Munk himself died of heart disease.) Munk's family experience was a starting point, but, Bob Bell, president of the University Health Network, added, "[Peter Munk] has embraced the idea that Canada needs a centre of global excellence … He wants to see Canadian health care recognized around the world."[19] Bell's statement is interesting because it implies that previously Toronto didn't have a global centre of cardiac excellence – but it has had one since Bigelow, and right at the General! And it is interesting because it correctly recognizes that Canadian contributions have been much underappreciated internationally. Internationally, in the cardiac area, many Canadian contributions have been quite ignored.

These funds were used in 2010 to outfit the Multi-Purpose Operating Room (MPOR), which unified all investigative aids in one place, obviating the need to push the patient about the hospital from cath lab for an angiogram to the Radiology Department to investigate a suspected ruptured aorta. "Time is of paramount importance in these instances," said Rubin. "With new technology, patients can come directly from the ER into the MPOR." In 2014 an even newer Guided Therapeutics OR was opened, with its two CT scanners, to make it possible to implant stents under X-ray guidance.[20] It was this 2010 donation that really changed Rubin's ability to exercise "leverage" on the competing cardiologists and cardiac surgeons.

There was much excitement about support devices for the left ventricle. The first was implanted in November 2001. It was followed by subsequent models, and, as mentioned earlier, on 31 October 2014, Robert Power, in advanced heart failure, became the first patient in Canada to be implanted with the latest mechanical heart device, the HeartMate III LVAD, under the aegis of Vivek Rao.[21] It was the Munk funds that helped endow the new LVAD (or simply VAD) program; this grant also helped establish the Melanie Munk Chair of Cardiac Surgery, and permitted nurses Betty Watt and Ann Tattersall to fly out to San Francisco to hear Tirone David's presidential address before the American Association of Thoracic Surgeons. Munk later said, "It was all Tirone's idea. I provide the tools to enable him to do what he does."[22]

By September 2016, two hundred such devices had been implanted – at more than $100,000 per device. Health Canada began picking up part of the tab in 2018, but until then private philanthropy and the provincial Ministry of Health had paid for the LVADs.

In addition, philanthropic support permitted PMCC to recruit and retain world-leading physicians such as cardiologists Harry Rakowski and Heather Ross, and such world-class surgeons such as Tirone David. As of 2019, the centre boasted twenty chairs and six professorships made possible by donors.[23]

Then finally in 2017, a year before his death, Munk donated a massive $100 million to the centre. It was Munk's friendship with Tirone David and Barry Rubin that greatly eased this flow of generosity, which turned out to have a bit of a downside for Rubin. Said Rao, "When Barry put his name in to be the new president of the hospital Peter was still alive. Peter said, 'If you're no longer the head of the Peter Munk Cardiac Centre, I'm not sure I want to support them anymore because I want you in this position.' So there was a bit of a conflict for Barry there. It never materialized, because someone else [Peter Pisters] got the job."[24] (Rubin later confirmed this story in an interview.[25])

For all the generosity of the Munk family, it was actually the province that funded the twenty-one ORs in the Munk Building. None was specifically dedicated to cardiac surgery, but pump surgery could be done in ten of the twenty-one. In 2018 Heidi Duringer was the nurse supervisor of all twenty-one ORs. She said, "It's not like there's a plaque outside of it that says 'cardiac only.'" A pump might be needed, for example, in endovascular aneurysm repair, where, said Duringer, "we always have a pump on standby in case something perforates and they may have to go on pump in there." There would be pumps every day in four of the ten, said Duringer. The Munk money paid for some of the equipment in these rooms, but the hospital, via the ministry, funded the brick and mortar and actually runs the rooms. It is Shaf Keshavjee, as professor of surgery, who leads the operative side of things, not Barry Rubin.[26]

The Donor World

The Munks had given $175 million, but 43,000 donors contributed a large additional chunk. In November 2014, the Rogers Foundation donated $130 million to UHN, SickKids, and the University of Toronto to create the Ted Rogers Centre for Heart Research. (They were going to call it the "Centre for Heart Failure," but the family said that Ted Rogers would never have his name associated with failure of any kind.[27]) The Rogers Centre was part of the Munk Centre. (The partner institutions themselves matched the grant.) Of this grant, $47 million went to the Foundation of the Toronto General and Western Hospital. The Rogers Centre's purpose was networking research to reduce heart failure and would bring together genomic research, stem cell experimentation, and cardiac treatment under a single roof.[28]

Of the five chairs the Rogers family funded, appointments had been made in two by the time of this writing (2019): the Ted Rogers Chair in Heart Function Outcomes (founding incumbent, Douglas Lee); and the Ted Rogers and Family Chair in Heart Function (founding incumbent, Heather Ross). Moreover, in January 2019, Ross became head of the Cardiology Division of UHN. Hanson said that after Ted Rogers died in 2008, "Loretta [Rogers] wanted to do something that was both in tribute to Ted and also in recognition of the incredible care that Heather

Ross had provided – as well as the whole team. She personally gave as well as the family foundation."[29]

Competing dynastic names? Hanson said there was never a hint of competition for attention between the two families, which had been close friends in life and were linked at the deaths of their founders in the prominent signage on University Avenue.

Tirone David's role in fundraising? David, in a sense, "saw himself as an arm of the fundraising department," said Hanson. "Advancing the ability of the centre to do more has always been important to him." Scully added, "People might ask 'Is there anything I can do to help?' and that is an entrée to say, 'Well, here are the kind of things where we do need assistance.' I think Tirone was a master at that." One member of the De Gasperis family had received surgery at the hospital and, said Hanson, "wanted to give back." David recommended establishing chairs, and the family went on to fund three chairs, the Alfredo and Teresa De Gasperis Chair in the Surgical Management of Heart Failure; the Angelo and Lorenza De Gasperis Chair in Cardiovascular Surgery Research (inaugural holder, Terrence Yau); and the Antonio and Helga De Gasperis Chair in Clinical Trials and Outcome Research (inaugural holder, Chris Feindel). They also funded cardiac cath equipment. And Jimmy De Gasperis, Fred's son, backed the lovely De Gasperis Conservatory in the hospital. The story goes that the De Gasperis family offered early support of the mechanical heart program. Said Hanson, "Fred got a lot of his colleagues together. They closed the doors." The idea was, said Scully, "you're not leaving until ..."[30]

Barry Rubin's Career

Rubin was born in 1960 in Montreal and earned a bachelor's degree in 1982 from McGill in physics and physiology. He graduated in medicine in 1986, then wanted to move on to train in surgery in Toronto.

But the Toronto program turned out to be very difficult to get into. He was interning at the Mount Sinai Hospital, where, he later said, "two people arrested simultaneously. They both happened to be Dr. [Robert] Ginsberg's patients, who was the surgeon-in-chief, and the next morning the chief resident said I saved two of his patients, so he [Ginsberg] said, 'What do you want to do?' and I said 'Surgery.' Really, that's why I got in."[31]

Rubin also enrolled in the surgeon-scientist stream of the Institute of Medical Science (and earned his PhD in 1991).

By his account, he sort of drifted into vascular surgery. "The truth is," he told an interviewer, "that I was a general surgery resident and I had done a straight internship before that. I didn't think anybody could be that tired and still be alive, so I thought that maybe I should go into a research lab and take a break. I tried to get into a transplant lab, because I thought transplantation sounded cool although I didn't know anything about it." But that spot was filled so he took a slot in vascular surgery. "After a year in the lab, my supervisor Paul Walker said, 'So you are going to be a vascular surgeon?' and I said 'Okay.' And that is the sum total." Rubin was head of vascular surgery from 2001 to 2010, becoming head of PMCC in that year.

Rubin remembered the big incisions involved in fixing aortic aneurysms. "I did big open operations, great anatomy – you just see everything. I loved that about it. Two-foot incisions, thoraco-abdominal stuff like that." But then this work dried up as stent grafts became available. "Now the most common operation we do is fixing aortic aneurysms and I rarely make an incision. It is all percutaneous [with a wire through a blood vessel in the groin] with the patient awake and they go home the next day."[32]

So changing technologies had been a big theme in Rubin's career. He joined the surgical faculty at UHN in 1995, headed the Division of Vascular Surgery at UHN from 2003 to 2010, and in 2010 became medical director of the Munk Centre, Canada's largest cardiovascular unit. After 2003 he also chaired the joint Mount Sinai–UHN Academic Medical Organization, which at this writing includes all physicians from Mount Sinai, TGH, the Princess Margaret Cancer Centre, Toronto Rehabilitation Institute, and the Michener Institute. Hugh Scully is currently the president of this organization.

Within the Munk Centre, there were seven centres of excellence. Cardiologist Heather Ross led the Ted Rogers Centre of Excellence in Heart Function (as well as being medical director of the Heart Failure and Transplant Clinic). There were, in addition, as of 2014, six other centres: a centre of excellence for aortic disease (Clinton Robbins, chair); heart rhythm disease (Kumaraswamy Nanthakumar, chair); multinational clinical trials (Michael Farkouh, chair); cardiac rehabilitation (Paul Oh, chair); valve disease (Vivek Rao, chair); and molecular medicine (Michael Gollob, chair).

The Centre for Rehabilitation was funded by GoodLife Fitness and its CEO, David Patchell-Evans. It was called the GoodLife Fitness Centre of Excellence in Cardiovascular Rehabilitation Medicine.[33] In September 2014 GoodLife Fitness launched "CardioStrong," a program to help cardiac patients transition into the community and maintain long-term commitments to their cardiac rehabilitation.[34]

Governance

What of the traditional department and division structure, once so
mighty, of the university and the hospitals? How does an intruder like
PMCC fit in? Money talks, and Barry Rubin has it. "The majority of
funding now runs through the programs," he said, "as opposed to the
Department of Medicine or the Department of Surgery." The departments look after education and academic promotion. But as for funding
the new cath labs, "There is nothing from the Department of Medicine
[cardiology] to fund that. Actually I didn't ask them. I went out and
raised the money, and then said, 'We really need to have new cath labs.
There's going to be this explosion in transitioning from open surgery to
no-incision repair of valves, holes in heart and things like that. We need
to build adequate facilities to manage that.'"

Rubin added, "Shaf [Keshavjee, hospital head of surgery] knows that
I respect the historical authority of the departmental structure. Shaf
also knows that I have access to who gets $100 million."[35]

We asked Vivek Rao, head of cardiac surgery at the General, whom
he reports to. He did not say "Shaf Keshavjee." He said simply, "Barry
Rubin."[36]

Governance of cardiac surgery within the university has always
been a rather touchy matter. The university chairs of cardiac surgery
for decades had little authority, unlike other university chairs. Why
was that? Scully said, in an interview, "The chair has come from Sick
Kids three times because no adult [surgeon] would take the position,
because they wouldn't be supported by Tirone or the other adult
hospitals. That's straightforward. And the others wouldn't agree to
have Tirone as the university chair. That's been going on for fifteen
to twenty years, so it's a very weak position, there's no money that
comes with it, there's no prestige that comes with it, no power to
make decisions that comes with it." Scully thought, however, that that
might be changing.[37]

Cardiac Surgeons and Cardiologists as a Team

Cardiologists are internists with a specialty interest in the heart. Cardiac
surgeons are, of course, trained as surgeons. Often the surgeons are
referred to as "cardiologists," but this is incorrect. The two fields have
entirely different backgrounds. Yet cardiac surgeons and cardiologists had always worked together, the cardiologists catheterizing the
patients in the cath lab, the surgeons making decisions in the OR on
the basis of the findings (if the cardiologist does not do PCI while the

patient is still on the cath table). But forging surgeons and cardiologists into a joint team began with Rubin.

We're in the cath lab. Rubin is talking to the head: "I'm very unhappy with this 'have an angiogram, independent operator decides what happens.' So I said, 'Going forward, I want to see a list of anatomic criteria, that if you have this coronary anatomy, the angiogram stops. You take out the catheters, and we have a heart team discussion between interventional cardiology, cardiac surgery, and, importantly, medical cardiology. And again, I said, 'If you don't want to do that, I'm just not paying for these advanced interventions.' I give them credit; they've embraced the heart team approach."[38] Big surprise.

What's the problem here? Rubin: "You are lying on the table having an angiogram. And the cardiologist doing the procedure alone makes the decision whether you should get a stent or not. Ninety-one per cent of the time the patient gets a stent. Take the exact same patient, with the heart team approach: 60 per cent of patients get a stent. Sixty!"[39]

The background: as surgery began to shift from the cardiac surgeons to the interventional cardiologists, it became apparent in some centres that cardiologists, responding to financial incentives, were installing far too many stents. In fairness, some were responding to the logic of the catheter. Medical historian David S. Jones writes, "Cardiologists complain that angiography initiates a clinical cascade that forces them to intervene whenever they find a plaque."[40]

Rubin said the PMCC lays great importance on the surgeons and cardiologists working together in teams. In 2005 they performed a Canadian "first" in repairing a leaky mitral valve with a catheter (the valve was permitting regurgitation, or backflow, from the left ventricle into the atrium). Previously, defective mitral valves had been treated in open-heart surgery. But a new, proprietary technology from Evalve Inc. in Menlo Park, California, made it possible to put a clip on a catheter, thread the catheter through a blood vessel to the left atrium ("percutaneous"), and lodge the clip in place between the leaflets of the valve, thus holding them together and greatly reducing regurgitation to manageable levels. In 2005 these were the first operations in a multicentre trial called EVEREST II (endovascular valve edge-to-edge repair study – meaning that the edges of the valve leaflets were clipped together). The trial at the PMCC unified cardiologists (Eric Horlick, and Leonard Schwartz), imagers (Melitta Mezody, an echocardiologist), and surgeons (Tirone David and Michael Borger), in addition to other specialists. By 2009, the four-year results of the EVEREST II trial as a whole (all centres included) were that surgery had an advantage over edge-to-edge repair. The mortality rate (at 17 to 18 per cent) was the same; but operations for re-repair of a continuously leaky valve in the edge-to-edge group were 20 per cent at one year and 25 per cent at four years (versus much lower rates for surgery).[41]

Much the same can be done for the aortic valve, and here Chris Feindel enters the story on the cardiac side. Feindel went to Vancouver in 2007 to learn the Transcatheter Aortic Valve Implantation (TAVI) procedure (a technique for implanting an aortic valve with a catheter rather than opening the chest) from interventional cardiologist John G. Webb. Later in 2007 Feindel imported TAVI to Toronto This was of particular utility in dealing with elderly patients, who often had stenotic aortic valves (the two-year mortality of symptomatic patients with aortic stenosis was more than 50 per cent.) There were two approaches: threading the catheter through the femoral artery, often impractical in the elderly; or inserting the catheter at the apex of the left ventricle, which involved a chest incision. The technique, presupposed that echocardiography and angiography equipment were present in the OR to steer the catheter so that it would expand the balloon that contained the new valve at exactly the right spot. Happily, the PMCC met these preconditions. According to Mitesh Badiwala, the then-resident who wrote up the Feindel story, "Dr. Feindel thinks that this is the future of cardiac surgery. He sees the future involving the adoption of this and other innovative catheter-based technologies in the operating room."[42] (In fact, in November 2014, Peter Munk had a TAVI, not having anticipated this course of events at all when he financed the centre named after him.[43])

As stated, the TAVI was introduced at the Peter Munk Centre in January 2007, with cardiac surgeon Chris Feindel running the procedure. Barry Rubin was the vascular surgeon, and Mark Osten, Eric Horlick, and others the cardiologists. By May 2009, forty-six patients had undergone TAVIs, either via the femoral artery or the apex of the left ventricle. Overall mortality at one month was 6 per cent. At two years, both TAVI approaches showed good valve durability with no cardiac-related deaths after discharge from hospital.[44] Said surgeon Maral Ouzounian, "We regularly perform TAVI on patients beyond the age of 90 – and most often, they go home within a day or two of the procedure."[45]

These new interventions carried a logic of their own. Previously, there had been some competition between surgeons and cardiologists, as the surgeons saw their bypass volumes drop because of stenting. Feindel said, "You are arguing and discussing and negotiating about certain patients with a certain kind of anatomy that could go for surgery or stenting. And out of that came the concept of what we called a heart team, which was basically surgeons and cardiologists looking at these cases rather than one individual who has a vested interest." Feindel said that Barry Rubin encouraged it, "but with the VAD and the TAVI program we automatically have a heart team sitdown every Wednesday." It started when Feindel himself directed the heart program, "It wasn't that well received back then because you are talking about people's turf and it gets very sensitive."[46] They didn't use the phrase "heart team" then, but that was the gist.

In Canada, regarding the balance between angioplasty (balloons, stenting, etc.) and bypass surgery in revascularization procedures (surgically bypassing blockages in the heart's arteries), angioplasty made steady progress, and by about 2004, represented some 63 per cent of the total of the two; then a slight retreat began. In 2007, the last year for which nationwide data are available, angioplasty stood at around 60 per cent of the total.[47]

A big step forward came in 2015 with ultra-rapid care for such conditions as aortic stenosis, now called aortic valve disease. In the community, such patients, often elderly, were quite at risk of sudden death and were often "stuck for weeks or months at the family doctor level" – as cardiologist Eric Horlick put it. At the PMCC they would be seen "by an aortic stenosis expert within 24 hours."[48]

In aneurysms of the aorta in the thorax and abdomen, the cardiac surgeons often collaborated with the vascular surgeons. Aortic dissections and aneurysms became the specialty of Maral Ouzounian (for more on Ouzounian, see "Maral Ouzounian" in chapter 23), who said, "We have a very collaborative approach and all complex cases are discussed as a team. Our goal is to be able to provide the best possible treatment of thoraco-abdominal aortic aneurysms right here at the Centre," rather than sending them, as before, to Houston.[49]

At the level of research, funds flowed easily back and forth between cardiology and cardiac surgery. Mitesh Badiwala led the team interested in "donation after circulatory death." This is called DCD transplantation: the stilled heart of the deceased is quickly removed and efforts undertaken to make it suitable for transplantation.[50] This research cost hundreds of thousands of dollars. Where did it come from? Initially from Shaf Keshavjee, the professor of surgery, said Badiwala. "I also got a big chunk from Heather Ross at the Ted Rogers. I got money from MOT [multi-organ transplant] from Atul Humar [TGH Research Institute], and recently it has been from Barry [Rubin]. It goes around."[51]

Patients at risk of sudden death can make you look bad on paper. Brows wrinkled when in 2018 PMCC staff took a look at mortality and found that at 1.9 per cent, it was almost twice what one conventional model might have predicted (1.03 per cent). Yet this result was not because the PMCC surgeons were incompetent but because the unit accepted the most difficult cases, patients who at all events were very much at risk of dying.[52] Barry Rubin said, "We want to be the place that takes care of the sickest. But we shouldn't be penalized for doing so." Journalist André Picard added, "Report cards are great, but what and how you measure matters a lot. That's an important caveat in an era where we are obsessively measuring, encouraging patients to use data to make wise choices."[53]

Cooperation between cardiologists and cardiac surgeons meant excellent patient care. "The whole thing is here for patients," said Tirone David, on whose watch the centre had arisen. "Research and teaching are linked to it, but our raison d'être is taking care of the patients. What's best for the patient? Medical therapy, an intervention done by the interventionist, or surgery? We're no longer competitive. We try to put the patient first. So if you come with an aortic stenosis, for example, the second most common cardiac disorder after heart attack. You're a ninety-year-old. You have just one kidney. The other kidney doesn't function normally, you had a mini-stroke last year, but you're dying now from the aortic stenosis. So a surgeon and two or three cardiologists discuss your case. Nobody's going to operate on you, because there is an alternative therapy now that is far less invasive than opening your chest and replacing your valve." David was referring to an aortic stent: the valve is inserted with a stent, not surgery. "So we work much more in a collaborative fashion."[54]

Thus, the culture changed. Unlike Bigelow, the single towering figure giving orders to his "boys," the Peter Munk Centre placed emphasis on multidisciplinary cooperation. Said Barry Rubin in 2015, "We believe that patients are best served in a team-based approach and that's how we try and manage patients – especially when we are using newer, more complicated technologies."[55] For a TAVI, the operating room, as reported by the *Toronto Star*, "is awash in fluorescent and LED lights. It's a hive of activity: rushing, buzzing, busy hands and beeps as more than a dozen medical staff tend to the patient."[56] Of course, surgeons and cardiologists had worked together since the days of Bigelow's Bungalow, but now many more specialists were in the mix: diagnostic imagers, urologists, and nephrologists (for the heart conditions involving the kidneys such as malignant hypertension), and immunologists for the transplants. The day of the titan in the white coat was past.

Congenital Heart Disease in Adults

A key event in the lives of congenital heart patients was the transition to adulthood around eighteen. That meant their care was transferred from the Hospital for Sick Children to the Toronto General Hospital; in adulthood, across Canada, the resources for these patients really were rather meagre. The attitude of many in the country as a whole was, "You've had your procedure, you're fixed." Yet continuous redos are often required, as, for example, adult women face pregnancy or adult patients acquire other cardiac risk factors such as coronary disease.

Bill Williams

The needs of adult congenital patients drew William ("Bill") Williams into the story.[57] Born in 1939 in Toronto, Williams grew up in the suburb of Etobicoke in the family of an orthopedic surgeon (his father operated at St. Joseph's Hospital); he attended high school in Etobicoke, then studied medicine at the University of Western Ontario. He graduated in 1964 and trained in cardiac and thoracic surgery at the Toronto Western Hospital under Ron Baird and Don Wilson.

Bigelow then beckoned to Williams to come over to the General. Why? Williams's father, C.D.G. Williams the orthopod, had been in the war together with Bigelow, first at the base at Basingstoke, then in Holland. That was a powerful bonding force. So, just as Chris Feindel, the son of William Feindel at the "Neuro" in Montreal, was looked after, so was the son of "C.D.G." In 1972 Bill Williams came on staff at the Children's Hospital, where he worked for "fifteen wonderful years" under Bill Mustard. (Said Williams, "He was a unique individual. Totally honest, embarrassingly so. He had no scruples about telling any story about anybody that was true, as long as it was true.")

At the Hospital for Sick Children, the care of congenital pediatric cases was highly collaborative between surgeons and cardiologists. Williams noted, "Children were not 'medical' or 'surgical' patients; they were the cardiac program patients." Joint weekly rounds were held; even though cardiologist John Keith and surgeon William Mustard were – as Williams notes – "polar opposites in personality, their mutual professional respect and collegiality set a high standard for future generations of cardiac program staff."

But what happened when these children who had been successfully operated on became adults? Around the time of the Second World War only 20 per cent survived to adulthood; today, 90 per cent do. Mustard, of course, had had a dramatic impact on children with transposition of the great vessels. Williams said, "It was just night and day in terms of the long-term prospect for these patients. Until 1963 [Mustard's first operation], an 80 per cent one-year life expectancy in mortality was changed to an 80 per cent 20-year survival." As cardiologist Louise Harris pointed out in 2011, "There are now more adults with congenital heart disease in Canada than children with this condition."[58]

In 1959 adult cardiologist John Evans, later president of the university, and pediatric cardiologist John Keith founded at the General a clinic for the care of adults with congenital heart disease. This was the first clinic in the world for congenital cardiac care in adults and became a hub for treatment and research. The goal was to formalize the transition from pediatric to adult. Even today, such programs remain the exception.[59] At the time there were not a lot of adults with congenital heart disease because, as we know, most died in childhood: the operations were risky, and many children succumbed without being operated on or died during the surgery. Yet with the revolution in pediatric cardiac surgery the transition from childhood to adulthood became increasingly common for heart patients. (After age seventeen, youth were no longer eligible for care at the Hospital for Sick Children.) Surgery on these adults slowly began tapping its way forward.

Williams at HSC quickly developed an interest in congenital defects. Mustard's transposition patients were just becoming teenagers as Williams came on staff. Williams spent three months in Europe at the main centres for treatment of congenital heart disease. At their eighteenth birthdays, congenital patients would be discharged from care at HSC. This group was becoming a new specialty, and Al Trimble was operating on some tetralogy of Fallot patients who were in their thirties. Most had already been operated on as children but now had developed new complications.

In 1973 Williams opened at the General a surgical service for adult congenital patients called the Congenital Cardiac Program. Trimble, who was already ailing, uncomplainingly acceded to this. Williams also tried his hand at general cardiac surgery in adults and in fact did twenty-nine bypasses. ("What?!" was the astonished reaction of Goldman and Scully upon hearing this.) Williams said, "It was kind of a way to ease into doing full-time congenital." It was actually one day a week. The rest of the time Williams was at HSC. From the mid-1970s on cardiologist Peter Laughlin and Williams held joint congenital-patient rounds.

Congenital patients were not like most adult cardiac patients: they needed to be followed continuously, often on a chronic basis. Williams said, "They become program patients rather than a surgical patient or a cardiology patient." In congenital, "the operation is done and the patient goes back to cardiology and is followed by cardiology and occasionally the surgeon, but mostly cardiology, and they often come back for more surgery. It's a captive audience that is lifelong."

At the General, the interventional program for adults started to shift to cardiology under McLaughlin. This began in 1983 with percutaneous interventions for ductus and other lesions. The care of congenital adult patients thus began to pass from the cardiac surgeons largely to the cardiologists. By 1999 it was clear that the transition was well underway. Richard Weisel, at this point university chair of the Division of Cardiac Surgery, noted that interventional cardiologists were "treating an ever-increasing proportion of patients with coronary artery disease and congenital heart defects, leaving only the more complex cases to be treated with surgery." But many of these cardiology patients do require surgery, which can "make cardiac surgery very challenging, particularly for academic surgeons." But our outcomes remain excellent, he noted.[60]

A more formal structure began in 2002 as a working group of pediatric and adult congenital nurses began meeting, and organized "Transition Evenings" and "Toronto Congenital Cardiac Centre" welcome letters. In September 2008 a formal task force was convoked, with a director of its own. Task force meetings were held every two to three months. The task force comprised nurses, cardiologists, cardiology fellows, and psychologists from both sides of Gerrard Street, the street that runs between the General and the Children's Hospital. In 2006 HSC organized a "Good to Go" program to prepare children with congenital heart disease for the passage across the street on their eighteenth birthday.[61]

At PMCC the clinic became the Adult Congenital Cardiac Clinic, after 2006 under the direction of Swiss-born cardiologist Erwin Oechslin. The surgery itself on adult congenital patients came to be performed by SickKids surgeons at the Toronto Congenital Cardiac Centre for Adults in the Munk Centre. By 2017, of the six hundred adult congenital heart patients treated at PMCC, about three hundred came from the Hospital for Sick Children, and another three hundred from other centres.[62]

The results of the clinic steadily improved between 1980, when a database was begun, and 2009. Over that period, 12,600 adults were followed. And of those involved in six specific "study cohorts" (specific diagnoses): from 1980 to 1989, of those who died, the average age at death was 30.8 years; from 1990 to 1999, 37.2 years; from 2000 to 2009, 38.8 years. (The average age on entry into the database was 21.1.)[63] So the clinic had added around seven years to the lives of these often desperately ill patients.

What disorders? Between 2008 and 2018, the congenital heart disease clinic at the General operated by far most often on tetralogy of Fallot patients (27 per cent of the total) – adults who were redos rather than those who had not been operated on in childhood at the HSC or elsewhere. Only atrial septal sinus venosus formed more than 6 per cent; other indications did not rise above 2 to 3 per cent of the total.[64] Eighty per cent of all congenital adult operations are, according to Williams, redos.

HSC and the General are now responsible for all congenital heart care from the Quebec border to Saskatchewan, with the exception of a few cases a year in Ottawa. Williams said, "Complex cases from Ottawa will come down here. Sometimes the surgeon will come and do the case here. The whole milieu has to be right. So you cannot do the occasional congenital cardiac patient and have a good outcome. You need the ICU, the cardiology, the intervention, the imaging capability. It is a whole package, it is not just doing an operation under anesthetic and saying, 'Okay, we are done.'"

It seems also true that congenital patients may be slower to get heart transplants. Regular transplant patients might well be admitted to hospital for the wait for a new heart and be put on a regimen of cardiac drugs. "Whereas if a congenital heart patient needs a transplant, [they are] probably at home waiting for a call. So they never get up to the priority they need to overcome all the ranks of the people ahead of them on the list." Nonetheless, there are heart transplants in congenital patients, and the outcomes – though superior to the conventional stereotype – are not as good as the outcomes in other transplant patients. Led by Vivek Rao, the Toronto surgeons compared transplantation results in thirty-five congenital patients over the years from 1988 to 2016, versus eighty-one non-congenital patients. At the first year, survival in the congenital group was 65 per cent; in the non-congenital group, 90 per cent.[65]

Indeed, Williams flagged several issues in the care of congenital patients. For one thing, there's a prejudice that, as he put it, "If you have a newborn that had an operation that was successful, do you have an obligation thirty-five years later not to say, 'Well, you've already had your chance, we've given you thirty-five years, we're going to give up on you now.'"

In addition, these complex congenital operations might well tie up an operating room for an entire day, whereas you could do three bypasses in the same OR – and earn much more income for the hospital.

GOLDMAN: So it was always an uphill struggle?
WILLIAMS: Yeah, and it still is.

Chris Feindel

Born in Montreal in 1946, Christopher Feindel grew up in the family of William Feindel, the third director of the Montreal Neurological Institute (the "Neuro").[66] Chris Feindel then embarked upon what must have seemed an endless program of training: He began a degree in electrical engineering at McGill in 1963 and completed it in 1968. He thereupon worked at the communications branch of the National Research Council of Canada in the intelligence area. This involved a stint from 1969 to 1970 as a computer engineer at the National Security Agency at Fort Meade in the United States.

Why medicine? Feindel had, of course, been influenced by his neurosurgeon father. (It was William Feindel who introduced modern neuroimaging to Canada.) But Chris's mother, having seen a surgeon's lifestyle from the inside, said, "Do anything but medicine." Nonetheless, Chris earned a McGill MD in 1976; after a surgical internship at the Montreal General Hospital, he did a residency in general surgery from 1977 to 1981 at the University of Western Ontario; then a year's fellowship at the Banting Institute in Toronto; then from 1982 to 1984 another residency, this time in thoracic and cardiovascular surgery at the General (Bigelow remembered him as a child); then a fellowship at the Western from 1984 to 1985. At this point Feindel finally won his cardiac fellowship from the Royal College, in a pathway of higher study that had started twenty years previously. He was at the Western from 1985 to 1989; there, he directed transplantation surgery from 1986 until leaving for the General; and he directed transplantation surgery at the General to 2002.

Why did he choose cardiac surgery rather than neurosurgery? On the licensing exams he did worst in neurology. "I thought it was a message, stay away. But I did like surgery."[67] When he did a surgical rotation as an intern, "I enjoyed that much more [than cardiology] because I thought you could really actually do something rather than just watch people and give a few pills and see what happens." He did a rotation with cardiac surgeon Tony Dobell at the Montreal Children's Hospital and really enjoyed that. Then off to the Western because people advised him against Toronto: If you were an outsider, they'd ship you off to the periphery. Resources at the English teaching hospitals had been curtailed by the Québécois government, and when Feindel made it to Ontario, he "was absolutely stunned at the resources, that people actually had something called an IV [intravenous] team, which was unheard of in Montreal. So we had nurses going around starting IVs. Of course when they couldn't, they would get a resident. Of course none of the residents could start an IV." But Feindel could.

Feindel was considered a master at a technique of reconstructing damaged hearts so risky and out-of-the-ordinary that it was called the "UFO" (Unidentified Flying Object). In 2015, Christopher Scott, age thirty-three, was admitted to PMCC with a raging infection he had picked up from a dialysis line; the infection had spread to his heart. Mitesh Badiwala, then on call, rushed Scott to the OR, opened him up and was appalled at what he saw: two badly damaged heart valves that were letting blood leak backwards into the lungs.

"We had to do something," said Badiwala. "He basically was drowning."

Worse, much of the myocardium was destroyed by the infection.

"Every time we tried to hold the valves, they just fell apart," Badiwala said. There was no tissue that new valves might be attached to. This called for a UFO, for sure. Feindel was called in.

"My first reaction," said Feindel, "was 'this poor guy's not going to survive this no matter what we do.'" Feindel said the damage was "spectacular." "I have to say my first response was 'There's no way this guy is going to get through surgery.' We're going to go through with it, but what do you do? He's a young man. You can't just walk away from him."

The UFO was not an operation done in most hospitals, Feindel said, "To be honest, a lot of these patients won't even get referred to surgery, because people basically give up on them."

But Feindel went to work and spent the next ten hours on the UFO (known in the United States as "a commando operation"). Using myocardium from a cow, Feindel constructed a patch into which he sewed two mechanical valves. This saved Scott's life. Scott spent the next four months in hospital, had several further procedures, but emerged grateful to be "hanging around the house, a family meal," preparing for Christmas. One of the stockings over the fireplace had Chris Feindel's name on it.[68]

(On Feindel's role in bringing transaortic valve implantation (TAVI) from Vancouver to Toronto, see "Cardiac Surgeons and Cardiologists as a Team," earlier in this chapter.)

Innovation

How do you fund innovation? Rubin said, "I wasn't happy with the way I was asked to fund things. The typical scenario would be someone would come to my office, arm on my shoulder, 'Barry, we go back a long time, I know you have some money, what do you think, this is a great project.' That was constant. It became apparent to me that we needed to develop a strategy to address those requests, and that's where the notion of having six people from the healthcare world and six people from the business world sit together on an innovation committee." He said the business people had the ability to "know a winner when you see it." They were also able to make decisions with incomplete information ("as opposed to us, who want to know every single thing about a patient before we say, 'Yeah, we're taking you to the operating room.'")[69]

So, in 2012 Rubin and cardiologist Harry Rakowski organized a Dragon's Den–style way of financing innovative, patient-centred cardiac research. (The term is the *Globe and Mail's*.[70]) The idea was to dodge the built-in conservatism of doctor-run grants committees and propel innovation at PMCC. Any of the thousand-plus employees of the PMCC was welcome to submit proposals, and the committee would meet four times a year. The Innovation Committee would finance eight innovative treatments from its $2 million Innovation Fund.[71] The point? To support small, promising projects that might otherwise be lost in the great mill of grant getting. Typical members of the Innovation Committee might include a frozen-food magnate, a real-estate developer, and a cardiologist. Said member William Charnetski, Ontario's chief health innovation strategist, "I truly believe that the optimal solutions to the challenges that face the health-care system will come from the collaboration of the public sector and the private sector."[72]

No Women's Chapter?

The reason there is no women's chapter in this volume is that the two main women cardiac surgeons – Lynda Mickleborough and Stephanie Brister – have never felt themselves discriminated against as women in any way. Putting them in a "women's chapter" would suggest that they had been included only because of their gender rather than because of their achievements.

Still, a couple of remarks about women in cardiac surgery might be appropriate, because their situation is not exactly comparable to that of men. First of all, Lorraine Rubis, the first female cardiac resident, rotated in 1975 through the division as she was completing her training in pediatric cardiac surgery. It was said that Tirone David was terribly hard on her. Scully reported, "It really was very embarrassing. I got involved several times, trying to get peace between them and telling Tirone to back off."[73] She went back to the United States.

The Cardiac Division did not sound like fertile territory for females. In Canada, as Glorianne Ropchan, a heart surgeon at Queen's, pointed out, "It seems as if there is one woman heart surgeon per centre across the country. I don't think any of us have ever had a female colleague for a very long period." It is true that Brister and Mickleborough over-lapped briefly at the General before Mickleborough retired in 2003. Otherwise, it was a singleton female.[74] (This is no longer true in Toronto today, where there are three women among the eight residents, and two women on the division's staff.)

Why was that? Ropchan continued, "What's bad about being a car-diac surgeon? Basically when you're working, you have no life." Rop-chan's days in Kingston started at seven-thirty and ended around eight or nine at night.[75] Many women shrank back from such a demanding schedule.

There is little evidence that women were actively discouraged from the field. But they were not encouraged either. Bigelow attached no particular importance to the presence of women in heart surgery, and always referred to colleagues as "men," and to his students as "boys." In 1984, the Canadian Society of Cardiovascular and Thoracic Surgeons launched an annual lecture series, "the Bigelow lecture." The first lec-turer would be John Callaghan, chief of cardiovascular and thoracic surgery at the University of Alberta Hospital in Edmonton, "referred to as one of 'the Bigelow boys.'"[76]

Stephanie Brister

It is a measure of Stephanie Brister's mettle that at some point she applied for astronaut training along with Roberta Bondar. As Terry Kieser a Toronto-trained cardiac surgeon in Calgary, comments, "Fortunately for all of us [she] decided on inner space rather than outer."[77] Brister was born in 1953 in the small prairie town of Rivers, Manitoba; her father in the military was stationed there; her mother taught primary school. After about nine months in Rivers, the Bristers moved on to other bases and other schools.

The advantages of this kind of itinerant education? "What the mili-tary was able to do for my family was give it access, as children, to resources that my parents could never have afforded otherwise. We learned to ski. You never had to buy equipment, you just signed it out of the base. So when I made the transition from a base school into an upper middle class school [in Calgary] that had very affluent people, I could ski as well, if not better than most people. So I could still be with those people and be included in the activities, swimming, sailing, curl-ing. I could do all of those things. Because of the army. It allowed that social acceptance to occur."[78]

The choice of medicine? It was because of her father. He wanted his daughter to be "completely independent. And for some reason being a doctor symbolized that." Her mother was not thrilled about medicine as a choice. "She just thought that medicine was going to be too hard on life. But she never told me."

Brister earned a medical degree at the University of Calgary in 1979, then wanted to come east for specialty training. "I perceived that some of the more academic institutions were here in the east and I just wanted to see what they were like." She was accepted at McGill as an intern in internal medicine. But in the middle of the program she decided to change to surgery and chose cardiac. "The majority of what you do actually helps people live a better life. And in many specialties you cannot say that. And there was a bit of drama to it. I mean, it is an exciting thing to do."

She spent the next seven years training as a general surgeon at McGill in the Montreal General Hospital. In 1986 she moved to Kingston, and passed two years training in cardiovascular and thoracic surgery at Queen's. Then in 1988 she undertook a fellowship year in cardiac surgery at the Toronto General Hospital, where she was mentored by Mickleborough. In 1989 she joined Hamilton General Hospital as a cardiac surgeon with a faculty appointment at McMaster.

Asked by a journalist in 2008 if she wanted to see more women cardiac surgeons, she gave a laugh. "That's like asking if I want to see Hillary Clinton be president. Yes, but it's not because they're better. You want good people doing it. And yes, you want more women doing it because I think they'll be good at it, but what you want is the best people doing it."

"It can be a tough life," Brister said, who had remained childless because the thirteen-hour days she regularly booked "wouldn't be fair to children." (But her husband Michael Buchanan, a professor of pathology and molecular medicine at McMaster, had two children from a previous marriage.) Her life was not, in fact, entirely dominated by surgery, and as a hobby she collected and restored carousel horses.

In 1998 she moved from Hamilton to Toronto. At McMaster, which then lacked a formal cardiac surgery training program, she had the feeling she had plateaued, and thought, "Well, given that I'm going to be in practice another 20 years, I'd like to move to something that's a bit more challenging." At the Munk Centre she played a capital role in training the six fellows who came from outside to hone their skills. This was in addition to the eight TGH fellows, two cardiac surgery residents and ten to fifteen medical students.[79] On the research side, Brister published widely on bypass, focusing on improving results in the elderly.[80] While in Hamilton, she scrubbed in on a procedure for pulmonary embolus (a thromboendarterectomy) in the pulmonary artery, the first performed in Canada – a challenging procedure for a condition that in the past almost invariably ended fatally.[81]

In Toronto, Brister was noted for her coolness under fire. She recalled, "It was just in the morning and I was doing rounds, and they gave a code in one of the rooms." It wasn't her patient, but she thought, "'Ah, maybe I should just go and have a look.' And I went in and the patient's blood pressure dropped. He had pulled what are called the pacemaker wires out, and when you pull the wire, it lacerates the heart and the patient bleeds and they have collapse. And they were calling for an echo and they were doing all of these things, and I said, 'Just get me a chest reopening set.' The patient was awake and they had called anesthesia, but they were not there yet. And so, I just opened the patient's chest while the patient was awake and put my finger on a hole and they came and they intubated him and then we went down to the operating room and closed it. And he went home in about ten days."[82]

How was it being a woman? "One of the boys?" to use Lynda Mickleborough's phrase? Brister said, "I never felt like I was one of the boys. Ever. Because I was treated differently. How to say it? You are always aware of whether or not you're speaking with men or with women. There's a different way that you related. And it's not good or bad, it's just different."

In the past Brister had suffered slights in cases of mistaken identity. When in Hamilton, they asked for an infectious diseases consult. "And the ID consultant came and he was assessing what he thought should be done and addressing me as if I was one of the nurse practitioners. Then he said, 'So you'll write the orders?' And I said, 'Well, I'm Dr. Brister, and I'm acting for Dr. Gustafson and this is what I want, so, this is what we're gonna do.' And he goes, 'Oh my god, I'm sorry.' [Laughter]." But this "never, never happened when I was [identified] as a physician."

Brister stopped doing pump surgery in 2012, although she continued with pacemaker surgery. She was appointed by Shaf Keshavjee as medical director of the operating rooms, working closely with Heidi Duringer, coordinator of the operating rooms at TGH, to make the best use of the resources available. Brister earned a reputation for open, honest, and diplomatic assignments of ORs to competing surgeons. She retired from the hospital and the university in 2016, having been for a decade the sole female cardiac surgeon at TGH (except for Lynda Mickleborough, who retired in 2003).

The biggest challenge? Staying up to date, she said. "We have gone from a specialty that was very hands-on, technical, skill-oriented with coronary artery bypass grafting and valvular surgery, which is very quote 'cut and sew,' to something that is much less invasive. It involves a lot of medical imaging, a lot of catheter skills which are really skills that traditionally-trained surgeons hadn't acquired in the past."[83]

Chapter Twenty-Three

The Next Gen

The younger and more recently recruited surgeons are already leaders in their specialties. After a certain scientific dormancy in the division, these energetic scientists and clinicians augur well for the future.

Maral Ouzounian

Maral Ouzounian joins the list of distinguished heart surgeons, male or female. She was a McGill student with a BSc in 1999 and an MD in 2003, then a resident at Dalhousie. In 2006, she came to Toronto as a trainee and scientist in the Clinician Investigator Program (Fellow of the Royal College of Physicians) in 2012

Then occurred one of those stages that one doesn't widely see: the division she was joining sent her off at their cost for further training. In 2012, after she had completed a PhD at the Institute of Medical Science, "we sent her to Texas to learn aortic surgery," said Rao. "[Tirone] was more than happy to have Maral take over the big thoracoabdominal cases." At the Texas Heart Institute at Baylor she studied thoracoabdominal aneurysms under Joseph Coselli, the foremost expert in this kind of work. When she returned in July 2013, Rao told her to "just settle in and take it easy." But on her first day back as a staff member, she found herself facing a twenty-six-year-old man with a ruptured thoracoabdominal aneurysm. "There was a litre of blood in his chest," Ouzounian said. Previously, such patients might have been sent to Coselli in Houston, but Ouzounian thought he wouldn't survive the trip, and she replaced much of his aorta on site. The operation went well. Welcome to the Division of Cardiac Surgery! Rao said, "Here she is flourishing and is probably one of the country's leaders in the big aortic cases.[1]

She told an interviewer of her focus on aortic disease, "We are seeing a rise in the number of cases of aortic diseases, particularly aneurysms and dissections. This may partially be due to better diagnostic techniques. In fact, now they are often detected when they are not even looked for. For example, a person may have a CAT scan for some other reason, and an aneurysm is detected." Not all are repaired. Stable aneurysms might not be. "If it's an appropriate size to treat [we] fix it – either through open surgery or with an endovascular stent." Treatments have greatly improved, not least because of the procedure that Tirone David introduced.[2]

Ouzounian and the vascular surgeons collaborate in the treatment of aneurysms of the descending aorta (thoracoabdominal aneurysms), a particular challenge because the blood supply to the spinal cord is at risk. "We have a very collaborative approach and all complex cases are discussed as a team. Our goal is to be able to provide the best possible treatment of thoracoabdominal aortic aneurysms right here at the [Peter Munk] Centre," Ouzounian said. The day of sending these patients to Houston was over.[3]

In scientific terms, Ouzounian was first author (Tirone David was a coauthor) on a paper in 2017 on the superiority of the Ross Procedure in treating aortic stenosis in the young. It was a procedure that David had reintroduced to surgery in 1990.[4]

At Toronto, David did most of the mitral valve operations. It remained for the two juniors, Maral Ouzounian and Mitesh Badiwala to divide up the work that David didn't touch. (For more on Badiwala, see "Mitesh Badiwala," later in this chapter.) Badiwala said in an interview, "Maral is developing herself as the aortic root surgeon, valve-sparing surgeon. I don't do any of those operations. They go to her. Similarly, she doesn't do any of the mitral valve repairs. They come to me, if he [David] is not going to do them. We develop silos of expertise internally. If I get a referral for an aortic problem, if it is a straightforward ascending aorta, I'll keep it, but if it's anything more, I send it to Maral. We share that way and we don't compete for that kind of thing."[5]

This third generation of Toronto cardiac surgeons, in other words, was struggling to come out from under the shadow of the great man. And what would happen to valve surgery after the great man retired remained an ongoing problem for the division and for the entire Peter Munk Cardiac Centre.

Mitesh Badiwala

Badiwala was born in Toronto in 1978, his parents having emigrated from India.[6] His father, trained as a chemist, ended up working in a motion-picture laboratory. Badiwala said, "He would take the reels and develop them overnight. He worked the nightshift." His mother was a housekeeper. The Badiwala family moved out to Mississauga, a city west of Toronto, where they bought a house and Mitesh went to high school. "While in high school" he said, "I got interested in medicine because I volunteered at the Mississauga Hospital in their emergency department." He did a three-year arts degree at McMaster University, then got into medical school at the University of Toronto and graduated in 2004.

As an undergraduate, he was mentored by Heather Ross and several of the surgeons. "I used to come in on Saturday mornings and follow her around the CCU, and when she would leave after the morning rounds, she would pair me with her fellow. I would watch them put the lines in, and it was all very exciting to me." Badiwala opted for cardiac surgery after his MD as he watched, during the summer, the surgeons of the division operate. "I remember going into the old ORs and watching Dr. Yao, Dr. Cusimano, Dr. Mickleborough, and Dr. Scully operate. I developed a very deep interest in trying to spend as much time as I could watching them. I remember spending late nights with Dr. Cusimano watching him do all sort of crazy things. With piles of blood bags on the ground." He also worked in Richard Weisel's lab. "I developed a fascination with heart surgery while doing that type of work. I used to spend two or three days shadowing in the operating room while I was doing research in the first two days."[7] He joined the staff of the Cardiac Division in 2014.

Did those arts courses he took at McMaster stand him in good stead in medicine?

Badiwala said, "Yes, It makes me believe that I'm a better-rounded person and I can think about patients' background from a non-scientific view. When we sit and talk to patients pre-operatively it's important to understand where they are coming from. For example, if I have a very elderly person who I sense is not really keen on surgery, we will engage in a deeper discussion of what their goals in life are, what their life has entailed and what they are looking forward to. On occasion, we'll conclude that surgery is not the right thing for a patient, and I'm completely comfortable with that."

And regarding the question whether to operate on ninety-two-year-olds? Badiwala said, "For a ninety-two-year-old who has lived a good life and really doesn't want to live another twenty years and does not want to go through a big operation ..."

GOLDMAN: You were offering them twenty years at ninety-two? [laughter]
SCULLY: Going back, the age where that discussion used to take place was about eighty. Sometimes they would elect to go ahead and sometimes they would elect not to.

It is a measure of the progress of cardiac surgery that this discussion now takes place at a much later age.

An interviewer observed, "It's interesting that the magnetic attraction of these storied figures was greater than Heather Ross's magnetic attraction because otherwise you would have gone into cardiology."

Badiwala agreed but said, "She still had an influence. Heart failure and transplant, which is what I do now."

Badiwala was asked if when he set foot in the division, did he have the feeling it was a historic kind of opportunity and that it was a fabled division that he was now part of?

Badiwala answered, "Yes. It was kind of hard not to because you look around and you see operations invented by surgeons here. You saw first implants of ventricular assist devices back then, when Viv [Rao] came back."

And how does he, as a third-generation member, carry on the division's traditions of global excellence? Badiwala pointed out that he doesn't have any "protected" rescarch time. All the research he does is on his own dime, not through released time. That said, he continued, "I am developing ex-vivo heart perfusion technologies in my laboratory with Viv to evaluate donor hearts that we typically don't use, to see if we can recover function, augment function, use hearts from brain-dead donors that don't have circulatory mechanisms of death. There is a whole line of investigation that I wish I could spend more time hands-on doing."

Badiwala then made a point that highlights the General's attractiveness as a scientific environment. "The problem here is that if I go home and tell my wife that I am going to spend my time in the lab and because of that I am going to take a significant pay cut, she knows what I'm worth elsewhere because she knows what was offered to me elsewhere."

For example, Badiwala fellowed at Northwestern University. They liked him a lot and wanted him to stay on, but he was indecisive.

"We were driving back home [to Toronto] and had stopped somewhere in Michigan, and he [the head of the division at Northwestern] had emailed me an offer right after I left. It was literally right after I left. So I showed it to my wife, and I said, 'Should we keep driving or drive back?'

"She goes, 'Just keep driving – what's wrong with you?'"

Terry Yau

Terrence M. Yau, or Terry as he is universally known, was born in Windsor, Ontario, in 1963, the son of an electrical engineer.[8] He is the elder of the newcomers – and he is currently the university chair of the Division of Cardiac Surgery. "We moved all over the globe," he said, "and I lived for ten years in Hong Kong." He finished high school there.

He earned a BA, basically in molecular biology, from Johns Hopkins University in 1984, and graduated MD from McGill in 1988. Why McGill? "That was the American love affair with McGill," he said, "from New England all the way down to Maryland. Who the hell knew where U of T was compared to McGill?" During his studies at McGill, he decided to do cardiac surgery. "I looked around at programs and I thought the U of T is where I would ultimately like to train." He came down to Toronto as a medical student for a cardiac surgery rotation and attended the Friday morning "triage" rounds (assessing new patients). "We would pass around the list of cases for the next week that we were seeing, and there would be 'R.J.B.' – Baird, this and that. I was in third-year medical at the time and I said to myself, 'Okay, one day I'm going to come back here, and it will be T.M.Y. on that list.' I jokingly said that. That actually never happened, because by the time I came back they changed it so that you just print the full name. There has never actually been a list that says T.M.Y."

But let's not get ahead of the story. Yau passed through the Gallie Residency Program in General Surgery at Toronto from 1989 to 1995, and finished the cardiovascular surgery residency program in 1997 as one of the last residents to do general surgery before cardiac. (After that, it was straight entry into cardiac.) He chose Toronto because, by that time, his family was back in Canada. During his training, he spent two years in the lab with Dick Weisel on "myocardial protection" and the use of "cardioplegia" to nourish the heart when its beating was stilled. (For more on this, see chapter 15.)

If Yau had stayed at McGill, would he have had the same academic success as in Toronto? Yau said, "Everybody that comes through the [Toronto] program has some initiative and drive, but if you don't have the opportunity it is very difficult and it is very hard to build something out of nothing. When the program is set up and it is literally a factory for producing academic surgeons, that makes it easy. It was Richard [Weisel] who came to me and said, 'Hey, let's go talk about what you want to do.'" At Montreal, Yau was handicapped because he didn't speak French fluently. And nobody took any particular interest in him.

For years in the division, Yau ran a lab, his interests shifting to stem cell research that he, Weisel, and Ren-Ke Li at St. Michael's Hospital undertook. Out of this collaboration came some important work.[9]

Why is stem-cell research important? "It's a miserable life," Yau told a journalist in 2008. The article explained, "Few patients are truly glad to see Terry Yau. He may be kind and thoughtful, but this heart surgeon is also many people's last hope. And all too often, he has to explain there's nothing he can do." A lack of donors means that most potential transplant recipients don't get a new heart. Yau said, "Instead of living, they're just waiting to die. That's the thing I hate most."[10]

Here stem cell transplantation enters the picture. In 1996, workers at the Research Institute of TGH showed that the heart's pumping action could be strengthened by transplanting stem cells.[11] After 1998 Yau and Weisel led stem-cell research in Toronto in cardiac disease. Weisel, who was also a senior scientist at the McEwen Centre for Regenerative Medicine at UHN, had helped develop the technique, which involved re-injecting into the patient's heart stem cells isolated from the patient's own bone marrow. In 2003 Yau, Weisel, Rao, and Ren-Ke Li gave an overview of this research,[12] which culminated with a large randomized multicentre study reported in 2016 of the kind of patients that were candidates for this procedure: bypass, damaged myocardium, stem cell treatment [13]

In January 2012, James Culross, a sixty-seven-year-old man from the Toronto suburb Etobicoke whose heart had been damaged in an infarct in November, became Ontario's first patient to receive a novel kind of stem cell therapy developed by Yau, director of the cardiac stem cell program at PMCC. On Mr. Culross, Yau first did a bypass graft, then injected the stem cells directly into the area of the damaged myocardium. The bone-marrow cells were processed at UHN's Organ Regeneration Laboratory.[14] "I thought it was great," Culross said of the procedure. "It's your stem cells, nobody else's."

Where Is the Division Going?

Where is the division going? Yau put on his university chair hat. "The wire" was changing things. "Certainly, the field of valve surgery is changing with the onset of TAVI [transcatheter aortic valve implantation]. We often hear that 'AVRs [aortic valve replacement] are going to go the way of the dodo.' That process is happening. It is one of those things we would certainly want our trainees to get some exposure to, wire skills." But in general, this was not for residents. "Wire skills is probably one of those things that you would need a dedicated fellowship to do." The field as a whole was heading toward micro "keyhole" surgery. Toronto, alas, not quite yet.

So caution here. Yau said, "Basically, in order to be a good minimally invasive surgeon you have to be an excellent mitral surgeon to begin with. We have that responsibility to train our residents and fellows in that way. I think the underlying responsibility of the program has always been to make our residents into excellent surgeons with that basic skill set and then to facilitate additional training and whatever other things they want to do." Yau said there was probably not going to be a hybrid interventional field. "If you take a trained cardiac surgeon, you can teach [them] wire skills in a few months in a cath lab. However, if you try to take an interventional cardiologist and you want to make them into a surgeon, it would be ..." His voice trailed off.

Chapter Twenty-Four

Conclusion

In 2019, *Newsweek* ranked the Toronto General Hospital as number seven in the ten top hospitals in the world.[1] Bigelow would not have been surprised. TGH went on to be ranked fourth in the world in 2020 and again in 2021. The rating singled out cardiac surgery as one of the hospital's key achievements. The Department of Surgery of the Faculty is Medicine is, as a recent review put it, "one of the top tier Departments in the world."[2] This assessment concurred with a global survey published by *U.S. News and World Report*, which ranked it in fourth place behind Harvard, Johns Hopkins, and Pittsburgh.[3] The clinical program overall, meanwhile, was rated sixth worldwide according to the prestigious *Times World University Rankings*.[4] So the story has had a favourable outcome. But it's not over yet.

We Learn That Cardiac Surgeons Are a Bit Different

When Richard Reznick was professor of surgery from 2002 to 2010, he resolved to have a sitdown interview with each of the surgeons in the academic department, and in fact he interviewed 150 of them. Maybe it was just because of Resnick's skills as a one-time aspirational psychiatrist, but many of the surgeons opened up. He said, "I got to understand a little bit about the complexities of what it means to be an academic surgeon and especially some of the stresses. After those 150 interviews, there was a tremendous sense of concern over the degree of unhappiness amongst our surgeons."

Why?

"Marital disharmony, substance abuse, and depression."

They opened up about substance abuse?

"Yes. Oh, yes; that, and about depression. There was a lot about marital disharmony. Probably the most interesting was 'not having achieved what I could have achieved. I thought I was going to achieve so much and it hasn't materialized.'"[5]

As the lead author of this volume, Shorter interviewed in depth almost all of the members of the Cardiac Division, and his overwhelming impression is that if Reznick's impressions of surgeons in general are correct, the cardiac surgeons are not like them at all. They are, insofar as one can tell, not haunted by domestic problems and have a great sense of fulfilment. In the Division of Cardiac Surgery, people have very much achieved what they set out to – and often much more, although, with this typical Canadian sense of modesty, they are not boastful about it. These pages are filled with the stories of men and women who have made great contributions to cardiac science and to the art and science of surgery. And this story continues.

The Captain of the Team?

In internal medicine and family medicine, cooperation among equals is now the preferred model. In training, that means one resident with several staff. Cooperation among equals is not the rule in cardiac surgery, where the hierarchical team model prevails in most places: chief, senior, junior, in that order.

> SCULLY: It takes guts to be a cardiac surgeon. You encounter things you
>   haven't done before and have to innovate, real time, on the fly ...
>   Sometimes that's a pretty tough decision. You are the leader in the room,
>   you don't go "Oh shit, now what am I going to do?" You've got to be the
>   leader.
> GOLDMAN: Or, you have an orderly plan in your mind because things are
>   moving quickly once you go on the pump and support the circulation,
>   especially in the early days. The patient's proteins were getting churned
>   up, red cells were getting banged around, and infection was always a
>   possibility. So you had to have a plan based on your experience that this
>   is how an aortic valve is done, and you had to be able to adhere to your
>   plan, and adapt, as Hugh says, to changes, and adapt quickly, but not get
>   spooked. And not let the team get spooked. Because the last thing you
>   need is everyone panicking and chaos. So you have to manage. You've
>   got to work with the anesthetist. I remember [Hugh] once restrained
>   me as I tried to reach out and punch the anesthetist. It was during the
>   unstable angina case, and he wasn't controlling the blood pressure. He
>   was afraid to give this and afraid to give that.
> SCULLY: I see him at the ballet all the time.
> GOLDMAN: Really, is he still alive? Punch him again.[6]

Yet the trend in cardiac care is away from the captain of the team and toward collaboration among a variety of specialists and heart-care personnel as equals. At PMCC, consensus on the team prevails. Cardiac surgeon Mitesh Badiwala, head of transplant surgery, described in 2017 a "culture of togetherness and communication" that he attributed to cardiologist Heather Ross. Ross said, "The transplant team is so big that it's important to create an environment where everyone knows that no member of the team is more important than anyone else. As they say in Africa, 'If you want to go fast, go alone. If you want to go far, go together.'"[7]

"The Desire to Make a Very Good Hospital into a Great Hospital"[8]

Some have the feeling that, today, a golden era might have passed. Is this just more Canadian self-effacement? Harry Rakowski said, "I have a vision of making us one of the best, the top five cardiovascular organizations in North America, which we are far from right now. Which we should be. And it is the same passion that the next head of cardiac surgery should have, making this one of the great surgical institutions because in the golden age of these gentlemen [pointing to Goldman and Scully] and Tirone, it was."[9]

Yet the old fire still burns. There is still the keenness of the surgeons to innovate. Shaf Keshavjee, the head of surgery at the General, was talking about the ability of surgeons here to make things happen, such as lung transplants. "What's special about [the General] is the innovative spirit, the ability to take innovation to the bedside. Like the cold-heart surgery, like a number of innovative investigations or research findings in the lab, people will be more able to bring it to the bedside."

Q: And that ability here is superior to other institutions?
KESHAVJEE: I think so.

Christopher Paige, vice-president today of research at the Toronto Hospital, echoes this. He says, "My vision for the Toronto Hospital Research Institute is for it to become the finest hospital-based research institute in the world."[10] An admirable goal, but an exact repetition of the hopes that Bill Bigelow held in the 1950s for the General. Bigelow's aspirations to make the General the number-one research hospital in the world are now long forgotten. But the feeling that the Big House – now the University Health Network, following the merger of the General, the Western, and the Princess Margaret Hospital (a cancer hospital) – should retain some kind of international primacy has not vanished. And these hopes are born by such yeoman flag-bearers as the staff of the Peter Munk Cardiac Centre at the General. Today, thanks to the generosity of such donors as the late Peter Munk, the funding picture is brighter.

But in the world there are a number of great hospitals. Is there anything distinctive about Canada's? Shorter thinks there is, and it gets back to the reticence that Bigelow complained about among Canadians: We are very British in our desire not to trumpet our achievements. Of course, the job of the hospital public relations department is to do exactly that, but when we look at the surgeons and scientists, a very British and un-American picture emerges: In the interviews that we did for this volume, with one or two exceptions, the senior figures were all *self-effacing*. They disclaimed personal triumphs and attributed success to group work, or good fortune, or something other than their personal brilliance. We asked Alan Hudson about this, who is also very self-effacing about his own achievements, caustic though he is in relations with others. "Most of us consider this a job of service. That's why we do the job, it's a privilege to do the job, you do your utmost to serve. People like John Wedge, Bryce Taylor, Bernie Langer, these are the salt of the earth, brilliant people who really built this place, and not one of them promotes themselves, ever."[11]

As noted, on 20 March 2019, the global ranking of the top ten of one thousand institutions reviewed worldwide was published in *Newsweek* magazine. The ranking was finalized by a panel of doctors, other medical professionals, and administrators across four continents. TGH was cited as one of the Top 10 (the seventh) elite hospitals in the world for transplant research and innovation, including triple organ transplant, and for *cardiovascular care at its Peter Munk Cardiac Centre*. It is the only Canadian hospital on the list.

The Story Continues

At this writing, in 2019, the story very much continues for some of the dramatis personae.

Bernie Goldman retired from surgery at age seventy-three, after more than forty years of cardiac work. With a career at the General and at Sunnybrook behind him, he "asked, am I hanging in or hanging on?"[12] Thus he made way for his colleague and student Steven Fremes to become head of cardiac surgery, and Goldman joined the surgical panel of the College of Physicians and Surgeons of Ontario.

From there he segued into the international cardiac care of children from developing countries. The story is this: in 1992 Martin Kamerow, Ami Cohen, and Ami's father Obadiah Cohen established the Wolfson Cardiac Surgery Foundation, the goal of which was to bring cardiac surgery to poor children across the globe whose lives would otherwise be much shortened.[13] In 1999 the foundation changed its name to Save A Child's Heart (SACH).

In 2001 SACH Canada was founded by philanthropist A.E. Diamond, with Bernie Goldman as its consultant surgeon, then leader. When Goldman visited the Wolfson Medical Center in Holon, Israel, where the SACH operations are performed, he said, "I was blown away by this project. SACH is almost unknown abroad and functions with no money for publicity. I had tears in my eyes when I saw what the operations did for the kids."[14] SACH sends teams of surgeons to various part of the developing world to assess children with cardiac conditions. The children are then operated on locally or flown to Israel. In 2014 SACH Canada launched a volume, *Mending Hearts, Building Bridges*, that tells this very moving story.[15] By 2018, more than 4,400 children from sixty-six countries had received free lifesaving heart surgery including pre- and post-operative care.[16] Said Goldman, "I believe this is one of the best global health initiatives there is."[17]

Hugh Scully is a leading figure in the world of motorsport medicine and safety. "Motorsport racing is a high-performance field, and I'm in a high-performance surgical specialty,"[18] he explained. In 1967 and 1968, Scully co-founded the Ontario Race Physicians (ORP) at the Mosport Park Circuit (then and still one of the most challenging race circuits in the world), while training in general surgery. ORP recently celebrated its fiftieth anniversary.

After a young Formula One driver friend, Helmuth Koinigg, was killed in a crash at Watkins Glen as a consequence of faulty safety equipment, Scully said to himself, "Scully, you must either walk away from this, or get more involved in motorsport safety and make a difference." *He got more involved!*

He became the national medical director for the Canadian Automobile Sports Clubs in 1975 and was the medical and safety director for Formula One racing in Canada from 1968 to 1972, for CART/IndyCar racing from 1984 to 2018, and for other series.

Working closely with his great friend, Professor Sid Watkins, a prominent London neurosurgeon and the official Fédération Internationale de l'Automobile (FIA) Formula One Medical Delegate, Sir Jackie Stewart, and others, has was a founding member of the FIA (World) Medical

Commission in 1981 and the FIA Institute for Motor Sport Safety and Sustainability in 2004, both based in Paris, representing Canada until 2018. He was also a founding member of the International Council of Motorsport Sciences (ICMS), established in Indianapolis in 1986, serving as its only Canadian chair, and chair emeritus to the present. He was the first physician elected to the Canadian Motorsport Hall of Fame in 2000 and has served as chair of the board since 2011.

In 1967, one Formula One driver in seven was killed each year. These organizations, focusing on expertise in emergency medical treatment and triage, driver fitness and nutrition, appropriate on-site medical facilities linked to communication and transport systems at major trauma centres, and working closely with engineers in car and circuit construction – with one unusual exception – reduced driver mortality in Formula One to zero by 1995. As one writer observed, "Their efforts have paid off. The ratio overall in motorsport today is 1 in 360."[19]

What do cardiac surgery and motorsport and have in common? In both arenas, quick decisions and actions are made under great pressure of time. In racing it is hot or wet, it is moderately dangerous, and there is intense publicity with worldwide television. In both, highly trained expert integrated teams make positive things happen and save lives.

Scully says, "I have always enjoyed the challenge of cardiac surgery, and am passionate about motorsport. I will say that it is more pleasant to walk through pit lane than through the cardiac surgical intensive care unit!"[20]

Tirone David, in 2011, stepped down from the chiefship at the General to head a new unit at the Peter Munk Centre focused on cardiac valve disease. (Munk had just donated $18 million to fund four new centres of excellence at the PMCC aimed at enlisting top talent.) David continues to be regarded in the division much as one would look at a kindly uncle, especially if that uncle happened to be Thomas Edison.

But there is an undercurrent of unease, and it is that David had failed to "ensure a proper transition" after his departure, as Hugh Scully puts it. "If we don't create a level playing field, we're going to lose because we won't have people in the lab, we won't be able to attract the brightest and the best anymore."[21] Only Badiwala, Rao, and Weisel had labs, which is the sine quo non of doing basic research in cardiac surgery. David retained surgery on the challenging mitral valve in his own hands. And in interviews, highers-up such as Keshavjee and Rubin expressed uncertainty about the division's ability to continue to contribute to the international research stream.

Elbowed Aside?

In Ontario, the number of angioplasties (mainly stents) increased by 66 per cent between 1998 and 2004, and the number of bypass operations decreased by 2.8 per cent. According to the Institute for Clinical and Evaluative Sciences, this surge was "chiefly due to the increased efficacy and declining price of stents, particularly drug-eluting [drug-coated] stents." Said cardiologist Jack Tu, co-author of the institute's report, "We need to stop training so many [cardiac surgeons]. They're not going to have a lot of work."[22]

Surgeons once lived on referrals from the cardiologists. Yet increasingly, the cardiologists themselves are doing procedures with "wires," as the catheters are called. For younger surgeons (willing to do night call), work increasingly comes from the Emergency Department. As Chris Feindel said, "Sixty per cent of the cases are triage cases; that is, they come in urgent."[23] Some of them are candidates for surgery, but not all of them. "The need for cardiac surgeons is to have a reset," said Bryce Taylor. "It's tough to be in cardiac. The toughest thing is to be in a specialty which has been compressed down to only the most complex of stuff, that only guys like Hugh [Scully] and Tirone [David] and others are capable of doing."[24]

Thus, unemployment has become a general problem in surgery. As the five-year review of the Department of Surgery noted in 2014, "Learners are fearful of the dire job market in … all surgical specialties. This has prevented talented medical students from considering career paths in surgery, and has created significant angst for residents who are about to enter the job market."[25] In cardiac surgery this has been a startling change. For most of our story, heart surgeons were in such short supply that the arrival of people such as Ray Heimbecker at the University of Western Ontario seemed like a gift from heaven. Yet of four of Stephen Fremes's newly trained cardiac surgeons at Sunnybrook in 2005, three had still not found work by October of that year.[26] By 2012, at least twenty new cardiac surgeons across Canada were unemployed. A report of the Canadian Society of Cardiac Surgeons said that if the failure to fill residency positions continued, there would be a "significant shortage of surgeons" in the future.[27]

Thus, in the rush of disciplines that started intervening in the heart, such as the investigational imagers and the investigational cardiologists, the surgeons found themselves increasingly elbowed aside. How do we sort this out? In the same way that, historically, ebb and flow problems have been sorted. Look at the decline of the old lithotomists and the rise of the urological surgeons. Old disciplines fall, new ones rise. Viv Rao foresaw in 2018 a reconfiguration of the discipline boundaries in ten years' time. People are regrouping on the basis of interest. "'I'm in heart failure.' So we've got a group of people who are interested in heat failure, or they're transplant cardiologists, or they're device guys, so they're putting in the pacemakers, the ICVs [interventional cardiac and vascular technology], or the transplant and the VAD guys. We've got structural guys that are interested in aortic valve disease. So, are you a surgeon? Are you a TAVI guy? And we've got people on both sides. So you're no longer going to be a heart surgeon or a cardiologist, or an interventional cardiologist; you're a heart failure specialist, you're an aortic valve specialist, you're a coronary [artery] specialist, and then you'll have access to all the technologies that deal with that disease."[28]

Lessons

"What can be learned from the history of cardiac therapies?" asks medical historian David S. Jones. "Historians have only just begun to scratch the surface."[29]

In the perennial debate about whether cardiac surgeons can also be scientists, and vice versa, there is a Canadian lesson that comes from Toronto: surgeons can also be scientists. Indeed, the dog lab is a precondition for innovation in the OR. The Toronto tradition, beginning with Bigelow and reinforced with Baird, is that innovation on the patient is pioneered by experimentation on the dog. The Toronto surgeons have paid their debt in full measure.

But cardiac surgery today is different from Bigelow's and Baird's day! Bryce Taylor said in 2018, "It's not like the old days, you're not getting straightforward cases anymore, everything is just complex and everything – the decision-making right from the beginning, the patients, even the investigations – are very high level and sometimes dangerous. The operations are different, the post-operative care is different, the selection of patients is totally different from what it used to be."[30] And this is a second lesson: Routine coronary bypass graft surgery can be done in a number of centres. The General is now a referral centre for the most difficult cases, and its surgeons are the leaders of the field. The surgeons we train must see themselves as up to this challenge.

There is another lesson here, and it regards the specialness of surgery. As Harry Rakowski said, "I think what cardiologists who do not go in the operating room don't understand is how hard it is to do cardiac surgery."[31] It is special.

Surgeons have a very intimate relationship with their patients. The surgeons are inside their bodies. This creates a special trust. John Wedge said, "It's the intrusion into one's body. It has to do with an ethos that you just can't pass patients from one surgeon to another. Continuity of care is our ensign. I remember working on a medical ward as a resident, and I said, 'Who is your doctor?' and he said, 'Well, I don't know – it's Monday now.' This would never happen in a surgical ward."[32]

Scully added, "Any time that I would be travelling, I would go around to my patients, say I was going to be away and so-and-so was going to be covering. I would identify another surgeon when I was not here."[33]

Wedge continued, "All surgeons do that. I think it's the fiduciary duty to the patient. Once you do an operation, only you know what went on in that operation, you and the people assisting you." Here, Wedge struggled to find words. He then said something directly opposed to the popular conception of surgeons. "It has to do with accountability, the autonomy, you know, surgeons I think are inwardly very self-critical, perhaps not outwardly. They can't stand failure. It is just a different personality set than an internist's."[34]

What we are dealing with here is a Toronto tradition of surgery, going straight back to William Gallie, who founded the surgery program in the 1930s. It is a tradition that puts the welfare of the patient above all else, and that includes the patient's sense of trust, confidence, and well-being. The people who pass through these pages have all been very mindful of this, and we must be careful not to lose it.

Appendix I: The Local, Regional, National, and International Impact of Residents and Fellows Who Trained and Studied at the Toronto General Hospital

From the early days with Bill Bigelow up to the present, residents and fellows from across Canada and around the world have gravitated to Toronto and the Toronto General Hospital to train in cardiovascular surgery and to pursue creative and productive research studies in cardiovascular science.

Residents have come from virtually every medical school in Canada to train as cardiovascular surgeons.

More than two hundred fellows from Canada, the United States, Mexico, South America, the UK, most European countries, Russia, the Middle East, India, Japan, Korea, Australia, and South Africa have honed their clinical and research skills at TGH and the Banting Institute.

As a tribute to the quality of the clinical and research environment at TGH, many of these trainees have gone forward to realize important leadership positions in cardiac surgery.

At TGH itself, following worldwide searches, the key position of chief of the Division of Cardiac Surgery has been awarded consecutively to TGH trainees: Ron Baird succeeded Bill Bigelow, followed by Tirone David and Viv Rao.

TGH "graduates" have dominated the position of chair of cardiovascular surgery at the University of Toronto: Bill Bigelow, Ron Baird, Bill Williams, Richard Weisel, and Terry Yau.

Bernie Goldman left TGH to establish a world-renowned cardiac surgical service at Sunnybrook Health Sciences Centre, where he was followed by Steve Fremes and Gideon Cohen.

At the Hospital for Sick Children, Bill Mustard created one of the foremost pediatric cardiac surgical services in the world, and was succeeded as chief by George Trusler, Bill Williams, Glen Van Arsdell, and Ed Hickey.

John Callaghan created a great cardiac surgical service in Edmonton, Alberta, as did Whit Firor in Saskatoon, Saskatchewan, and Paul Field in Sudbury, Ontario. Wilbert Keon was senior resident in cardiac surgery at TGH one day, then chief of cardiac surgery in Ottawa the next. He went on to create what is today a world-class cardiac surgical centre.

Cardiac surgical centres in Vancouver (Frank Tyers, Sam Lichtenstein), New Westminster (Tim Latham), Calgary (Paul Fedak), Edmonton (Ivan Rebeyka, pediatric), Hamilton (Kevin Teoh), Kingston (Gloria Ropchan), Mississauga (Gopal Bhatnagar), Newmarket (Charles Peniston), Sherbrooke (Claude Labrosse), Halifax (Stacey O'Blenes, pediatric), and St. John's, Newfoundland (Kevin Melvin) are or have been headed by "graduates" of the TGH program.

In the United States, Steve Plume at the University of Vermont and Dave Charlesworth in Manchester, New Hampshire, headed up thoracic surgical units where both focused more on cardiac surgery. Bob Kormos in Pittsburgh became a world leader in cardiac transplantation and mechanical hearts. Glen van Arsdell has been appointed head of cardiac surgery at UCLA in Los Angeles. Focusing more on the noncardiac side of cardiothoracic surgery, David Sugarbaker at Harvard in Boston and Alec Patterson at Washington University in St. Louis enhanced previously established world-class thoracic units.

In all the countries to which they have gone, TGH graduates have quickly risen to leadership positions. Particularly outstanding have been Michael Borger, a Canadian, in Leipzig, the first-ever non-native German appointed as professor of cardiac surgery anywhere in Germany; Ehud Raanani as director of cardiac surgery at the Leviev Heart Centre in Israel.

It is fair to say that our TGH cardiovascular surgical graduates have made great contributions in Canada and worldwide, one of the reasons the Toronto General Hospital is recognized as the best in Canada and fourth best in the world.

Appendix II: TGH Cardiac Surgeons Who Have Been Honoured by Awards and Elective Leadership Positions for Their Outstanding Contributions to Heart and Healthcare

American Association of Thoracic Surgery (AATS)

Celebrating a one-hundred-year legacy of education, scholarship, and research leadership in cardiothoracic health, the AATS is composed of 1,500 leading cardiothoracic (CT) surgeons from forty-two countries.

The majority of CT surgeons from TGH have had the honour of being elected to AATS membership, reflecting the high regards worldwide for the quality of education, research, and patient care at TGH.

At the international level, election to the presidency of AATS is the highest honour that can be realized by a CT surgeon.

TGH-Trained Surgeon Presidents of the AATS

CARDIAC

Wilfred (Bill) Bigelow – 1974–5
Tirone David – 2004–5
Pedro del Nido – 2014–15

THORACIC

Robert Janes – 1952–3
Frederick Kergin – 1966–7
Griffith Pearson – 1989–90
Joel Cooper – 2003–4
Alec Patterson – 2009–10
David Sugarbaker – 2013–14

Canadian Medical Association (CMA)

The CMA, founded in 1867, represents approximately 85 per cent of the physicians in Canada. There are awards recognizing outstanding leadership in several categories.

FNG Starr Award: The top award given to a CMA member in recognition of outstanding and inspiring lifetime achievement.

First awarded: 1936 – Sir Frederick Banting, Charles Best, J.B. Collip
TGH-trained CV Surgeon recipients:

Wilfred (Bill) Bigelow (TGH) – 1992
Wilbert (Will) Keon (Ottawa Heart) – 2007

Medal of Service: Awarded to a CMA member who has made exceptional contributions to the advancement of healthcare in Canada.

First awarded: 1964
Hugh E. Scully – 2010

Canadian Cardiovascular Society

The national voice for cardiovascular clinicians and scientists promoting cardiovascular health and care excellence through knowledge translation, professional development, and leadership in health policy and advocacy.

Founded: 1947 – Now more than two-thousand members

Surgeons Elected as CCS Presidents

Since 1947, only four surgeons have been elected to the position of CCS president, reflecting the very high esteem in which they were held by their colleagues in cardiology.
All four were TGH trained.

Wilfred (Bill) Bigelow (TGH) – 1971–2
Ronald J. (Ron) Baird (TWH) – 1976–8
Wilbert (Will) Keon (Ottawa Heart) – 1988–90
Hugh E. Scully (TGH/UHN) – 1998–9

CCS Achievement Award

This lifetime achievement award was created in 1992 to recognize Canadian physicians who have made outstanding contributions during their careers within the cardiovascular field.

Five of the six surgeon recipients were TGH trained.

Wilfred (Bill) Bigelow – 1995
Wilbert (Will) Keon – 1997
Raymond (Ray) Heimbecker – 1999
Tirone David – 2000
Hugh Scully – 2010

Canadian Society of Cardiac Surgeons (CSCS)

The CSCS was founded in 2012 to support the interests of CV surgeons in Canada in training, research, and career development.

It is an affiliate of the CCS.

TGH/UHN Presidents of the CCS

Christopher Feindel – 2014
Vivek (Viv) Rao – 2018

CCS/CSCS Wilfred G. Bigelow Lecture

Beginning in 1984, a distinguished speaker was invited to deliver a keynote address to the CCS/CSCS at the annual Canadian Cardiovascular Congress.

The list of speakers reads like a "who's who" of leading cardiac surgeons from Canada, the United States, the UK, and Europe.

TGH-trained Bigelow Lecturers at the CCS AGM:

John (Jack) Callaghan (Alberta) – 1984
Raymond (Ray) Heimbecker (Western) – 1985
Wilbert (Will) Keon (Ottawa Heart) – 1986
Tirone David (TWH, TGH, UHN) – 1997
Richard Weisel (TGH, UHN) – 2004
Bernie Goldman (TGH, Sunnybrook) – 2006
Hugh Scully (TGH, TWH, UHN) – 2010
Chris Feindel (TGH, UHN) – 2012
Pedro del Nido (Children's, Boston) – 2017

Canada International Gairdner Award

Awarded annually to residents of any country in the world for out-standing discoveries or contributions to medical science. (Receipt of the Gairdner is traditionally considered a precursor to winning the Nobel Prize in Physiology or Medicine.)

First awarded: 1959
Wilfred G. (Bill) Bigelow – 1959
Gordon D.W. Murray – 1964
William T. (Bill) Mustard – 1975

Canadian Medical Hall of Fame

Recognizes, honours, and celebrates Canadian heroes who have made outstanding contributions to our country's rich medical history and heritage and to world health.

First awarded: 1994
William T. (Bill) Mustard – 1995
Wilfred G. (Bill) Bigelow – 1997
Wilbert (Will) Keon – 2007

Order of Canada

The Order of Canada is the centrepiece of Canada's honours system. It recognizes a lifetime of outstanding achievement, dedication to the community, and service to the nation from people in all sections in Canadian society.

Officer (OC): Recognition for "achievement and merit of a high degree, especially service to Canada or to humanity at large."
TGH-trained CVT surgeon recipients:

Gordon Murray (TGH) – 1967
William T. (Bill) Mustard (HSC) – 1976
Wilfred (Bill) Bigelow (TGH) – 1981
Wilbert (Will) Keon (Ottawa Heart) – 1984
Tirone David (TWH, TGH, UHN) – 1996
Raymond (Ray) Heimbecker (Western) – 1997
Shaf Keshavjee (TGH, UHN) – 2014

Member (CM): Recognition for "distinguished service in or to a particular community, group or field of activity."
TGH-trained CVT surgeon recipients:

Berrnard Goldman (TGH, Sunnybrook) – 2009

Order of Ontario

The Order of Ontario is the province's highest honour, which may be awarded to an Ontarian who has shown outstanding qualities of individual excellence and achievement in any field.

Established: 1986
TGH-trained CVT surgeon recipients:

Wilbert (Will) Keon (Ottawa Heart) – 1990
Tirone David (TGH, UHN) – 1993
Raymond (Ray) Heimbecker (TGH, Western) – 2002
Shaf Keshavjee (TGH, UHN) – 2013

Appendix III: Leadership Other than Awards

The profile of TGH and its Cardiac Division provincially, nationally, and internationally is enhanced when individual members of the division are elected to leadership positions in major organizations that address health and healthcare not directly involved with cardiovascular science and surgery.

In his numerous positions as president of the OMA and CMA, member of the councils/boards of the Royal College of Physicians and Surgeons of Canada, the Canadian Medical Hall of Fame, the Canadian Medical Foundation, and the World Medical Foundation, Hugh Scully has always been recognized as coming from one of the world's great hospitals and universities. The same is true of many provincial, national, and international positions he has held in the high-stress world of motorsport racing and safety.

Participation in these arenas by cardiac surgeons has generally been very rare, and has not been supported by fellow cardiac surgeons or other colleagues. That said, cardiac surgeons are generally highly intelligent, articulate, disciplined, focused, and comfortable with the concept and application of the team approach. They can and should be recognized and supported as potential leaders in the changing world of health, healthcare, and related education and research.

Notes

Preface

1 Bigelow to McNab, 4 Jan. 1977, Bigelow Papers.
2 Dwight C. McGoon of the Mayo Clinic, originator of a heart valve (the quote was found on a single loose leaf in Bigelow Papers), evidently written in 1950s.
3 Interview with Bernard Goldman and Hugh Scully, 4 Apr. 2018.
4 Interview with Bernard Goldman and Hugh Scully, 4 Apr. 2018.
5 Bigelow, "Meeting of May 24, 1967 ... to discuss some admitting problems of the Cardiovascular Surgical Division," Bigelow Papers.
6 Bigelow to J.A. McNab, executive director, TGH, 14 June 1971, Bigelow Papers.
7 See David S. Jones, *Broken Hearts: The Tangled History of Cardiac Care* (Baltimore: Johns Hopkins University Press, 2013), 218–22.
8 OECD, *Health at a Glance 2011: OECD Indicators* (Paris: OECD Publishing, 2011), 91, tab 4.6.1.
9 "Surgical Triumph Arouses Interest," *Globe and Mail*, 13 Apr. 1914, 8.
10 Edward Shorter, *Partnership for Excellence: Medicine at the University of Toronto and Academic Hospitals* (Toronto: University of Toronto Press, 2013).
11 Myunghyun M. Lee, Juglans Alvarez, and Vivek Rao, "History of Cardiovascular Surgery at Toronto General Hospital," *Semin Thorac Surg* 28(3) (Autumn 2016), 700–4.
12 Bigelow, "Meeting of May 24, 1967 ... to discuss some admitting problems of the Cardiovascular Surgical Division," Bigelow Papers.
13 Goldman in Stephanie Brister interview, 29 Nov. 2018.
14 David Wright, *SickKids: The History of the Hospital for Sick Children* (Toronto: University of Toronto Press, 2016).
15 Wilfred G. Bigelow, *Cold Hearts: The Story of Hypothermia and the Pacemaker in Cardiac Surgery* (Toronto: McClelland and Stewart, 1984), 9.

Introduction

1 See, for instance, James Peto, ed., *The Heart* (New Haven and London: Yale University Press / London: Wellcome Collection, 2007), companion to an exhibition at the Wellcome Collection, which examines the evolution of our understanding of the heart and its anatomical and symbolic significance from the earliest written and visual images to the present.

2 Stephen L. Johnson, *The History of Cardiac Surgery, 1896–1955* (Baltimore: John Hopkins Press, 1970), 5.

3 The early history of heart surgery, focusing mainly on American and British developments, is covered in Stephen L. Johnson, *The History of Cardiac Surgery, 1896–1955* (Baltimore and London: Johns Hopkins Press, 1970). For Canadian developments, one of the present authors put together an anthology, *Heart Surgery in Canada: Memoirs, Anecdotes, History and Perspective*, ed. Bernard S. Goldman and Susan Bélanger (Philadelphia: Xlibris, 2009), though this is not a detailed review of cardiac surgery in Canada. Some material on the pioneer generation of Canadian cardiac surgeons, along with cardiologists, is also provided in Harold Segall, *Pioneers of Cardiology in Canada, 1820–1970: The Genesis of Canadian Cardiology* (Willowdale: Hounslow Press, 1988).

4 J.T.H. Connor, *Doing Good: The Life of Toronto's General Hospital* (Toronto: University of Toronto Press, 2000), 15–31.

5 Connor, *Doing Good*, 85.

6 Connor, *Doing Good*, 62–4.

7 Cynthia Macdonald, "A New Era in Medicine: How a Historic $250 Million Gift to U of T Will Transform Medical Education – and Improve Patient Care," *University of Toronto Magazine*, 14 Dec. 2020.

8 Edward Shorter, *Partnership for Excellence: Medicine at the University of Toronto and Academic Hospitals* (Toronto: University of Toronto Press, 2013), 18–22.

9 Shorter, *Partnership for Excellence*, 623–6.

10 Shorter, *Partnership for Excellence*, 243–4.

11 University of Toronto, Faculty of Medicine, https://medicine.utoronto.ca/about-faculty-medicine/fully-affiliated-hospitalsresearch-institutes, accessed 22 Jan. 2020, and https://medicine.utoronto.ca/about-faculty-medicine/community-affiliated-hospitals-and-sites, accessed 22 Jan. 2020.

12 Shorter, *Partnership for Excellence*, 52–5.

13 W.G. Bigelow, *Mysterious Heparin, the Key to Open-Heart Surgery* (Toronto: McGraw-Hill, 1990); Shorter, *Partnership for Excellence*, 48–9.

14 W.G. Bigelow, *Cold Hearts: The Story of Hypothermia and the Pacemakers in Heart Surgery* (Toronto: McClelland and Stewart, 1984).

15 Shorter, *Partnership for Excellence*, 168–70.

16 University Health Network Archives, description for the Toronto Hospital, https://www.archeion.ca/toronto-hospital, accessed 24 Jan. 2020.

17 University Health Network, Our History, https://www.uhn.ca/corporate /AboutUHN/OurHistory, accessed 25 Jan. 2020.

18 Noah Miller, "The 10 Best Hospitals in the World," *Newsweek*, 5 Apr. 2019; https://www.newsweek.com/2019/04/05/10-best-hospitals-world-1368512 .html. The 2020 rankings appear in "The World's Best Hospitals," http:// www.newsweek.com/best-hospitals-2020, and those for 2021 in "The World's Best Hospitals," http://www.newsweek.com/best-hospitals-2021.

1. Gordon Murray

1 Bigelow, "Donald Walter Gordon Murray, C.C., 1897–1976," Bigelow Papers. The eulogy bore not a trace of the ill will that Murray was so quick to show to others.

2 Gordon Murray, *Medicine in the Making* (Toronto: Ryerson, 1960), 2–3.

3 Hannah Institute for the History of Medicine, Oral History Interviews, vol. 24 (Dr. William S. Keith), 60, University of Toronto Archives and Records Management Service (UTARMS).

4 Bigelow, Murray eulogy.

5 Hannah Institute for the History of Medicine, Oral History Interviews, vol. 24 (Dr. William S. Keith), 59, UTARMS.

6 Murray, draft letter to Mr. Franken, Secretary of the Association of Surgeons of Great Britain and Ireland, 22 Sept. 1926, Library and Archives Canada (LAC), MG 30, B110, vol. 28.

7 See Murray to Sister Superior, St. Michael's Hospital, 12 Jan. 1927; LAC MG 30, B110, vol. 28.

8 Murray, *Medicine in the Making*, 46.

9 See "Donald Walter Gordon Murray, University of Toronto Staff Report," UTARMS, A 1981–0047, box 12.

10 Elsinore Macpherson Haultain to Mrs. Hindmarsh, 4 Jan. 1968; LAC MG30, B110, vol. 28. Elsinore Haultain had been at Havergal, a private girls' school, with Ruth Atkinson, and was appealing to her former classmate. The Atkinsons and Hindmarshs were among the five families to whom, in the Atkinson Charitable Foundation, the *Toronto Star* was bequeathed in 1948. Elsinore Haultain, married to N.R. Hindmarsh, was requesting the intervention of the foundation on behalf of Murray, now under siege for his improbable discovery of a "cure for paralysis."

11 Murray, *Medicine in the Making*, 55.

12 Hannah Institute for the History of Medicine, Oral History Interviews, vol. 33 (Dr. William T. Mustard), 157, UTARMS.

13 Bryce Taylor to Edward Shorter, personal communication, 15 Nov. 2018.

14 Hugh Scully to Susan Bélanger, personal communication, 30 Jan. 2020.

15 Hannah Institute for the History of Medicine, Oral History Interviews, vol. 19 (Dr. John Drennan Hamilton), 12–13, UTARMS.

16 Murray to Elias Rodriguez Asopurus, Caracas; LAC, MG30, B110, vol. 31.

17 Heimbecker to Bigelow memo, undated, attached to which was a list: "General Surgery in P.O.R. Jan + Feb 1965"; on "half," see Bigelow to R.A. Mustard, 14 July 1962; both documents in Bigelow Papers.

18 The work was published in 1933, by which time Markowitz was back in Toronto. Yet the title page gives Markowitz's institutional affiliation as the Physiologic Laboratory of Georgetown University School of Medicine. Although not the senior author of the paper, Markowitz led the cardiac work. Frank C. Mann, James T. Priestley, J. Markowitz, Wallace M. Yater, "Transplantation of the Intact Mammalian Heart," *Arch Surg* 26 (1933), 219–24.

19 See J. Markowitz, "Curriculum Vitae," 12 June 1964; UTARMS, B2004–0021–001–07.

20 Jacob Markowitz, *Textbook of Experimental Surgery* (Baltimore: Wood, 1937), 333, 344.

21 Shelley McKellar, *Surgical Limits: The Life of Gordon Murray* (Toronto: University of Toronto Press, 2003), 218n74.

22 University of Toronto, *President's Report for the Year Ended June 1933*, 56.

23 D.W.G. Murray, L.B. Jacques, T.S. Perrett, and C.H. Best, "Heparin and Vascular Occlusion," *CMAJ* 35(6) (Dec. 1936), 621–2.

24 Ronald James Baird, "The Development of Cardiac and Vascular Surgery in Canada: Personal and Anecdotal Reflections of an Era, 1854 to 1994," undated ms.,] 37–8; Bernard S. Goldman and Susan Bélanger, eds., *Heart Surgery in Canada: Memoirs, Anecdotes, History and Perspective* (Philadelphia: Xlibris, 2009), 69; the original reference is D.W.G. Murray. L.B. Jacques, T.S. Perrett, and C.H Best, "Heparin," *Surgery* 2 (1937), 163–87.

25 Murray, *Medicine in the Making*, 98.

26 W.G. Gallie, memo on "heparin," see 12 Jan. 1938, Bigelow Papers, box 5.

27 "Paper and Proceedings of the Gallie Club Meeting, Mayo Clinic, 10–12 May, 1948," Bigelow Papers.

28 University of Toronto, *President's Report for the Year Ended June 1938*, 79.

29 "English Surgeon Is Sure Air Raids Will Come," *Globe and Mail*, 12 Oct. 1939, 4.

30 Bigelow, "Notes on the History of the Cardiovascular Service: A Memorandum for Dr. W.G. Cosbie," Bigelow Fonds, TGH, 0094–13–0-23.

31 Gordon D.W. Murray, "Heparin in Thrombosis and Embolism," *Brit J Surg* 27 (1940), 567–98.

32 "Toronto Doctor Reveals Heparin Saved 149 Here," *Toronto Star*, 19 Dec. 1946, 1.

33 W.E. Gallie to Murray, 7 June 1933, LAC, MG 30, B110, vol. 28.

34 TGH, Surgical Staff Meeting, 6 Jan. 1938, LAC MG30, B110, vol. 28 (Murray's talk was number three in the programme); Gordon Murray, F.R. Wilkinson, and R. MacKenzie, "Reconstruction of the Valves of the Heart," *CMAJ* 38(4) (Apr. 1938), 317–19. See also McKellar, *Surgical Limits*, 54.

35 Murray, *Medicine in the Making*, 135.

36 Murray, *Medicine in the Making*, 169–70.

37 Donald R. Wilson interview, Hannah Oral History, 32–3, vol. 46, UTARMS.

38 Gordon Murray, "Surgical Treatment of Coarctation of the Aorta," *CMAJ* 62(3) (March 1950), 241–3.

39 Stephen J. Evelyn and Iain MacKay, "Anesthetic for Cardiac Surgery," *Current Researches in Anesthesia and Analgesia*, 33 (1954), 186–94.

40 Murray, *Medicine in the Making*, 202–3. Alfred Blalock and Helen B. Taussig, "The Surgical Treatment of Malformations of the Heart," *JAMA* 128(3) (19 May 1945), 189–202.

41 Murray, *Medicine in the Making*, 208–9.

42 Murray, *Medicine in the Making*, 212–14.

43 James Vipond, "Death Follows Canada's First 'Blue' Operation," *Globe and Mail*, 11 Mar. 1946 It was not in fact Canada's first blue baby operation but rather Toronto's. See also McKellar, *Surgical Limits*, 58–9. The exact nature of Isabel's cardiac pathology was unclear.

44 "Toronto Doctor Gives Blue Baby 'New Heart,'" *Globe and Mail*, 4 July 1946, 5.

45 "Historic Blue Baby Awaits First Child," *Globe and Mail*, 5 Dec. 1967, 10.

46 See Frontenac Programme Continuity, sponsor, Albert's Hardware, 29 Sept. 1946. "An Orchid This Week to Doctor Gordon D.W. Murray – Famed for His 'Blue Baby' Operations," LAC MG 30, B110, vol. 28.

47 Baird, "Remarks for the Academy of Medicine Gold Symposium," 1 Nov. 1994, 2, Scully personal archive.

48 Murray, *Medicine in the Making*, 215.

49 Alfred Blalock to Murray, 3 Oct. 1946, LAC MG 30, B110, vol. 28.

50 "'Blue Babies' Stream to Toronto Hospital," *Toronto Star*, 1 Mar. 1947, 3; *Toronto Star*, 28 Apr. 1947, 7.

51 George Bain, "Heart Operation Opens New World for Billy," *Globe and Mail*, 19 June 1948, 4.

52 "Birthday Eve Ends in Death of 'Blue Baby,'" *Globe and Mail*, 22 Jan. 1949, 5.

53 Stephen J. Evelyn and Iain MacKay, "Anesthetic for Cardiac Surgery," *Current Researches in Anesthesia and Analgesia* 33 (1954), 186–94.

54 Gordon Murray, "Surgical Treatment of Congenital Heart Disease (Tetralogy of Fallot)," *CMAJ* 58(1) (Jan. 1948), 10–12.

55 Dorothy B—— to Murray, 9 Sept. 1947, LAC MG30, B110, vol. 31.

56 Peter Y—— to Murray, 22 Aug. 1948; LAC MG30, B110, vol. 31.

57 Murray, *Medicine in the Making*, 219.

58 Gordon Murray, "Surgical Treatment of Mitral Stenosis," *CMAJ*, 62(5) (May 1950), 444–7. Bigelow asserted that Murray began mitral valvuloplasty in 1948. Bigelow, "Cardiovascular Statistics," 15 Feb. 1966. It was Edouard Gagnon in Montreal who pioneered commissurotomy on the mitral valve. Gagnon said the "valvuloplasty using a venous graft" that Murray did in Toronto "would seem to require greater technical skill than we possess." Edouard D. Gagnon, "Commissurotomy in Mitral Stenosis," *CMAJ* 63(6) (Dec. 1950), 537–40.

59 Gordon Murray, "Surgical Treatment of Mitral Stenosis."

60 For an overview, see Lorenzo Gonzalez-Lavin, "Charles P. Bailey and Dwight E. Harken – The Dawn of the Modern Era of Mitral Valve Surgery," *Ann Thorac Surg* 53(5) (May 1992), 916–19. One overview of the history of pediatric cardiac surgery omits entirely any reference to Murray's work. Robert M. Freedom, J. Lock, and Ti. Bricker, "Pediatric Cardiology and Cardiovascular Surgery: 1950–2000," *Circulation* 102 (20 suppl. 4) (14 Nov. 2010), lv-58–lv-68.

61 Murray, *Medicine in the Making*, 136–7.

62 Roy Greenaway, "Renews Valve in Heart – Murray 10 Years Ahead – U.S. Specialist Admits," *Toronto Star*, 1 Feb. 1950, 21.

63 Gordon Murray, "Closure of Defects in Cardiac Septa," *Annals of Surgery* 128(4) (Oct. 1948), 524–34. Murray explained his development of the VSD closure in *Quest in Medicine* (Toronto: Ryerson, 1953), 39–45, and the first successful operation, 45–50.

64 Gordon Murray, *Quest in Medicine*, 49–50.

65 "Had 3 Months to Live but See Years Added by Delicate Operation," *Toronto Star*, 14 Jan. 1950, 1.

66 Murray, *Quest in Medicine*, 91.

67 Charles A. Hufnagel et al., "Surgical Correction of Aortic Insufficiency," *Surgery*, 35(5) (May 1954), 673–83.

68 Gordon Murray, Walter Roschlau, and William Lougheed, "Homologous Aortic-Valve-Segment Transplants as Surgical Treatment for Aortic and Mitral Insufficiency," Angiology, 7(5) (Oct. 1956), 466–71.

69 Raymond O. Heimbecker, "Heart Valves 1955," *Can J Cardiol* 10(5) (June 1994), 571–2.

70 Baird, "Development," 48–9.

71 A.J. Kerwin, S.C. Lenkei, and D.R. Wilson, "Aortic-Valve Homograft in the Treatment of Aortic Insufficiency: Report of Nine Cases, with One Followed for Six Years," *NEJM* 266 (26 Apr. 1962), 852–7.

72 Murray to V.K. Saini, 16 Aug. 1957, LAC MG30, B110, vol. 28.

73 Bigelow … Murray, "Clinical Homograft Valve Transplantation," *J Thoracic and CV Surg* 48 (Sept. 1964).

74 "Blue Baby Expert, Dr. G.D.W. Murray, Leaves for U.K.," *Globe and Mail*, 22 June 1949, 5.

75 Hannah Institute for the History of Medicine, Oral History Interviews (Dr. Donald R. Wilson), vol. 46, 33, UTARMS.

76 Hugh Scully, interview, 23 Feb. 2018.

77 Gordon Murray, "The Pathophysiology of the Cause of Death from Coronary Thrombosis," *Annals of Surgery* 126 (1947), 523–34. The erroneous view has crept in that it was investigators at Northwestern University who in 1959 first induced a heart attack in a laboratory animal. See, for example, David S. Jones, *Broken Hearts: The Tangled History of Cardiac Care* (Baltimore: Johns Hopkins University Press, 2013), 34.

78 Murray, "Pathophysiology." See Murray's chronicle of these dramatic events in his *Quest in Medicine*, 36–7.

79 Murray, *Quest in Medicine*, 38.

80 Baird, "Development," 42.

81 Jean Kunlin, "Le traitement de l'arterite obliterante par la greffe veineuse," *Arch Mal Coeur* 42 (1949), 371–2.

82 Baird, "Development," 40.

83 See the "Notice of Appointment," 23 June 1959, LAC MG30, B110, vol. 29.

84 Murray to Gordon A. Donaldson, Boston, 4 Aug. 1960, LAC, MG30, B110, vol. 29. The actual statistics were scrawled on a scrap of paper next to the letter, and evidently Murray forwarded these at some later point.

85 Goldman, private communication to Shorter, 1 Mar. 2018.

86 Hannah Institute for the History of Medicine, Oral History Interviews, vol. 28 (Dr. Robert Laidlaw MacMillan), 34, UTARMS.

87 Douglas Robb to Ethel Kerr, 30 Jan. 1958, LAC MG 30, B110, vol. 28.

88 W.G. Bigelow, *Mysterious Heparin: The Key to Open Heart Surgery* (Toronto: Ryerson, 1990), 78.

89 Bigelow to Drucker, 4 July 1968, Bigelow Papers; see also McKellar, *Surgical Limits*, 59.

90 Murray to Lorne Pierce, Ryerson Press, 20 Oct. 1959, LAC MG30, B110, vol. 29.

91 R.M. Taylor to M.J. Grimes, 14 Aug. 1969, LAC MG30, B110, vol. 30.

92 Rowan Nicks, "The Auckland Hospital Board Meeting 9/2/53/ Report of Mr. Rowan Nicks, Thoracic and Cardiac Surgeon on His Activities During Study Leave Overseas," LAC, MG 30, B110, vol. 28, 19–20.

93 Murray to W. Eric Phillips, 8 May 1947, LAC MG 30, B110, vol. 28.

94 Robert Janes to Murray, 30 Sept 1947, LAC MG 30, B110, vol. 28.

95 Hugh J. McLaughlin to Murray, 21 May 1954, LAC MG30, B110, vol. 28.

96 For details, see McKellar, *Surgical Limits*, 119, 161.

97 McKellar, *Surgical Limits*, 81–4.

98 University of Toronto, *President's Report for the Year Ended June 1948*, 12.

99 Goldman, *Heart Surgery in Canada*, 120.

100 Hannah Institute for the History of Medicine, Oral History Interviews, vol. 30 (Dr. Ernest McCulloch), 16–17, UTARMS.

101 George Trusler, interview, 27 Nov. 2018.

102 Baird, "Development," 14.

103 For Baird's discussion of Murray, see Baird, "The Story of Heparin," *J Vasc Surg* 11 (1990), 4–18, 14–16.

104 Memo, 27 Dec. [1960], LAC MG30, B110, vol. 29.

105 Goldman, *Heart Surgery in Canada*, 105n.

106 Draft "Dear Dr," [Dec. 1957]; attached to Murray to Neil A. Watters, 6 Dec. 1957, LAC MG30, B110, vol. 28.

107 John Oille to Ethel Kerr, 26 Nov. 1957, LAC MG30, B110, vol. 28.

108 See McKellar, *Surgical Limits*, 105–32.

109 Gordon Murray, Eva Ugray, and Aileen Graves, "Regeneration in Injured Spinal Cord," *Am J Surgery* 109 (Apr. 1965), 406–9, 408.

110 "Doctor Gives Hope Paraplegic May Still Walk," *Toronto Star*, 16 Nov. 1965, 45.

111 Gordon Murray, "Surgical Treatment of Paraplegia," *Panminerva Medica*, 14 (1972), 296–303.

112 McKellar, *Surgical Limits*, 138–9.

113 McKellar, *Surgical Limits*, 133–60.

114 This controversy is marginal to the story of cardiac surgery and will not be followed here, but it was avidly chronicled in the *Toronto Star* in many news stories and columns beginning with Marilyn Dunlop, "Dr. Murray Clashes with Hospital over Effect of Spinal Surgery," *Toronto Star,* 22 Nov. 1967, to "Nothing New Found in Murray's Surgery," *Toronto Star*, 23 Jan. 1968, C1. McKellar's coverage of the story is exhaustive and exemplary.

115 McKellar, *Surgical Limits,* 146.

116 Bryce Taylor, interview, 15 Nov. 2018.

117 Murray, obituary, *Globe and Mail*, 9 Jan. 1976, 2.

118 James C. Fallis, letter, *Globe and Mail*, 21 Jan. 1976; see also Arthur E. Parks's outraged letter, which enumerated some of Murray's accomplishments, 21 Jan. 1976, 7.

119 Bigelow, "Notes on the History of the Cardiovascular Service: A Memorandum for Dr. W.G. Cosbie" (1972), Bigelow Fonds, TGH, 0094–13–0-23.

2. Uncle Bill

1 "A Message to Ruth from Her Lonely Lover," 4 Mar. 2000, Bigelow Papers.

2 Bruce West, "The Midwife's Quill," *Globe and Mail*, 27 Oct. 1968, 17.

3 Bigelow does use the phrase "a pioneer horse and buggy doctor" in *Cold Hearts* (13). But W.A. Bigelow was not at all typical of the genre.

4 Wilfred Abram Bigelow, *Forceps, Fin and Feather* (Altona, MN: Friesen, 1969), 16.

5 Wilfred Abram Bigelow, *Forceps*, 11.

6 Wilfred G. Bigelow, preface, in Wilfred Abram Bigelow, *Forceps*, xviii.

7 Tim McNab, interview of Bigelow, undated. Ms. in Bigelow Papers.

8 Philip Mascoll, "Dr. Wilfred Bigelow, 91, Was a Giant of Medicine," *Toronto Star*, 29 Mar. 2005, A20. See Bigelow, *Cold Hearts,* for some detail on this period, 32–4.

9 Bigelow to Charles Tator, 5 July 1997, Bigelow Papers. This account differs from that in *Cold Hearts*, 35.

10 University of Toronto, *President's Report for the Year Ended June 1945*, 108.

11 Bigelow to Kergin, 17 July 1963, Bigelow Papers.

12 Bigelow, *Cold Hearts*, 39.

13 Alfred Blalock and Helen B. Taussig, "The Surgical Treatment of Malformations of the Heart," *JAMA* 128 (19 May 1945), 189–202.

14 Ron Baird, 1995, "Reflections on the Heart," talk to Aesculapian Club, in Scully Papers.

15 On this chronology, see Bigelow to W.G. Cosbie, 23 June 1971, Bigelow Fonds, TGH, 0094–13–0-23.

16 Bigelow, "Intellectual Humility in Medical Practice and Research," *Surgery* 65 (1969), 1–9, 1.

17 Baird, "Development," 2.

18 Bigelow to Murray, 21 Feb. 1951, Bigelow Papers.

19 Bigelow to R.W. Janes, 6 Jan. 1953, Bigelow Fonds, TGH, 0094–13–0-34; on Murray in Ward C, see McKellar, *Surgical Limits*, 64.

20 "Average Length of Present Hospitalization, Ward 'C,'" 21 Apr. 1954, loose leaf, Bigelow Papers.

21 Bigelow to J.E. Sharpe, superintendent TGH, 17 Apr. 1959, Bigelow Papers.

22 Ray Heimbecker to H. Doyle, assistant superintendent, TGH, 14 Apr. 1959, Bigelow Papers.

23 Bigelow to J.R.F. Mills, 1 Apr. 1968, Bigelow Papers.

24 Bigelow to Bengt Johansson, 26 Jan. 1962, Bigelow Fonds, TGH, 0094–8–0-32.

25 Bigelow, *Cold Hearts*, 67.

26 Arthur J. Snider, "Groundhogs' Secret Gives Surgeons Hope," *Chicago Daily News*, 5 Oct. 1953, 8.

27 W.G. Bigelow, "Cold Hearts and Vital Lessons," *Bulletin, American College of Surgeons* 69, no. 6 (June 1984), 12–20, 16–17.

28 Bigelow, "Medical Research: A Triple Responsibility," address to the Canadian Heart Foundation, 4 Nov. 1964, unpaginated. Address reprinted in *Varsity Graduate*, 12 (Spring, 1966).

29 Goldman, "The Real End of the 'Hibernin' Story," ms., 2018.

30 Goldman, quoted in Ivan Oransky, Bigelow obituary, *Lancet* 365 (7 May 2005), 1616.
31 Scully and Goldman, in Stephanie Brister interview, 29 Nov. 2018.
32 Bigelow to M.S.A. Woodside, 13 June 1966, Bigelow Papers.
33 Bigelow to Weisel, 9 Apr. 1999, Bigelow Papers.
34 Scully, in interview with Heather Ross, 30 Nov. 2018.
35 Bigelow, "Creative Advances in Cardiovascular Surgery," International Conference on History of Cardiovascular Surgery, Moscow, 24–25 Sept. 1996; Bigelow, "Intellectual Humility in Medical Practice and Research," *Surgery* 65 (1969), 1–9; see also Bigelow, *Cold Hearts*, 173–7.
36 Edward Najgebauer, "I Remember," *Globe and Mail*, 7 Apr. 2005, S9.
37 Bryce Taylor, interview, 15 Nov. 2018.
38 Goldman, *Heart Surgery in Canada*, 24.
39 Wayne Johnston, interview, 12 Dec. 2018.
40 Goldman, personal communication, 15 Apr. 2019.
41 Bigelow to Lowy, 1 Dec. 1986, Bigelow Papers.
42 Wilbert Keon, "I Remember," *Globe and Mail*, 7 Apr. 2005, S7.
43 Scully, in Wayne Johnston interview, 12 Dec. 2018.

3. "Bigelow's Boys"

1 Goldman, *Heart Surgery in Canada*, 23.
2 Loose-leaf, "Surgical Publications," Bigelow Papers.
3 The information in this paragraph comes from Alan Stephen Trimble: Academic Staff Record, UTARMS, A 1981–0047, box 010; see also Bigelow, "Cardiovascular Division, Toronto General Hospital: An Outline of the Background, Activities and Requirements," undated (1967?), Bigelow Papers.
4 A.S. Trimble, R.O. Heimbecker, and W.G. Bigelow, "The Implantable Cardiac Pacemaker," *CMAJ* 90(3) (18 Jan. 1964), 106–10; the paper was delivered in 1963 at a meeting.
5 Joan Hollobon, "Surgeons Here Say Transplants Depend on Rejection Findings," *Globe and Mail*, 13 Jan. 1968, 5. "3 Worked Years Toward Operation," *Globe and Mail*, 21 Oct. 1968, 12.
6 Bigelow to Trimble, 11 July 1968, Bigelow Fonds, TGH, 0094-8-0-14.
7 Scully, note to Edward Shorter, 28 Jan. 2019.
8 Goldman, "Fall of a Giant," ms, 2018; personal communication, 11 Aug. 2018.
9 Bigelow to Kergin, 10 Nov. 1960, Bigelow Papers.
10 Bernard Goldman to H.S. Doyle, assistant director, medical, TGH, 10 Jan. 1966, Bigelow Papers. Goldman gave a carbon to Bigelow, "Dear Sir, thought I'd send you a copy in case I get fired."

11 Bigelow to John Hamilton, 25 July 1967, Bigelow Papers.

12 Bigelow to Ian Macdonald, 5 July 1962; letter in Goldman's possession.

13 Goldman to Shorter, 23 Jan. 2019.

14 Bernard Langer, present at Bernard Goldman interview, 30 July 2018.

15 Goldman, *Heart Surgery in Canada*, 453.

16 Sources of this paragraph are Baird, "Development," and Goldman, personal communication.

17 Salem Alaton, "Mr. Levy Has a Bypass," *Globe and Mail*, 18 June 1994, D1.

18 As with a number of quotes in this section, this quote is from an interview with Scully, 10 Dec. 2018.

19 Hugh Scully, interview, 20 June 2018.

20 Scully, interview, 4 Apr. 2018.

21 Sarah Hampson, "Dr. Fix-it," *Globe and Mail*, 27 Jan. 2000.

22 Scully, personal communication, 29 Jan. 2020.

23 Heimbecker to Murray, 1 Mar. 1955, LAC MG30, B110, vol. 28.

24 Heimbecker to Ethel Kerr (Murray's secretary), 23 Oct. 1957, LAC MG30, B110, vol. 28.

25 R.O. Heimbecker and W.G. Bigelow, "Intravascular Agglutination of Erythrocytes (Sludged Blood) and Traumatic Shock," *Surgery* 28(3) (Sept. 1950), 461–73.

26 R.O. Heimbecker et al., "Experimental Studies of the Production of Deep Hypothermia by Means of a Pump Oxygenator and Heat Exchanger," *Canad J Surg* 79 (1959), 465–72; Heimbecker et al., "The Heat Exchanger in Extracorporeal Circulation," *J Thorac and Cardiovasc Surg* 43 (April 1962), 465–72; "Kitchen Idea Aids Science," *Globe and Mail*, 1 Jan. 1960, 4.

27 Gordon Murray, "The Pathophysiology of the Cause of Death from Coronary Thrombosis," *Annals of Surgery* 126(4) (Oct. 1947), 523–34.

28 R.O. Heimbecker and Gordon Murray, "A Curette for Embolectomy," *American Journal of Surgery* 99 (June 1960), 918–20.

29 Murray to Heimbecker, 9 Apr. 1959, LAC, MG30, B110, vol. 29.

30 Goldman, personal communication, 15 Apr. 2019.

31 See Stuart Vandewater, "A Personal Experience," in Robert J Byrick, ed., *A Commemorative History of the Department of Anaesthesia* (Toronto: University of Toronto, Department of Anaesthesia, 2004), 102.

32 Bigelow to Kergin, 21 Oct. 1961, TGH, Bigelow Fonds, 0094–8-0–12.

33 Bigelow to Heimbecker, 7 July 1961, Bigelow Papers.

34 Kergin, "Memo, Discussion with Dr. W.G. Bigelow, June 17, 1963," UTARMS, A1989–0030, box 002.

35 Kergin, "Memorandum, Discussion with Dr. W.G. Bigelow, Sept. 6, 1963," UTARMS, A1989–0030, box 002.

36 Honor G. Nivin, letter, *Globe and Mail*, 12 Mar. 2014, S6.

37 For an early report on a series of twenty, all without a death, see James A. Key, "The Symptomless Abdominal Aneurysm – What Should Be Done about It?" *CMAJ* 82(18) (30 Apr. 1960), 924–5.

38 Nicol Kingsmill, "A Valve Gave Them Life …," *Telegram* [no date preserved] (1968).

39 Scully, interview, 20 June 2018.

40 Goldman, personal communication, 15 Apr. 2019.

41 Bigelow, "Jim Key's Eulogy," 13 July 1996, Bigelow Papers.

42 "Salad, Scotch, Sex: Tongue-in-Cheek Advice Is Given to Prevent Heart Diseases," *Globe and Mail*, 14 Mar. 1963, 5.

4. Hypothermia Discovered

1 John H. Talbott and Kenneth J. Tillotson, "The Effects of Cold on Mental Disorders: A Study of Ten Patients Suffering from Schizophrenia and Treated with Hypothermia," *Diseases of the Nervous System* 2 (1941), 118–26.

2 See Peter Ziegelroth, *Handbuch der physikalisch-diätetischen Therapie (Natur-Heilverfahren)* (Leipzig: Garms, 1906), 77.

3 Bigelow, *Cold Hearts* (1984), 11–12.

4 Meeting with Bernard Goldman and Hugh Scully, 4 Apr. 2018.

5 See W.G. Bigelow and E.C.G. Lanyon, "Some Uses for Dry Cold Therapy, and a Proposed Cooling Cabinet," *British Medical Journal* 1 (12 Feb. 1944), 215–17.

6 Among the sources for this material are W. Gerald Rainer, interview, 22 June 1973, "Wilfred Bigelow, MD," Bigelow Papers; Bigelow to W.G. Cosbie, 19 Aug 1971, Bigelow Fonds, TGH, 0094–13-9-23.

7 Bigelow, "Medical Research: A Triple Responsibility," address to the Canadian Heart Foundation, 4 Nov. 1964, unpaginated. Address reprinted in *Varsity Graduate* 12 (Spring, 1966).

8 University of Toronto, *President's Report for the Year Ended June 1948*, 113.

9 W.G. Bigelow, W.K. Lindsay, R.C. Harrison, R.A. Gordon, and W.F. Greenwood, "Oxygen Transport and Utilization in Dogs at Low Body Temperatures," *American Journal of Physiology* 160(1) (Jan. 1950), 125–37; the paper was received for publication in July 1949.

10 Bigelow to L.W. Billingsley, 7 Aug. 1950, Bigelow Papers.

11 Ron Kenyon, "Heart Shut Off, Dog Lives, Use 'Cold' Anesthesia," [Toronto] *Telegram*, 5 Dec. 1949.

12 W.G. Bigelow, J.C. Callaghan, J.A. Hopps, "General Hypothermia for Experimental Intracardiac Surgery," *Ann Surg* 132(3) (Sept. 1950), 531–9: this was the paper presented at Colorado Springs. W.G. Bigelow, W.K. Lindsay, and W.F. Greenwood, "Hypothermia: Its Possible Role in Cardiac Surgery: An Investigation of Factors Governing Survival in Dogs at Low

Body Temperatures," *Annals of Surgery,* 132(5) (Nov. 1950), 849–66: this paper was submitted in Nov. 1949.

13 Bigelow, "Hypothermia in Surgery (for Ontario Centennial Project)," undated paper, Bigelow Papers.

14 W.G. Bigelow, W.T. Mustard, and J.G. Evans, "Some Physiologic Concepts of Hypothermia and Their Applications to Cardiac Surgery," *J Thorac Surg* 28(5) (Nov. 1954), 463–80.

15 Goldman, quoted in Ivan Oransky, obituary of Bigelow, *Lancet* 365 (7 May 2005), 1616.

5. The First Operations

1 Bigelow, *Cold Hearts,* 61.

2 Meeting, "Cardiovascular Surgical Division, Toronto General Hospital," 24 May 1967, UTARMS, A1989–0030, box 002.

3 Steven G. Friedman, "The 50th Anniversary of Abdominal Aortic Reconstruction," *J Vascular Surg* 33(4) (Apr. 2001), 895–8.

4 The information in this paragraph is from Baird, "Development," 41.

5 Dwight E. Harken and Paul M. Zoll, "Foreign Bodies in and in Relation to the Thoracic Blood Vessels and Heart, III: Indications for the Removal of Intracardiac Foreign Bodies and the Behavior of the Heart During Manipulation," *American Heart Journal* 32 (July 1946), 1–19.

6 Hannah Institute for the History of Medicine, "Oral History Interviews (Dr. Donald R. Wilson)," UTARMS, 38.

7 William G. Williams and Bernard S. Goldman, "Wilfred Gordon Bigelow, MD, 1913–2005," *Trans Amer Surg Assn* 124 (2006), 301–2.

8 Claude S. Beck, "The Development of a New Blood Supply to the Heart by Operation," *Annals of Surgery* 102(5) (Nov. 1935), 801–13.

9 Arthur A.M. Vineberg, "Development of an Anastomosis between the Coronary Vessels and a Transplanted Internal Mammary Artery," *CMAJ* 55(6) (June 1946), 117–19.

10 Arthur M. Vineberg, "Development of Anastomosis between the Coronary Vessels and a Transplanted Internal Mammary Artery," *Journal of Thoracic Surgery* 18(6) (Dec. 1949), 839–50.

11 Arthur Vineberg and Gavin Miller, "Internal Mammary Coronary Anastomosis in the Surgical Treatment of Coronary Artery Insufficiency," *CMAJ* 64(3) (March 1951), 204–10.

12 Arthur Vineberg et al., "Four Years' Clinical Experience with Internal Mammary Artery Implantation in the Treatment of Human Coronary Insufficiency," *J Thorac Surg* 29(1) (Jan. 1955), 1–35, 31.

13 Bigelow to Donald B. Effler, 31 Mar. 1990, in Bigelow Papers.

14 Ron Baird, "Remarks for the Academy of Medicine Gold Symposium,"
    1 Nov. 1994, 4, Scully Papers.
15 Bigelow to J.S.W. Aldis, Ontario Health Services Insurance Plan, 29 Dec.
    1970, Bigelow Fonds, TGH, 0094–13–0-8.
16 Bigelow, "Cardiovascular Statistics," 15 Feb. 1966.
17 Donald B. Effler, Laurence K. Groves, F. Mason Sones, Jr., and Earl K.
    Shirey, "Increased Myocardial Perfusion by Internal Mammary Artery
    Implant," *Ann Surg* 158(4) (Oct. 1963), 526–34; the paper was first
    presented in April 1963 at a meeting of the American Surgical Association.
18 Bigelow to W. Bruce Fye, 24 Nov. 1993, Bigelow Papers.
19 Bigelow, "Surgery of Coronary Heart Disease," Moynihan Lecture, ms.,
    April 1968, 2, Bigelow Papers.
20 W.G. Bigelow, H. Basian, and G.A. Trusler, "Internal Mammary Artery
    Implantation for Coronary Heart Disease," *J Thorac Cardiovasc Surg* 45
    (Jan. 1963), 67–78.
21 Bigelow to J.S.W. Aldis, Ontario Health Services Insurance Plan, 29 Dec.
    1970, Bigelow Fonds, TGH, 0094–13–0-8.
22 On Sones's work, see David S. Jones, Visions of a Cure: Visualization,
    Clinical Trials, and Controversies in Cardiac Therapeutics, 1968–1998,"
    Isis 91(3) (Sept. 2000), 504–41, 511–12, which notes none of the Canadian
    contributions to the story.
23 F.M. Sones, "Cinecardiography," in *Clinical Cardiopulmonary Physiology*,
    2nd ed., ed. B.L. Gordon (New York: Grune and Stratton, 1960),
    130–44; see also F. Mason Sones, Jr., and Earl K. Shirey, "Cine Coronary
    Arteriography," *Modern Concepts of Cardiovascular Disease*, 31 (1962), 735–8.
24 Copies of both papers in Bigelow Papers.
25 F. Mason Sones, Jr., "Increased Myocardial Perfusion by Internal
    Mammary Artery Implant: Vineberg's Operation," *Annals of Surgery* 158
    (Oct. 1963), 526–36.
26 Bigelow to J.S.W. Aldis, Ontario Health Services Insurance Plan, 29 Dec.
    1970, Bigelow Fonds, TGH, 0094–13–0-8.
27 Joseph B. Shrager, "The Vineberg Procedure: The Immediate Forerunner
    of Coronary Artery Bypass Grafting," *Ann Thorac Surg* 57(5) (May 1994),
    1354–64.
28 Shrager, letter, *Ann Thorac Surg* 58(6) (1994), 1793–94.
29 See the Goldman letter in response to Shrager article, *Ann Thorac
    Surg*. Goldman said that Bigelow "persisted with this frustrating and
    unpredictable procedure partly from a sense of loyalty to a fellow
    Canadian's concept and partly as a reflective counterpoint to the more
    evangelical Arthur Vineberg ... I believe Bigelow's gentle personality,
    integrity, and long-term assessment are what prompted Mason Sones
    to invite a Toronto patient (as well as Vineberg's Montreal patients) to

Cleveland for IMA angiography." Bigelow incorporated into the procedure a resection of the left stellate ganglion to prevent mammary artery spasm. Shrager, in response, said, "Since publication of the article, I have heard from a large number of surgeons ... The overall sense I get ... is that many agree that the operation was of far greater benefit than generally has been credited." Goldman and Schrager letters, *Ann Thorac Surg* 58(6) (Dec. 1994), 1793–4.

30 Baird, ms., "Remarks for the Academy of Medicine Gold Symposium," 1 Nov. 1994, 5, Scully Papers.

31 See René Favaloro, "Critical Analysis of Coronary Artery Bypass Graft Surgery: A 30-Year Journey," *JACC* 31 (No. 4 Suppl B [15 Mar 1998]), 1B–63B, 4B–5B.

32 David Schechter, office in General Motors Bldg, NYC, to Bigelow, 30 May 1983, in Bigelow Papers.

33 Bigelow to W.G. Cosbie, 19 Aug. 1971, Bigelow Fonds, TGH, 0094–13–0-23.

34 George Trusler, interview, 27 Nov. 2018.

35 Lauder Brunton, "Preliminary Note on the Possibility of Treating Mitral Stenosis by Surgical Methods," *Lancet* 1 (8 Feb. 1902), 352.

36 Henry Souttar, "The Surgical Treatment of Mitral Stenosis, *BMJ* 2 (1925), https://www.bmj.com/content/2/3379/603.

37 Henry Souttar, *A Surgeon in Belgium* (1915), http://www.gutenberg.org /files/11086/11086-h/11086-h.htm.

38 Dwight E. Harken et al., "The Surgical Treatment of Mitral Stenosis," *NEJM* 239 (25 Nov. 1948), 801–9.

39 Charles Philamore Bailey, "The Surgical Treatment of Mitral Stenosis (Mitral Commissurotomy)," *Diseases of the Chest* 15(4) (April 1949), 377–93. The paper was originally presented at a meeting of the American College of Chest Physicians in Chicago, 20 June 1948.

40 Baird, "Development," 50.

41 Bigelow said he did his first mitral valvoplasty in 1950. "Cardiovascular Statistics," 15 Feb. 1966.

42 [Toronto] *Telegram*, "New Surgical Success," 8 Sept. 1951.

43 Edouard D. Gagnon and Paul David, "Traitement chiriurgical de la sténose mitrale: Commissurotomie," *L'Union Médicale du Canada* 79 (1 Oct. 1950), 1142–7; Gagnon, "Commissurotomy in Mitral Stenosis," *CMAJ* 63 (Dec. 1950), 537–40.

44 Goldman, personal communication, 1 Mar. 2018.

45 Bigelow to Blalock, 23 Aug. 1953, Bigelow Papers.

46 Joan Hollobon, "Heart Patient Regards Life As Gift of Fortune and Science," *Globe and Mail*, 9 Feb. 1967, W3. Bigelow dates the operation as "1953." *Cold Hearts*, 124.

47 Bigelow, *Cold Hearts*, 56.

48 Case record in Bigelow Papers.
49 Ron Kenyon, "Refrigerated for Surgery," [Toronto] *Telegram*, undated clipping from 1953.
50 This account is based on *Globe and Mail*, "Need Much Equipment to Chill Patient," 25 July 1953, 3; Bigelow, "Cardiovascular Statistics," 15 Feb. 1966. The patient's chart is also in the Bigelow Papers.
51 J.E. Sharpe to Harold C. Casper, Sales Manager, *Encyclopaedia Britannica*, 26 Nov. 1953, Bigelow Papers.
52 Lotta Dempsey, "Person to Person," *Globe and Mail*, 2 Oct. 1953.
53 Bigelow, *Cold Hearts*, 56.
54 David Spurgeon, "Find Heart Surgery Now Is Much Safer," *Globe and Mail*, 13 June 1959, 11.
55 W.G. Bigelow, W.F. Greenwood, A.D. McKelvey, and J.K. Wilson, "The Surgical Treatment of Mitral Stenosis," *CMAJ* 69 (1953), 588–97, 594.
56 These operative reports are all in the Bigelow Papers.
57 James Y. Nicol, "Girl, 15, 'Dies' Twice Is Given New Life by Rare Operation," *Toronto Star*, 23 Dec. 1955, 1.
58 W.G. Bigelow, W.F. Greenwood, "Mitral Stenosis with and without Surgery," *Surgical Clinics of North America* 34 (Aug. 1954), 1–28, 27.
59 "Much Progress in 20 Years, but Still Need Heart Funds," *Globe and Mail*, 16 Oct. 1959, 13.
60 David Spurgeon, "Child Crippler: Specialist Sees Rheumatic Fever Wiped Out," *Globe and Mail*, 4 Oct. 1960, 15.
61 Meeting, "Cardiovascular Surgical Division, Toronto General Hospital," 24 May 1967, UTARMS, A1989–0030, box 002.
62 See B.J. Miller, J.H. Gibbon, Jr., and Charles Fineberg, "An Improved Mechanical Heart and Lung Apparatus: Its Use during Open Cardiotomy in Experimental Animals," *Med Clin. North America* (Nov. 1953), 1603.
63 C. Walton Lillehei et al., "Mitral, Aortic, and Tricuspid Replacement with the Ball Valve," *J Thorac Cardiovasc Surg* 157 (Jan. 1965), 184–204.
64 Bigelow to Charles Hufnagel, 14 Dec. 1953, Bigelow Papers.
65 Mrs. A.A.'s case record is the Bigelow Papers.
66 Case record in Bigelow Papers.
67 Doyle to Janes, 15 Dec. 1952; Janes to Bigelow, 18 Dec. 1952; Bigelow to Janes, 6 Jan. 1953, Bigelow Papers.
68 Baird, "Development," 51.
69 Mentioned in Bigelow to Edouard D. Gagnon, 7 Aug. 1963, Bigelow Fonds, TGH; 0094–7-0–6/.
70 W.G. Bigelow, J.K. Yao, H.E. Aldridge, R.O. Heimbecker, and G.D.W. Murray (by invitation), "Clinical Homograft Valve Transplantation," *J Thoracic and Cardiovasc Surg* 48 (Sept. 1964), 333–45.
71 Goldman to Shorter, 29 Jan. 2019.

72 Bill Trent, "Help from the Dead for a Human Heart," *Weekend Magazine*, 1966.

73 Daniel A. Goor, *The Genius of C. Walton Lillehei and the True History of Open Heart Surgery* (New York: Vantage, 2007), 201. Henry Swan et al., "Surgery by Direct Vision in the Open Heart," *JAMA* 153(12) (21 Nov. 1953), 1081–5.

74 Bigelow to W.B. Kouwenhoven, 16 May 1955, Bigelow Papers.

75 Bigelow to Jaroslav Barwinsky, Winnipeg, 29 Apr. 1991, Bigelow Papers.

76 Operative notes on Mrs. C. in Bigelow Papers.

77 Bigelow to W.F. Lumsden, 23 Mar. 1962, Bigelow Papers.

78 Chart in Bigelow Papers.

79 Bigelow to Janes, 19 Feb. 1954, Bigelow Papers.

80 Bigelow to R.M. Janes, 6 Apr. 1954, Bigelow Papers.

81 R.O. Heimbecker, R.J. Baird, T.Z. Lajos, A.T. Varga, and W.F. Greenwood, "Homograft Replacement of the Human Mitral Valve," *CMAJ* 86(18) (5 May 1962), 805–9. On the first homograft replacement of the aortic valve see Donald Ross, "Homograft Replacement of the Aortic Valve," *Lancet* 2 (8 Sept. 1962), 487.

82 A.J. Kerwin, S.C. Lenkei, and D.R. Wilson, "Aortic-Valve Homograft in the Treatment of Aortic Insufficiency: Report of Nine Cases, with One Followed for Six Years," *NEJM* 266 (26 Apr. 1962), 852–7; "Report New Ways to Repair Hearts," *Toronto Star*, 14 May 1962, 2.

83 Baird, "Development," 49.

84 Goldman, in interview with Chris Feindel, 11 Dec. 2018.

85 See David S. Jones, *Broken Hearts: The Tangled History of Cardiac Care* (Baltimore: Johns Hopkins University Press, 2013), 128–31.

86 Sidney Katz, "Transplants Are a Blessing," *Toronto Star*, 17 Jan. 1968, 18.

87 Faculty of Medicine, *Annual Report, 1954*, 51.

88 "Toronto Doctor Wins Heart Surgery Award," *Globe and Mail*, 6 Dec. 1949, 4.

89 Joan Hollobon, "New Surgery Method Saves Life of Boy, 15," *Globe and Mail*, 12 Nov. 1960, 5.

90 R.O. Heimbecker and T.Z. Lajos, "Ice-Chip Cardioplegia," *Arch Surg* 84 (Jan. 1962), 148–58.

91 Ghislaine Lawrence, "Design Solutions for Medical Technology: Charles Drew's Profound Hypothermia Apparatus for Cardiac Surgery" in *Manifesting Medicine: Bodies and Machines*, eds. Bud, Finn, and Trischler (1999), 62–77.

92 Bernard Goldman, personal communication, 28 Jan. 2020.

93 Scully, in interview with George Trusler, 27 Nov. 2018. But see Samuel V. Lichtenstein et al., "Warm Heart Surgery: Experience with Long Cross-Clamp Times," *Ann Thorac Surg* 52(4) (Oct. 1991), 1009–13, who demonstrated that hypothermia may be dispensed with.

6. Homes

1 Bigelow to Carl Burton, Ontario Heart Foundation, 2 Apr. 1955, Bigelow Papers.
2 Bigelow, "Cardiovascular Service: Information for the Board of Trustees. Personal and Confidential," Oct. 1957, Bigelow Papers.
3 Baird, "Development," 5.
4 The 1956 date is given in Bigelow, "Cardiovascular Division, Toronto General Hospital: An Outline of the Background, Activities and Requirements," undated, Bigelow Papers.
5 See W.F. Greenwood to Bigelow, 1 Nov. 1967, Bigelow Papers.
6 H.E. Pugsley and W.F. Greenwood, to Janes and Farquharson, "Requirements of Space for a Cardio-respiratory Investigation Unit," Feb. 6, 1952; Bigelow memo, 5 Mar. 1952, Bigelow Fonds, TGH, 0094–13–0-24.
7 Bigelow to Janes, 2 Jan. 1954, Bigelow Fonds, TGH, 0094–13–0-24.
8 Bigelow, "Requirements for Cardiovascular Surgery, Toronto General Hospital," 12 Sept. 1957, Bigelow Papers; H. Barrie Fairley, "Recollections of the Toronto General Hospital," in *A Commemorative History of the Department of Anaesthesia*, ed. Robert J. Byrick (Toronto: University of Toronto, Department of Anaesthesia, 2004), 121.
9 Bigelow to Janes, 22 Feb. 1955, Bigelow Fonds, TGH, 0094–13–0-24.
10 Bigelow to J.A. McFadyen, 17 June 1955; John T. Frame and John A. McFadyen to the Trustees, TGH, 21 June 1955, Bigelow Fonds, TGH, 0094–13–0-24. In *Cold Hearts*, 121–2, Bigelow gives an account of the dinner where he invited "McFayden" [sic] aside to discuss contributing to such a unit.
11 Bigelow to Greenwood, 25 Jan. 1973, Bigelow Fonds, TGH, 0094–8–0-102.
12 Viking Olov Björk et al., "Left Auricular Pressure Measurements in Man," *Annals of Surgery* 138 (1953), 718–25.
13 David Spurgeon, "New Toronto General Unit Aids Heart Disease Study," *Globe and Mail*, 11 Sept. 1956, 1.
14 David Spurgeon, "Conferences Decide on Surgery," *Globe and Mail*, 28 Sept. 1957, 3.
15 Goldman to Shorter, personal communication, 12 Dec. 2018.
16 Goldman to Shorter, personal communication, 12 Dec. 2018.
17 David Spurgeon, "TGH Leads Nation in New Heart Surgery Techniques," *Globe and Mail*, Sept. 27, 1957, 7.
18 Bigelow to Kergin, 3 Sept. 1957, Bigelow Papers.
19 Bigelow to W.G. Cosbie, 23 Feb. 1972, Bigelow Fonds, TGH, 0094–13–0-23.
20 Bigelow, *Cold Hearts*, 129.
21 "Set X-ray Unit Unveiling," [TGH] *Monitor*, Oct. 1974.
22 This paragraph relies on information in "25 Years for CVIU," [TGH] *Monitor*, Aug. 1981, 2.

23 Lisa Fitterman, "Gifted with a Stethoscope" [obituary], *Globe and Mail*, 12 July 2013, S8.

24 E.D. Wigle, R.O. Heimbecker, and R.W. Gunton, "Idiopathic Ventricular Septal Hypertrophy Causing Muscular Subaortic Stenosis," *Circulation* 26 (Sept. 1962), 325. But see Russel C. Brock, "Functional Obstruction of the Left Ventricle (Acquired Aortic Subvalvular Stenosis)," *Guy's Hosp Report* 106(4) (1957), 221–38.

25 Bigelow to Greenwood, 25 Jan. 1973, Bigelow Fonds, TGH, 0094–8-0–102.

26 Joan Hollobon, "Toronto Heart Team Proves Controversial Disease Exists," *Globe and Mail*, 9 Nov. 1967, W3. See E. Douglas Wigle, Alan S. Trimble, Allan G. Adelman, and W.G. Bigelow, "Surgery in Muscular Subaortic Stenosis," *Progress in Cardiovascular Disease* 11(2) (Sept. 1968), 83–112.

27 On the US debates, see David S. Jones, "Visions of a Cure: Visualization, Clinical Trials, and Controversies in Cardiac Therapeutics, 1968–1998," *Isis* 91(3) (Sept. 2000), 504–41.

28 See David S. Jones, *Broken Hearts: The Tangled History of Cardiac Care* (Baltimore: Johns Hopkins University Press, 2013).

29 Baird, "Development," 52.

30 Baird, "Development," 52.

31 Bigelow, "Requirements for Cardiovascular Surgery," 12 Sept. 1957; attached to Medical Advisory Board Minutes, 21 Nov. 1957, TGH Fonds, TH 7.2.5.

32 [Fred Kergin], "Memorandum of Discussion with Dr. Bigelow about the Future of Cardiovascular Surgery in the Toronto General Hospital," 14 Aug. 1957, UTARMS, A1989–000, box 002.

33 See Bigelow, "Cardiovascular Surgery: Immediate Requirements," 8 Oct. 1957, Bigelow Papers.

34 Bigelow, "Cardiovascular Surgery: Immediate Requirements," 8 Oct. 1957, Bigelow Papers.

35 Mentioned in TGH Trustees Minutes, 1957–9, [date?], 4, TGH Archives, TH 8.1.16.

36 Medical Advisory Board Minutes, 21 Nov. 1957, 6, TGH Archives, TH 7.2.5.

37 Bigelow to R.H. Gourlay, St. Paul's Hospital, Vancouver, 1 Apr. 1960, Bigelow Papers.

38 Joan Hollobon, "Girl, 19, Stakes Life to Win at Heart Unit," *Globe and Mail*, 20 Jan. 1962, 5.

39 See Shorter, *Partnership for Excellence: Medicine at the University of Toronto and Academic Hospitals* (Toronto: University of Toronto Press, 2013), 219; Bigelow to W.G. Cosbie, 19 Aug. 1971, Bigelow Fonds, TGH, 0094–13–0-23.

40 Bigelow to J.E. Sharpe, 15 Nov. 1957, Bigelow Papers.

41 Kergin, "Memorandum of discussion with Dr. Bigelow about the future of Cardiovascular Surgery in the Toronto General Hospital," 14 Aug. 1957, Bigelow Papers.

42 Bigelow to R.M. Janes, 17 Jan. 1957, Bigelow Papers.

43 Bigelow to Kergin, 18 Sept. 1957, Bigelow Papers.

44 Bigelow to Kergin, 1 Apr. 1959, Bigelow Papers.

45 Bigelow, "Cardiovascular Division, Toronto General Hospital: An Outline of the Background, Activities and Requirements," undated (1967?), Bigelow Papers. He dated the move as "1956," but it seems actually to have occurred two years later.

46 Bigelow, "Notes on the History of the Cardiovascular Service: A Memorandum for Dr. W.G. Cosbie" (1972), Bigelow Fonds, TGH, 0094–13–0-23.

47 Bigelow to J.E. Sharpe, Superintendent, 15 July 1958, Bigelow Papers.

48 Key to John E. Sharpe, 17 May 1961, Bigelow Papers.

49 James A. Key, brochure, "Official Opening of the Cardiovascular Surgical Unit of the Toronto General Hospital, January 19th, 1962." Copy in Bigelow Papers.

50 M.M. Lee et al., "History of Cardiovascular Surgery at Toronto General Hospital," *Seminars in Thoracic and Cardiovascular Surgery* 28(3) (autumn 2016), 700–4; Shorter, *Partnership for Excellence*, 168–70.

51 Budget item note (C), Fall 1967, Bigelow Papers.

52 Trimble to Bigelow, 10 July 1968, Bigelow Papers.

53 Memo from Jane C.D. Channell to Bigelow, 20 Feb. 1968, Bigelow Papers.

54 Nancy Howard, psychiatric social worker, to Bigelow, 11 Dec. 1969, Bigelow Papers.

55 Bigelow to Kergin, 15 Feb. 1960, Bigelow Papers.

56 Bigelow to Drucker, 7 Feb. 1969, Bigelow Papers.

57 Kergin, "Memorandum of discussion with Dr. Bigelow about the future of Cardiovascular Surgery in the Toronto General Hospital," 14 Aug. 1957, Bigelow Papers.

58 See on this Hannah Institute for the History of Medicine, Oral History Interviews (Dr. E. Bruce Tovee), vol. 42, 80, UTARMS.

59 Marilyn Dunlop, "Heart-stopping Medical History for 50 Years," *Toronto Star*, 21 Nov. 1980, A16.

60 Bigelow, "Cardiovascular Research (The Need for a Heart Laboratory, 1959)," Bigelow Papers.

61 Bigelow to E.R. Yendt, Department of Medicine, 24 Dec. 1964, Bigelow Papers.

62 Bigelow to E.R. Yendt, 12 July 1966, Bigelow Fonds, TGH, 0094–8-0–20.

63 Bigelow to Charles H. Hollenberg, 31 Jan. 1973, Bigelow Papers.

7. The Pacemaker

1 Albert S. Hyman, "Resuscitation of the Stopped Heart by Intracardiac Therapy," *Archives of Internal Medicine* 46 (1930), 553–68.

2 Albert S. Hyman, "Resuscitation"; see also Hyman, "Resuscitation of the Stopped Heart by Intracardial Therapy, II. Experimental Use of an Artificial Pacemaker," *Archives of Internal Medicine* 50 (1932), 283–305.

3 David C. Schechter, "Background of Clinical Cardiac Electrostimulation," *New York State Journal of Medicine* 72(8) (April 1972), 953–61, 957–8.

4 Schechter, "Background," 958.

5 "Pilot, Toronto Doctor Survive Artic Ordeal," *Globe and Mail*, 9 Dec. 1948, 1.

6 Bigelow to David C. Schechter, 9 May 1969, Bigelow Papers.

7 Bigelow ms., "Hypothermia," not in *Cold Hearts*, Mar. 1983, 59–60, Bigelow Papers.

8 See Richard Cairney, "Pioneering Alberta Cardiac Surgeons Walked into Uncharted Territory 40 Years Ago," *CMAJ* 156(4) (15 Feb. 1997), 549–51.

9 J.A. Hopps to Bigelow, 26 Jan. 1983, Bigelow Papers.

10 Bigelow to Dwight C. Harken, 17 Mar. 1993, Bigelow Papers.

11 Bigelow to Jack Hopps, 6 Nov. 1950, Bigelow Papers.

12 Bigelow to Harken, 17 Mar. 1992, Bigelow Papers.

13 Bigelow, *Cold Hearts*, 90.

14 Bigelow, *Cold Hearts*, 90.

15 1949: Bigelow wrote the director of the electrical division of the NRC in November. "Mr. Jack Hopps of your division at N.R.C has been with us in the Banting Institute this week, testing an experimental machine which he has put together for radio frequency rewarming of animals at low body temperature." Bigelow was so pleased with Hopps's work that he asked if "it is possible for Mr. Hopps to return to Toronto with an oscillator, which he is attempting to assemble and stay with us for several weeks to continue his work on the machines." Bigelow to B.G. Ballard, 18 Nov. 1949, Bigelow Papers.

16 Hopps wrote in 1963, "Callaghan first used artificial stimuli for intracardiac bipolar excitation of the S-A node during hypothermia. Exponential decay pulses of 3-millisecond duration and 1 volt amplitude were applied. The inter-electrode impedance was calculated to be about 1000 ohms. The current requirement was therefore 1 milliampere and the pulse energy 3 microjoules." (J.A. Hopps, "Cardiac Resuscitation – the Present Status of Defibrillation and Stimulation Techniques," paper no. 3070, session no. 11 [NRC?], 66–7.)

17 Hopps told Bigelow in a subsequent communication that it was the technician J.R. Charbonneau who "actually constructed the unit." (Hopps to Bigelow, 4 Mar. 1983, Bigelow Papers.)

18 This account from Bigelow, "The Pacemaker Story: A Cold Heart Spinoff," *PACE* 10 (Jan.–Feb. 1987), 142–50; and from Bigelow, "The Pacemaker Story: A Cold Heart Spin-off," *CMAJ* 131(8) (15 Oct. 1984), 943–5.

19 Bigelow, "Creative Advances in Cardiovascular Surgery," International Conference on History of Cardiovascular Surgery, Moscow, 24–5 Sept.

1996, in Bigelow Papers; a slightly different version of this text is in Bigelow's *Cold Hearts*, 148–9.

20 W.G. Bigelow, J.C. Callaghan, and J.A. Hopps, "General Hypothermia for Experimental Intracardiac Surgery: The Use of Electrophrenic Respiration, an Artificial Pacemaker for Cardiac Standstill, and Radio-Frequency Rewarming in General Hypothermia," *Annals of Surgery* 132 (1950), 531–9. Radio-frequency rewarming turned out to be an idea without a future and it was permitted to lapse. See W.G. Bigelow, J.A. Hopps, and J.C. Callaghan, "Radio-Frequency Rewarming in Resuscitation from Severe Hypothermia," *Canadian Journal of Medical Sciences* 30 (1952), 185–93.

21 William L. Laurence, "Start Stopped Hearts by Toronto Machine," *NYT*, 24 Oct. 1950, 1. This account of the discovery of the pacemaker from Bigelow, "The Pacemaker Story: A Cold Heart Spinoff," *PACE* 10 (1987), 142–50.

22 See, for example, Lester Allen, "Toronto Doctors Make 'Life-saving' Device, Mends Ailing Hearts," *Toronto Star*, story dateline Boston, 24 Oct. 1950.

23 John C. Callaghan and Wilfred G. Bigelow, "An Electrical Artificial Pacemaker for Standstill of the Heart," *Annals of Surgery* 134(1) (July 1951), 8–17.

24 Dwight E. Harken and Paul M. Zoll, "Foreign Bodies in and in Relation to the Thoracic Blood Vessels and Heart, III. Indications for the Removal of Intracardiac Foreign Bodies," *American Heart Journal* 32 (1 July 946), 1–19.

25 Goldman memo to Shorter, 1 Mar. 2018.

26 Paul Zoll to J.C. Callaghan for pacemaker information, 30 Oct. 1950, Bigelow Papers.

27 See Callaghan to Dwight Harken, 11 Sept. 1991. (Hopps wrote the "very annoyed" comment on a copy of the Boston "abstract"; this and the Zoll letter were dated 1950, but they were enclosures to this 1991 letter.)

28 Zoll stipulated that the machine he borrowed from Krayer ["Kreyer" sic] was a Grass physiologic stimulator and said that Grass personally expressed uninterest in Zoll's suggestion that Grass Instrument Company in Quincy, Massachusetts, "develop and manufacture pacemakers for clinical use in the treatment of cardiac arrest." Paul Zoll note, in Dwight E. Harken, "Pacemakers, Past-Makers, and the Paced: An Informal History from A to Z," *Biomedical Instrumentation & Technology*, July–Aug. 1991, no vol. nr., 319. The Toronto group gets short shrift in this account, even though a graph shows their priority (313).

29 Paul M. Zoll, "Resuscitation of the Heart in Ventricular Standstill by External Electric Stimulation," *NEJM* 247 (11 Nov. 1952), 768–71.

30 Bigelow to Harold N. Segall, 15 Feb. 1989, Bigelow Papers.

31 "Proceedings of the Seventy-Second Meeting of the Committee on Patents of Canadian Patents and Development Limited," 18 Feb. 1953, Bigelow Papers.

32 See Bigelow to F.E. Tricerri, 26 Apr. 1955, Bigelow Papers.

33 Hopps to Bigelow, 20 Oct. 1953, Bigelow Papers.

34 Paul M. Zoll to J.A. Hopps, 13 Feb. 1953, Bigelow Papers.

35 Paul M. Zoll. "Treatment of Stokes-Adams Disease by External Electric Stimulation of the Heart," *Circulation* 9(4) (April 1954), 482–93.

36 Hopps to Bigelow, 4 Sept. 1964, Bigelow Papers.

37 William W.L. Glenn to Bigelow, 13 Dec. 1960, Bigelow Papers. In 2015 Ivan Cakulev and Albert Waldo at the Case Medical Center in Cleveland challenged an adulatory biography of Zoll by Stafford J. Cohen on the grounds that Zoll did not, in fact, merit some of the "firsts" that had been accredited him. Review of Cohen, *Paul Zoll MD: The Pioneer Whose Discoveries Prevent Sudden Death* [Salem NH: Free People Pub, 2014]. Review in *Circulation* 31(7) (2015), e421.

38 Bigelow to Measurement Engineering Company, 26 Apr. 1955, Bigelow Papers.

39 See G.W. MacDonald at Measurement Engineering Ltd., 4 May 1955, and Bigelow's reply, 9 May 1955, Bigelow Papers.

40 Hopps to Bigelow, 18 Mar. 1974, Bigelow Papers.

41 Paul M. Zoll to Bigelow, 20 Aug. 1964, Bigelow Papers.

42 Bigelow to Hopps, 31Aug. 1964, Bigelow Papers.

43 Undated Electrodyne promotional brochure, in Bigelow Papers. The flysheet said in large type, "developed by Paul M. Zoll, M.D."

44 Paul M. Zoll, letter, *PACE* 10 (1987), 1388.

45 See also Furman to Bigelow, 21 July 1987, Bigelow Papers.

46 Bigelow to Hopps, 2 Oct. 1987, Bigelow Papers.

47 Zoll's role in the development of the pacemaker is discussed at further length in Kirk Jeffreys, *Machines in Our Hearts: The Cardiac Pacemaker, the Implantable Defibrillator, and American Health Care* (Baltimore and London: Johns Hopkins Press, 2001).

48 Bigelow to Henry Swan, 10 Jan. 1951, Bigelow Papers.

49 Bigelow to James F. Dickson III, 9 Oct. 1951, Bigelow Papers.

50 Bigelow talk, "Cardiac Resuscitation," Hamilton, 14 Nov. 1955; Bigelow to B.G. Ballard, 24 June 1950, Bigelow Papers.

51 Bigelow to Hopps, 9 Oct. 1951, Bigelow Papers.

52 Bigelow to James F. Dickson III, 9 Oct. 1951, Bigelow Papers.

53 For this chronicle, see J.A. Hopps to F.R. Charles, Patents Office, 19 Feb. 1953, Bigelow Papers.

54 Bigelow to Janes, 2 July 1952, Bigelow Papers; see J.A. Hopps and W.G. Bigelow, "Electrical Treatment of Cardiac Arrest: A Cardiac Stimulator-Defibrillator," *Recent Advances in Surgery* 16(4) (Oct.1954), 833–49. The paper was received for publication on 23 Dec. 1953 but prepared at least a year in advance.

55 Hopps to C.F. Pattenson, 2 Mar. 1953, Bigelow Papers.

56 See J.A. Hopps, "Evaluation of Council [NRC] on Medical Physics' Report on 'Electrical Apparatus for Cardiac Resuscitation,'" 13 Jan. 1961, Bigelow Papers.

57 Bigelow to Hopps, 16 May 1955, Bigelow Papers.

58 Measurement Engineering Ltd., "New Product Release," attached to Hopps to Bigelow, 14 Mar. 1962, Bigelow Papers.

59 Trimble to J.C. Fortin (manager operating rooms), 2 Sept. 1969, Bigelow Papers.

60 John C. Callaghan, "Early Experiences in the Study and Development of an Artificial Electrical Pacemaker for Standstill of the Heart: View from 1949," PACE 3(5) (Sept. 1980), 618–19.

61 Callaghan to David C. Schechter, 16 May 1969, Bigelow Papers.

62 Callaghan note, in Dwight E. Harken, "Pacemakers, Past-Makers, and the Paced: An Informal History from A to Z (Aldini to Zoll)," Biomedical Instrumentation & Technology, no vol. nr. (1991), 318.

63 Bigelow to Carl V. Hays, General Electric Company, 27 July 1964, Bigelow Papers.

64 Bigelow to N.P. Hill, 16 Mar. 1962, Bigelow Papers.

65 Bigelow to Michael E. DeBakey, 7 Feb. 1974, Bigelow Papers.

66 Michael E. DeBakey to Bigelow, 30 Mar. 1974, Bigelow Papers.

67 "Award of the Heart," Time, 26 Nov. 1973.

68 John C. Callaghan to Bigelow, 18 Mar. 1974, Bigelow Papers.

69 Bigelow to Harold N. Segall, 15 Feb. 1989. Segall had been writing "Pioneers of Cardiology," Bigelow Papers.

70 Bigelow to Robert E. Beamish, 8 Nov. 1995, Bigelow Papers.

71 Hopps to Bigelow, 22 Aug. 1995, Bigelow Papers.

72 Elizabeth Callow to Bigelow, 18 Nov. 1965, Bigelow Papers.

73 Bigelow to Callow, 19 Nov. 1963, Bigelow Papers.

74 Bigelow ms., "Pacemaker," not in Cold Hearts, Mar. 1983, 54–7, Bigelow Papers.

75 On the triumph of the US "research" model, at least in Toronto, see Shorter, Partnership for Excellence, 286–8.

76 Bigelow, "Medical Research: A Triple Responsibility," address to the Canadian Heart Foundation, 4 Nov. 1964. Address reprinted in Varsity Graduate 12 (Spring, 1966).

77 Bigelow to H. Brodie Stephens, 22 Nov. 1954, Bigelow Papers.

78 J.W.B. to Bigelow, 18 July 1954, Bigelow Papers. Patient's full name not revealed.

79 Bigelow to J.W.B., 26 Sept. 1954, Bigelow Papers.

80 Bigelow to P.E. Bernatz, 14 Mar. 1956, Bigelow Papers.

81 Bigelow to W.L.C. McGill, 17 May 1955, Bigelow Papers.

82 Bigelow to H.K. Nancekivell, 12 Sept. 1958, Bigelow Papers.

83 Bigelow to William W.L. Glenn, 5 Dec. 1960, Bigelow Papers.
84 Bigelow talk on the occasion of the "Distinguished Scientist Award," North American Society of Pacing and Electrophysiology, Toronto, 10 May 1985. See also Bigelow to Dickson, 9 Oct. 1951, Bigelow Papers.
85 Bigelow to Earl E. Bakken, 2 Nov. 1977, Bigelow Papers.
86 Bigelow talk, "Distinguished Scientist Award," 1985.
87 Bigelow to Lawrence Burr, 14 Feb. 1998, Bigelow Papers. The cardiovascular surgeons soon abandoned the diathermy rewarming device, a blanket with heating coils, in Canada. See Bigelow to R.H. Patterson, Cornell Medical Center, 24 Nov. 1962, Bigelow Papers.

8. Bypass

1 Elizabeth N., "Operation Record," 15 May 1957, Bigelow Papers.
2 Goldman, *Heart Surgery in Canada*, 528–9.
3 Richard Cairney, "Pioneering Alberta Cardiac Surgeons Walked into Uncharted Territory 40 Years Ago," *CMAJ* 156(4) (15 Feb.1997), 549–51.
4 Goldman, *Heart Surgery in Canada*, 529.
5 Mary Nersessian, "John Carter Callaghan, 1923–2004," *Globe and Mail*, 24 July 2004, F10.
6 This account is based on Goldman, *Heart Surgery in Canada*, 117, and H. Barrie Fairley, "Recollections of the Toronto General Hospital," in Robert J. Byrick, ed., *A Commemorative History of the Department of Anaesthesia* (Toronto: Department of Anaesthesia, 2004), 120–1.
7 W.T. Mustard et al., "Clinical Experience with the Artificial Heart Lung Preparation," CMAJ 76 (4) (15 Feb. 1957), 265–8.
8 George Trusler, ms. memoir, Jan. 2019.
9 Bigelow to H.S. Doyle, 12 Nov. 1956, UTARMS, A 1981–0047/007.
10 Heimbecker to Murray, Mar. 28, 1957, LAC, MG30, B110, vol. 28.
11 Heimbecker, untitled ms. on dog research, Dec. 1957, LAC, MG30, B110, vol. 28.
12 Bigelow to John C. Coles, London, ON, 10 Jan. 1958, Bigelow Papers.
13 Heimbecker, memoir, in Goldman *Heart Surgery in Canada* 118–19; Barrie *Advance*, 30 June 2009. The pump in question was evidently the one he had assembled out of parts. See Ron Csillag, Heimbecker obituary, *Globe and Mail*, 3 Mar. 2014, S8. It is unclear what happened to Heimbecker's pump-oxygenator. In a survey of oxygenators that he drafted in March 1957 for the Ontario Heart Foundation, he makes no reference to his own work (which indeed might not yet have been ready at that point), and recommends the Lillehei apparatus. Heimbecker, "Open Heart Surgery Performed by Extra-corporeal Circulation through Pump-Oxygenators," UTARMS, A1989–0030, box 002.

14 Bigelow to Eric M. Nanson, 24 Oct. 1958, Bigelow Papers.

15 [Heimbecker], "Pump mort," 14 Oct. [1958?], LAC MG30, B110, vol. 28.

16 Bigelow patient records, Miss L.B. Her final operation occurred on 30 Jan. 1964.

17 Key to F.G. Pearson, chairman, operating room committee (and head of thoracic surgery), 14 Dec. 1970, Bigelow Papers.

18 See Bigelow to Doyle, 17 Feb. 1961, Bigelow Papers.

19 Society for Vascular Surgery, "An Interview with Ronald J. Baird" [interviewer Walter J. McCarthy], transcript of an interview on YouTube. https://www /youtube.com/watch?v=54G_gqpwQ18&feature=youtu.be, p 8.

20 Bigelow, "Requirements for Cardiovascular Surgery," 12 Sept. 1957, attached to Medical Advisory Board Minutes, 21 Nov. 1957, Bigelow Fonds, TGH, TH 7.2.5.

21 Baird, "Development," 52.

22 Baird, "Development," 52.

23 Bigelow to Kergin, 21 Oct. 1961, Bigelow Fonds, TGH, 0094-8-0-1.

24 Donald R. Wilson interview, Hannah Oral History, no. 46, 51, UTARMS.

25 Donald R. Wilson interview, Hannah Oral History, no. 46, 2, UTARMS.

26 John R. Evans, "Biographical Material on Donald R. Wilson," 22 Jan. 1996, UTARMS, B2006–0027, box 39, file 17.

27 Donald R. Wilson, interview, Hannah Oral History, vol. 46, 50, UTARMS.

28 The information in this paragraph comes largely from Donald Richards Wilson, Faculty of Medicine, Academic Staff Record, UTARMS, A 1987–0047, box 011.

29 "Cardiovascular Society," notice of meetings for 1959–60, LAC MG30, B110, vol. 29.

30 John Morch et al., "Late Results of Aortocoronary Bypass Grafts in 100 Patients with Stable Angina Pectoris," *CMAJ* 111(6) (21 Sept. 1974), 529–32.

31 D.C. MacGregor to Bigelow, 27 Nov. 1970, Bigelow Fonds, TGH, 0094-13-0-29.

32 D.C. MacGregor to Bigelow, 5 July 1972, Bigelow Fonds, TGH, 0094-13-0-29.

33 R.J. Baird, A.S. Trimble, and J. Yao, "The First 1000 Coronary Artery Repair Operations in Toronto," *CMAJ* 111 (21 Sept. 1974), 525–8.

34 H.E. Aldridge to W.F. Greenwood, 19 Feb. 1971, Bigelow Fonds, TGH, 0094-13-0-29.

35 Bigelow to J.A. McNab, executive director, TGH, 26 May 1971, Bigelow Papers.

36 See on this Daniel A. Goor, *The Genius of C. Walton Lillehei and the True History of Open Heart Surgery* (New York: Vantage, 2007), 276–85.

37 R.J. Baird, A.S. Trimble, and J. Yao, "The First 1000 Coronary Artery Repair Operations in Toronto," *CMAJ* 111 (21 Sept. 1974), 525–8.

38 *Tablet*, Winter 1984, 3.
39 Bigelow to R.W. Harris, 1 June 1965, Bigelow Papers.
40 Heimbecker to Bigelow, 27 May 1965, Bigelow Papers.
41 Bigelow, minutes, meeting of the "Cardiovascular Surgical Division," 24 May 1967, Bigelow Papers.
42 W.G. Bigelow to F.G. Kergin, 16 Dec. 1964, UTARMS, A1989/0030/002.
43 See, for example, J.H. Collins memo to Bigelow, 31 Mar. 1967, Bigelow Papers.
44 Trimble to Bigelow, 26 Oct. 1966, Bigelow Papers.
45 Bigelow to R.A. Mustard, 20 Apr. 1965, Bigelow Papers.
46 Ray Heimbecker to L.R. McCloskey, director of personnel, TGH, 31 Aug. 1967, Bigelow Papers.
47 Manuscript tabulations with cover sheet "Jan. 68–June 68," Bigelow Papers.
48 Heimbecker to Bigelow, 15 Dec. 1970, Bigelow Papers.
49 Alan Trimble to Bigelow, 10 May 1971, Bigelow Papers.
50 Key to Bigelow, 21 May 1971, Bigelow Papers.
51 B.S. Goldman, A.S. Trimble et al., "Functional and Metabolic Effects of Anoxic Cardiac Arrest," *Ann Thorac Surg* 11 (1971), 122–32.
52 Al Sokol, "Handball Helps Victim of Heart Attack," *Toronto Star*, 16 Feb. 1982, F5.
53 Jack V. Tu, C. David Naylor ... and the Steering Committee of the Cardiac Care Network of Ontario, "Coronary Artery Bypass Graft Surgery in Ontario and New York State: Which Rate Is Right?" *Ann Int Med* 126 (1997), 13–19.
54 Marvin L. Murphy et al., "Treatment of Chronic Stable Angina," *NEJM* 297 (22 Sept. 1977), 621–7. For a critique of the study see "Special Correspondence: A Debate on Coronary Bypass," *NEJM* 297 (29 Dec. 1977), 1464–70.

9. Moving On

1 "Blaiberg Will Die, Edmonton Surgeon Says," *Globe and Mail*, 10 Jan. 1968, 10.
2 Joan Hollobon, "Bricklayer Satisfactory in 1st Toronto Heart Switch," *Globe and Mail*, 21 Oct. 1968, 1.
3 Baird, "Development," 35.
4 W.R. Drucker to members, Cardiovascular Surgical Division, 10 May 1968, UTARMS, Department of Surgery, A 1998–0030, Department Chair files, box 001, file 25. It is interesting that Drucker, the only chair of surgery not from Toronto and plainly ill at ease in this new environment, had not succeeded in getting the first name right of one of his main lieutenants.

5 Goldman note to Shorter, 15 Apr. 2019.

6 Joan Hollobon, "Two City Hospitals Set for Heart Transplant," *Globe and Mail*, 3 Oct. 1968, W4.

7 Joan Hollobon, "Two Heart Patients Assessed for Possible Transplants by Toronto General," *Globe and Mail*, 2 Oct. 1968, 1. See also Drucker memo on the "unfortunate article," 11 Oct. 1968, UTARMS, A 1998 – 0030, box 001, file 25.

8 Baird, "Development," 53–5.

9 "Cape Town Transplant Terrific Advance, Surgeon Says," *Globe and Mail*, 7 Dec. 1967, 8.

10 "Western to Get Heart Transplant Centre," *Toronto Star*, 7 Dec. 1967, 12.

11 Bigelow, "Cardiovascular Units in University of Toronto Hospital Complex," personal report to Prof. W.R. Drucker, 1967, Bigelow Papers.

12 Baird, "Development" (unpaged section).

13 Drucker memo, 11 Oct. 1968, UTARMS, A 1998 – 0030, box 001, file 25.

14 Bigelow to Drucker, 16 Oct. 1968, UTARMS, A 1998 – 0030, box 001, file 25.

15 "Drucker Is Pleased," *Globe and Mail*, 21 Oct. 1968, 12.

16 Joan Hollobon, "Bricklayer Satisfactory in 1st Toronto Heart Switch," *Globe and Mail*, 21 Oct. 1968, 1.

17 Goldman, ms., "Personal TGH history."

18 Goldman, ms., "Personal TGH history."

19 "Transplant Doctor Meets Press," *Globe and Mail*, 21 Oct. 1968, 12.

20 Bigelow to Drucker, 15 Oct. 1968, UTARMS, A 1998 – 0030, box 001, file 25.

21 In addition to the superb journalism of Joan Hollobon, this account in based on the memoirs of Goldman and Baird.

22 "Boy Dies in Toronto Western and 5 Get Heart, Kidneys, Eyes in Multiple Transplants," *Toronto Star*, 29 Oct. 1968, 1, 4.

23 These details from Don Delaplante, "Surgeons Apply a New Technique for Metro's Third Heart Transplant," *Globe and Mail*, 14 Nov. 1968, 1.

24 Don Delaplante, "Surgeons Apply a New Technique for Metro's Third Heart Transplant," *Globe and Mail*, 14 Nov. 1968; on Gagnier's death see *Globe and Mail* note, 21 Nov. 1968.

25 Meeting with Bernard Goldman and Hugh Scully, 4 Apr. 2018.

26 "4th Heart Recipient Reported Progressing," *Globe and Mail*, 20 Nov. 1968, 11.

27 Joan Hollobon, "Quiet Dinner Marks End of 2 Years with New Heart," *Globe and Mail*, 17 Nov. 1970, 1.

28 Marilyn Dunlop, "Canada's 2 Living Transplants Doing Fine," *Toronto Star*, 25 Oct. 1989, 6.

29 Baird, "Development," 55.

30 Marilyn Dunlop, "Calgary Man Gets Heart of Woman," *Toronto Star*, 5 Apr. 1969, B1.

31 Joan Hollobon, "Suitable Transplant Age Argued by Heart Doctors," *Globe and Mail*, 7 June 1969, 1.

32 Bigelow to Drucker, 17 Dec. 1968, UTARMS, A 1998–0030, box 001, file 25.

33 See Bigelow to Drucker, 3 Feb. 1969, and attached memo, 13 Jan. 1969, "Confidential. Heart Transplantation – Statement of Policy."

34 W.G. Bigelow, "Heart Transplantation: Quiet Progress," *Globe and Mail*, 15 May 1972, 7.

35 Goldman in Mickleborough interview, 21 Nov. 2018.

36 Marilyn Dunlop, "24 Transplant Cases Died Awaiting Hearts Two Metro Doctors Say," *Toronto Star*, 19 Feb. 1971, 29.

37 "Minutes: Inter-Hospital Cardiovascular Surgical Committee," 19 May 1970, UTARMS, Department of Surgery, A 1998–0030, Department Chair files, box 001, file 25.

38 M.D. Silver, "Autopsy Report: Joseph M." The dates in this report differ from those in Bigelow's note to Silver.

39 Bigelow to M.D. Silver, 15 Sept. 1970, Bigelow Papers.

40 Bigelow et al. to McNab, attached to Trimble to Bigelow, 4 July 1972, Bigelow Papers.

41 Bigelow et al. to McNab, attached to Trimble to Bigelow, 4 July 1972, Bigelow Papers.

42 Mrs. P. Clark to Bigelow, 12 Sept. 1973; explanation for Review Committees, considered at meeting of Review Committee, 22 May 1973 is attached, Bigelow Papers.

43 See Matthias Barton et al., "Balloon Angioplasty – The Legacy of Andreas Grüntzig, M.D. (1939–1985)," *Front Cardiovasc Med* 1 (2014), doi: 10.3389/fcvm.2014.00015.

44 Heimbecker to Greenwood, 29 June 1971, Bigelow Papers.

45 John Gunstensen, Bernard S. Goldman, Hugh E. Scully, Victor F. Huckell, and Allan G. Adelman, "Evolving Indications for Preoperative Intraaortic Balloon Pump Assistance," *Annals of Thoracic Surgery* 22(6) (Dec. 1976), 535–46.

46 Goldman's letter is mentioned in R.A. Mustard to Bigelow, 10 July 1973, Bigelow Papers.

47 Bigelow to R.A. Mustard, 17 Aug. 1973, Bigelow Papers.

48 Bigelow to R.J. Baird, Ontario Heart Foundation, 30 Apr. 1973, Bigelow Papers.

49 Harold E. Aldridge note, "re: Program – Emergency Surgery for Heart Attack," 25 Oct. 1972, appendix A, Bigelow Papers.

50 Bigelow to Goldman, 30 May 1974, Bigelow Papers.

51 Goldman memo to Bigelow, 18 Feb. 1974, Bigelow Papers.

52 Ed Wigle to Bernard Goldman, 1 Aug. 1973, Bigelow Papers; as late as June, however, the cardiologists were rejecting the notion of a second

balloon pump and said they would acquire one only if cardiac surgery didn't. Wigle to Bigelow, 5 June 1973, box 7.

53 Samuel Campbell, "'Fantastic' Device Helps Saves Heart Patients' Lives," *Toronto Star*, 25 Feb. 1975, B7.

54 Goldman to Shorter, 22 Apr. 2018.

55 Interview with nursing supervisors, 14 Nov. 2018.

56 Goldman, in Stephanie Brister interview, 29 Nov. 2018.

57 Lynda Mickleborough, interview, 21 Nov. 2018.

58 Goldman, in Mickleborough interview, 21 Nov. 2018.

59 Joe O'Connor, "Meet the Ace Canadian Heart Surgeon," *National Post*, 20 Jan. 2016.

60 Dwight E. Harken, "The Emergence of Cardiac Surgery, I: Personal Recollections of the 1940s and 1950s," *J Thorac Cardiovasc Surg* 98 (1989), 805–13, 811.

61 Bigelow to Wolf Sapirstein, 19 Apr. 1960, Bigelow Papers.

62 Division of Cardiovascular Surgery, Memo: Operative Notes and Final Notes," (attached to Bigelow to Heimbecker, 7 Sept. 1967), Bigelow Papers.

63 Bigelow to Robert M. Hosler, 21 Aug. 1951, Bigelow Papers.

64 Chaplain Peter Tink to Bigelow, 23 Nov. 1971, Bigelow Papers.

65 Judy Wass to J. Drennan, assistant director nursing services, 29 Nov. 1971, Bigelow Papers.

66 Toronto General Hospital, Department of Medical Records, *Annual Statistical Report, 1968*, Bigelow Papers.

67 Bigelow to Wigle, 2 Jan. 1972, Bigelow Fonds, TGH, 0094–13–0-30.

68 George Trusler, interview, 27 Nov. 2018.

69 Alan Trimble to J.B. Wallace, executive director TGH, 17 Sept. 1969, Bigelow Papers.

70 Bigelow to McNab, 26 May 1971, Bigelow Papers.

71 TGH *Annual Report 1983/84*, 14.

72 "Dr. W.G. Bigelow Resigns as Chief of Cardiovascular Surgery at TGH," [TGH] *Monitor*, 1 July 1977, 2.

73 Manjula Maganti, Stephanie J. Brister, Terrence M. Yau, Susan Collins, Mitesh Badiwala, and Vivek Rao, "Changing Trends in Emergency Coronary Bypass Surgery," *J Thorac Cardiovasc Surg* 142(4) (Oct. 2011), 816–22.

74 Bigelow to McNab, 26 May 1971, Bigelow Papers.

75 Trimble to McNab, 27 June 1972, Bigelow Papers.

76 Al ——. to Trimble, 1 June 1971; see also Trimble to McNab, 27 June 1972, Bigelow Papers.

77 Al ——. to Brian Magee, 10 May 1971, Bigelow Papers.

78 Bigelow to Greenwood, 25 Jan. 1973, Bigelow Fonds, TGH, 0094–8-0-102.

79 J.A. McNab to all staff doctors, 13 Apr. 1973, Bigelow Papers.

80 W.G. Bigelow, "Medical Research: A Triple Responsibility," *Varsity Graduate* 12(3) (Spring 1966), unpaginated; the talk was given to the Canadian Heart Foundation on 4 Nov. 1964.

81 See Bigelow to McNab, 24 Nov. 1971; W.B. Drucker to Bigelow, 26 June 1969, UTARMS, A1981–0047/003.

82 Bigelow to J.W.R. Rennie, Manitoba, 23 Nov. 1966, Bigelow Papers.

83 Bigelow to McNab, 24 Nov. 1971, Bigelow Papers.

84 R.K. Magee to Bigelow, 22 Jan. 1964, Bigelow Papers.

85 John C. Coles to Bigelow, 5 Nov. 1962, Bigelow Papers.

86 Key to Bigelow, 27 Dec. 1963, Bigelow Papers.

87 Drucker to Bigelow, 13 May 1968, UTARMS, A 1998–0030, box 001, file 25.

88 Goldman in William Williams interview, 27 Nov. 2018.

89 Claudia Koropecki, "Cardiovascular Report," Apr. 1968, Bigelow Papers. Koropecki, cardiovascular head nurse in Toronto, was part of a team sent to observe cardiovascular nursing services at several US centres.

90 Goldman to Bigelow, 1 Apr. 1968, Bigelow Papers.

91 June Callwood, "Putting Hearts through Their Paces," *Globe and Mail*, 7 Nov. 1985, E13.

92 Bigelow to G.R. Paterson, head of Hannah Institute for the History of Medicine, 19 Aug. 1975, Bigelow Fonds, TGH; 0094–7-0–9.

93 John Wedge, interview, 28 Nov. 2018.

94 Goldman, in Trusler interview, 27 Nov. 2018. Bigelow was sixty-four. It is true that the university had a retirement-at-sixty-five rule, but Bigelow could have stayed on at the hospital. Murray was seventy-three when he finally resigned his hospital appointment in 1967.

95 Bigelow to R.A. Mustard, 24 Nov. 1976, Bigelow Fonds, TGH, 0094–7-0–9.

96 Bigelow to D.C. Robertson, Chair, Interdepartmental Planning Committee, 25 Sept. 1968, Bigelow Papers.

10. The Pacemaker Clinic

1 Samuel F. Lasky (Electrodyne) to Bigelow, 16 Jan. 1961. See the product description attached to Norman H. Simon (Electrodyne) to Bigelow, 18 Apr. 1961, Bigelow Papers.

2 Bigelow, "Cardiovascular Statistics," 15 Feb. 1966, Bigelow Papers.

3 A.S. Trimble, R.O. Heimbecker, and W.G. Bigelow, "The Implantable Cardiac Pacemaker," paper presented at the Canadian Medical Association Meeting, June 1963, ms. in Bigelow Papers.

4 W.B. Firor and B.S. Goldman, "Initial Experience with the Permanent Implantable Transvenous Pacemaker: A Report of 33 Patients," *CMAJ* 96(3) (Jan. 1967), 1–4.

5 Marvin Schiff, "Setting the Pace for Weak Hearts," *Globe and Mail*, 2 Nov. 1963, 5A.

6 E.D. (Doug) Wigle to Goldman, 11 Nov. 1969, Bigelow Papers.

7 W.F. Greenwood to James Key, 19 Nov. 1969, Bigelow Papers.

8 See Goldman to Bigelow, 15 Oct. 1971, Bigelow Papers.

9 Bigelow, *Cold Hearts*, 142.

10 Seymour Furman to Goldman, 2 Dec. 1969, Bigelow Papers, box 5.

11 Seymour Furman to Goldman, 2 Dec. 1969; Bigelow to Goldman, 12 Dec. 1969, Bigelow Papers.

12 James A. Key to F.G. Pearson, 4 Mar. 1970, Bigelow Papers.

13 B.S. Goldman, L.L. Black, and I.H. Lipton, "Implantable Transvenous Cardiac Pacemakers: Indications, Complications and Management," *CMAJ* 103(11) (21 Nov. 1970), 1163–7.

14 "TGH Doctor Implants Nuclear Heart Pacemaker," TGH *Monitor*, 1 Nov. 1973, 2.

15 See Goldman to Bigelow, 18 Aug. 1970, Bigelow Papers.

16 Bigelow ms. of Mar. 1983 on "Pacemaker," 57–8 of material not in *Cold Hearts*, Bigelow Papers.

17 F.G. Pearson to Bigelow, 27 Oct. 1971, Bigelow Papers.

18 J.A. McNab to Goldman, 13 Mar. 1972, Bigelow Papers.

19 Eileen D. Strike to Goldman, 2 Nov. 1972, Bigelow Papers.

20 "Canada Dependent on U.S. for Heart Pacers, Doctor Says," *Globe and Mail*, 27 Jan. 1973, 11.

21 Joan Hollobon, "Champagne Follows Nuclear Pacer Implant," *Globe and Mail*, 9 Oct. 1973.

22 Meeting with Bernard Goldman and Hugh Scully, 4 Apr. 2018.

23 Goldman message to Shorter, 9 Feb. 2009.

24 "Pacer Abuse Cited by MD," *Globe and Mail*, 28 Jan. 1972, 12.

25 Marilyn Dunlop, "Pacemaker Patients Are Victims of Indifference – MD," *Toronto Star*, 28 Jan. 1972, 61.

26 Joan Hollobon, "100 May Lose Chance for Heart Pacers, MD Warns," *Globe and Mail*, 24 Feb. 1975, 1.

27 B.S. Goldman, E.J. Noble, et al., "The Pacemaker Challenge," *CMAJ*, 110 (5 Jan. 1974), 28–30.

28 "Canadian Survey of Cardiac Pacing," World Symposium on Cardiac Pacing, Montreal, 2–5 Oct. 1979, entry for the Toronto General Hospital, in Bigelow Papers. See also Michael Moore, "New Heart Pacer with 8-year Life Implanted in Man," *Globe and Mail*, 4 Jan. 1979, 4.

29 D.C. MacGregor et al., "The Porous-Surfaced Electrode – A New Concept in Pacemaker Lead Design," *Journal of Thoracic and Cardiovascular Surgery* 78(2) (Aug. 1979), 281–91.

30 Andrea Jones to Bigelow, undated note [1995]. Bigelow Papers.

11. Ron Baird

1 Heidi Duringer, interview, 31 Oct. 2018. Leda Parente and Hugh Scully participated.
2 Society for Vascular Surgery, "An Interview with Ronald J. Baird" [interviewer Walter J. McCarthy], transcript of an interview on YouTube, p 3. https://www.youtube.com/watch?v=54G_gqpwQl8.
3 Goldman, *Heart Surgery in Canada*, 121.
4 Bigelow to R. Beverley Lynn, 29 Mar. 1963, Bigelow Papers.
5 Lynda Mickleborough, interview, 21 Nov. 2018.
6 Hugh Scully, interview, 20 June 2018, 7.
7 Baird, "Development," 10.
8 Baird, "Remarks for the Academy of Medicine Gold Symposium," 1 Nov. 1994, 5, in Scully Papers.
9 Baird, "Development," 11.
10 Lynda Mickleborough, interview, 21 Nov. 2018.
11 Baird, "Developments," 16.
12 Interview with nursing supervisors, 14 Nov. 2018.
13 See, for example, Ronald J. Baird et al., "An Improved Method of Myocardial Revascularization with a Vascular Implant," *AMA Arch Surg* 95(5) (Nov.1967), 724–35.
14 R.J. Baird, "The Reasons for Patency and Anastomosis Formation of the Internal Mammary Artery Implant," *Ann Roy Coll Phys and Surg of Canada* 1 (July 1969), 172–96; see also Baird, "The Reasons Why an Internal Mammary Implant Stays Patent and Why It Forms Anastomoses," *J Cardiovasc Surg* 11 (1970), 195–8.
15 Baird, "Development," 8.
16 See Baird, "Development," 5; T.E. Starzl et al., "A Technique for Bicuspidization of the Aortic Valve," *J Thorac Cardiovasc Surg* 38 (Aug. 1959), 262–70.
17 R.J. Baird et al., "An Evaluation of the Late Results of Aortic Valve Repair," *J Thorac Cardiovasc Surg* 49 (Apr. 1965), 562–73.
18 Aron M. Rappaport, R. Brian Holmes, Harold O. Stolberg, James L. McIntyre, and Ronald J. Baird, "Hepatic Venography," *Gastroenterology* 46 (1964), 115–27.
19 Ronald J. Baird et al., "Saphenous Vein Bypass Grafts to the Arteries of the Ankle and Foot," *Annals of Surgery* 172 (1970), 1059–63.
20 R.J. Baird et al., "Ascending Aorta to Bilateral Femoral Artery Graft via a Ventral Subcutaneous Route," *Annals of Surgery* 186 (1977), 210–12.
21 Society for Vascular Surgery. "An Interview with Ronald J. Baird," transcript of an interview on YouTube, p. 5.
22 Baird, "Development," 44.

23 Richard D. Weisel, Irving H. Lipton, Robert N. Lyall, and Ronald J Baird, "Cardiac Metabolism and Performance Following Cold Potassium Cardioplegia," *Circulation* 58, suppl. 1 (Sept. 1978), 217–26.

24 Ron Baird, "Reflections on the Heart, Remarks for the Aesculapian Club Dinner, Friday, 20 Jan. 1995," in Scully Papers.

25 Lillian Newberry, "Heart Patients Waiting 'Too Long' for Surgery," *Toronto Star,* 13 Jan. 1983, A1, 4; Marilyn Dunlop, "Plans for Extra Heart Surgery Units Praised," *Toronto Star*, 14 Jan. 1983, A4.

26 Rosie DeManno, "Did Health System Kill Man," *Toronto Star*, 13 June 1988, C1. The drumbeat of stories about waiting-list deaths did not, however, abate. "Second Heart Patient Dies as Surgery Delayed 9 Times," reported the *Toronto Star* on 6 Jan. 1989, A7.

27 Marilyn Dunlop, "Father, 37, Has Toronto's First Heart Swap Operation in 10 Years," *Toronto Star*, 8 Mar. 1985, A14.

28 *Globe and Mail*, 2 Mar. 2014. See Heimbecker's account in Goldman, *Heart Surgery in Canada*, 124–5.

29 Richard Reznick, interview, 3 Dec. 2018. See G.N. Craddock, S. Nordgren, and R.K. Reznick, "Small Bowel Transplantation in the Dog Using Cyclosporin A," *Transplantation* 35 (1983), 284.

30 Baird, "Development," 55.

31 Christie McLaren, "New Life," *Globe and Mail*, 5 Apr. 1985, 11.

32 "Financing Sought for Transplant Unit," *Globe and Mail*, 8 July 1985.

33 Erika Rosenfeld, "95-Minute Transplant a Record Operation," *Globe and Mail*, 12 July 1985, M1.

34 Baird, "Development," 55.

35 Chris Feindel interview, 11 Dec. 2018; Michael Valpy, "Transplant Patients Given Unapproved Drug," *Globe and Mail*, 10 May 2002.

36 Goldman letter to Shorter, 12 Dec. 2018.

37 Bernard Langer and Bernard Goldman comments in interview of 30 July 2018.

38 Baird, "Development," 12.

39 Bernard Langer, Bernard Goldman, interview, 30 July 2018.

40 Scully, in Wayne Johnston interview, 12 Dec. 2018.

41 "Wayne Johnston Elected President of the Society of Vascular Surgeons," [Department of Surgery], *Surgical Spotlight*, Fall, 2007, unpaginated.

42 "Vascular Surgery Division," [Department of Surgery] *Surgical Spotlight*, Spring 2004, 10.

43 "Celebrating a Decade of Excellence," *PMCC Clinical and Research Report* 11(2) (Winter 2016), 4; Richard Reznick, "The Vascular Saga: From Chaos to Emerging Calm," [Department of Surgery], *Surgical Spotlight*, Spring 2006, 3–4.

44 Scully, Goldman, in Stephanie Brister interview, 29 Nov. 2018.

45 A.W. Harrison, head of surgery at Sunnybrook, to Bigelow, 17 Dec. 1969, UTARMS, Department of Surgery, A 1998–0030, Department Chair files, box 001, file 25.

46 "Minutes: Inter-hospital Cardiovascular Surgical Committee," 10 Feb. 1970, UTARMS, Department of Surgery, A 1998–0030, Department Chair files, box 001, file 25, Cardiovascular Service, 1968–72.

47 Rene G. Favaloro, Donald B. Effler, et al., "Acute Coronary Insufficiency (Impending Myocardial Infarction): Surgical Treatment by the Saphenous Vein Graft Technique," *Am J Cardiology* 28 (1971), 598–607.

48 A.W. Chisholm to Wigle, 27 Mar. 1972, Bigelow Papers.

49 Matt Maychak, "Heart Surgery Is Only the Tip of Medical Crisis," *Toronto Star*, 5 Jan. 1989, A18. Authorities denied any link between the delay and Coleman's death. Maychak, "Improved Heart Surgery System Urged," *Toronto Star*, 1 Mar. 1989, A1.

50 Merrill L. Knutson and Hugh Scully, "Indications for and Access to Revascularization," Canadian Cardiovascular Society, 1995, https://www.ccs.ca/images/Guidelines/Guidelines_POS_Library/Revasc_CC_1995.pdf.

51 Shaf Keshavjee, interview, 30 Aug. 2018.

52 Keshavjee, interview, 30 Aug. 2018.

53 Scully, interview, 10 Dec. 2018.

54 Scully to Goldman, 8 July 2018.

55 S.E. Fremes, G.A. Patterson, W.G. Williams, B.S. Goldman, T.R. Todd, J. Maurer, "Single Lung Transplantation and Closure of Patent Ductus Arteriosus for Eisenmenger's Syndrome. Toronto Lung Transplant Group," *J Thoracic & Cardiovasc Surgery* 100(1) (July 1990), 1–5.

56 Goldman ms., "Some More Recall of TGH Cardiovascular History," 2018.

57 Regina Hickl-Szabo, "Heart-Lung Patient Improving," *Globe and Mail*, 5 July 1984, M3.

58 Marilyn Dunlop, "Pioneering Toronto Team Performs One of First Double-Lung Transplants," *Toronto Star*, 28 Nov. 1986, 1, 5.

59 Joan Hollobon, "Pump Takes Patient from Brink of Death," *Globe and Mail*, 7 May 1984, M6. The surgeons reported on this at the 21st annual meeting of the Society of Thoracic Surgeons, 21–3 Jan. 1985. The paper is referenced "Mechanical Right Ventricular Support after Cardiac Surgery," R.L. Kormos, M.J. Henderson, H. Rakowski, L.L. Mickleborough, and H.E. Scully, Toronto, Ont., Canada.

60 "Heart Month: Double Heart Surgery Survivor 84-Years-Young," http://www.uhn.ca/corporate/News/Pages/double_heart_surgery_survivor.aspx.

12. The Damaged Heart

1 Goldman to Shorter, 12 Aug. 2018.

2 Comments by Lynda Mickleborough are from Mickleborough, interview, 21 Nov. 2018.

3 Goldman, in Mickleborough interview, 21 Nov. 2018.

4 Raymond O. Heimbecker, Guy Lemire, and Charles Chen, "Surgery for Massive Myocardial Infarction," *Circulation*, suppl. II, 37–8 (Apr. 1968), II-3–II-11.

5 "Heart Repair Technique Described," *Globe and Mail*, 20 Jan. 1967, 10.

6 Raymond O. Heimbecker, Guy Lemire, and Charles Chen, "Surgery for Massive Myocardial Infarction," *Circulation*, suppl II, 37–8 (Apr. 1968), II-3–II-11.

7 Marilyn Dunlop, "Man With 'No Future' Recovers after 'Dead' Heart Muscle Cut Out," *Toronto Star*, 17 Feb. 1970.

8 See Eugene Downar, Lynda Mickleborough, et al., "Intraoperative Electrical Ablation of Ventricular Arrhythmias: A 'Closed Heart' Procedure," *J Am Coll Cardiol* 10(5) (Nov. 1987), 1048–59; Lynda L. Mickleborough et al., "Balloon Electric Shock Ablation," *J Thorac Cardiovasc Surg* 108(5) (Nov. 1994), 855–61; Mickleborough et al., "Balloon Electric Shock Ablation," Effects on Ventricular Structure, Function, and Electrophysiology," *J Thorac Cardiovasc Surg* 97(1) (Jan. 1989), 135–46.

9 Goldman, in Mickleborough interview, 21 Nov. 2018.

10 See Bigelow to W.G. Cosbie, 23 June 1972; see also Bigelow, "Notes on the History of the Cardiovascular Service: A Memorandum for Dr. W.G. Cosbie" (1972), Bigelow Fonds, TGH, 0094–13–0-23.

11 Lynda L. Mickleborough et al., "Late Results of Operation for Ventricular Tachycardia," *Ann Thorac Surg* 54 (1992), 832–9.

12 Terry Kieser, "Lynda Mickleborough," in Goldman, *Heart Surgery in Canada*, 493–6.

13 Lynda L. Mickleborough, Naeem Merchant, Joan Ivanov, Vivek Rao, and Susan Carson, "Left Ventricular Reconstruction: Early and Late Results," *J Thorac Cardiovasc Surg* 128(1) (July 2004), 27–37.

14 L.L. Mickleborough et al., "Is Sex a Factor in Determining Operative Risk for Aortocoronary Bypass Surgery?" *Circulation* 92 (9 Suppl) (Nov. 1995), 1180–4.

15 Lisa Priest, "Heart Surgery No Riskier for Women, Study Says," *Toronto Star*, 8 Dec. 1994. Their study itself appeared a year after the interview.

16 Vivek Rao, interview, 27 Aug. 2018.

17 Goldman, in Vivek Rao interview, 27 Aug. 2018.

18 Vivek Rao, interview, 27 Aug. 2018.

19 Goldman, in Lynda Mickleborough interview, 21 Nov. 2018.

13. Valves

1 Goldman to Shorter, note, 29 Jan. 2019.

2 Baird, "Development," 5.

3 The Scully quotes in this section are mainly drawn from a Scully memo of 28 Jan. 2019.

4 For these statistics, see Bigelow, "Cardiovascular Statistics," 15 Feb.1966, Bigelow Papers.

5 Arnold Brunner and Joan Hollobon, "Artificial Valve Has a Flaw, 47 Heart Patients Told," *Globe and Mail*, 12 July 1978, 1.

6 Bigelow to L.R. McCloskey, director of personnel, TGH, 29 Mar. 1967, Bigelow Papers.

7 A.S. Trimble and F.N. Metni, "The Use of Autologous Fascia Lata for Cardiac Valve Replacement: Preliminary Results," *CMAJ* 105(7) (9 Oct. 1971), 715–17; John Gunstensen, Malcolm D. Silver, et al., "The Late Results of Cardiac Valve Replacement Using Autologous Fascia Lata," *CMAJ* 110(10) (18 May 1974).

8 Editorial, "Obituary for Fascia Lata Heart Valves," *BMJ* 1 (17 Jan. 1976), 115–16.

9 Kergin to Doyle, 31 Aug. 1965, Bigelow Papers.

10 Heimbecker to Kergin, 20 Aug. 1965, Bigelow Papers.

11 Trimble to Fortin, 10 Sept. 1969, Bigelow Papers.

12 Heimbecker to R.C. Ritchie, Department of Pathology, 6 Dec. 1965, Bigelow Papers.

13 Joan Hollobon, "Hail Heart-graft Triumph," *Globe and Mail*, 23 June 1966, 5.

14 H.E. Scully, A. Damle, B.S. Goldman, C. Tong, J. Azuma, L.L. Mickleborough, L. Schwartz, and R.J. Baird, "Clinical Performance of Bjork-Shiley Mechanical Heart Valves: A Perspective on Outlet Strut Fractures in the 60 Degrees and 70 Degrees Convexo-concave Disc Models," *Can J Cardiol* 41(7) (1988), 386–92.

15 The world panel's report appeared as Anders Ericsson, Dan Lindblom, Gudmund Semb, Hans A. Huysmans, Christian Olin, Lars I. Thulin, Jan Kugelberg, Hugh E. Scully, Graeme Bennett, Jörg Ostermeyer, Nancy R. Davis, and Gary L. Grunkemeier, "Strut Fracture with the Björk-Shiley 70° Convexo-Concave Valve: An International Multi-Institutional Follow-Up Study," *European Journal of Cardio-Thoracic Surgery* 6(7) (1992): 339–46. The North American panel report was published as Loren F. Hiratzka, Nicholas T. Kouchoukos, Gary L. Grunkemeier, Craig Miller, Hugh E. Scully, and Andrew S. Wechsler, "Outlet Strut Fracture of the Björk-Shiley 60° Convexo-Concave Valve: Current Information and Recommendations for Patient Care," *Journal of the College of Cardiology* 11(5) (1988): 1130–7.

16 Hugh E. Scully, Cathy P. Tong, Leonard Schwartz, Lynda L. Mickleborough, and Ronald J. Baird, "The Monostrut Björk-Shiley Valve: Successful Successor to the Welded-Outlet-Strut Generation," presented

at the 44th Annual Meeting of the Canadian Cardiovascular Society, Calgary, Alberta, 18 Oct. 1991.

17 J. Butany, H.E. Scully, and C. Feindel [some authors' names have been omitted], "Pathologic Analysis of 19 Heart Valves with Silver-Coated Sewing Rings," *J Card Surg* 21(6) (Nov.–Dec.2006), 530–8.

18 Butany's and Scully's comments were recorded at an interview, 24 Oct. 2018.

19 David Israelson, "Pathologists' Puzzle: Mystery of the Silver-Coated Heart Valve," *PMCC Report*, Winter 2018, 34–5. This story broke in the media in Jesse McLean and Robert Cribb, "Faulty and Unproven Medical Devices Implanted in Canadian Patients Despite Known Risks," *Toronto Star*, 25 Nov. 2018.

20 Interview with Goldman and Scully, 10 Dec. 2018.

21 A. Maganti, V. Rao, S. Armstrong, H.E. Scully, and T.E. David, "Redo Valvular Surgery in Elderly Patients," *Ann Thorac Surg* 87(2) (2009): 521–5; Hugh E. Scully, Bernard Goldman, John Fulop, et al., "Five-Year Follow-up of Hancock Pericardial Valves: Management of Premature Failure," *Journal of Cardiac Surgery* 3(3 Suppl) (1988): 397–403; Hugh E. Scully and C. Susan Armstrong, "Tricuspid Valve Replacement: Fifteen Years of Experience with Mechanical Prostheses and Bioprostheses," *Journal of Thoracic and Cardiovascular Surgery* 109(6) (1995): 1035–41.

22 See Tirone E. David, "Aortic Valve Replacement with the Toronto SPV Bioprosthesis," *Operative Techniques in Thoracic and Cardiovascular Surgery* 6 (2001), 60–9.

23 Tirone David, interview, 23 Aug. 2018, 9.

24 Jagdish Butany, Mauro de Sa, Christopher M. Feindel, and Tirone E. David, "The Toronto SPV Bioprosthesis: Review of Morphological Findings in Eight Valves," *Seminars in Thoracic and Cardiovascular Surgery* 11 (Suppl. 1 (Oct. 1999), 157–62; N.D. Desai et al., "Long-term Results of Aortic Valve Replacement with the St. Jude Toronto Stentless Porcine Valve," *Ann Thorac Surg* 78 (2004), 2076–83.

25 Tirone E. David, Glorianne C. Ropchan, and Jagdish W. Butany, "Aortic Valve Replacement with Stentless Porcine Bioprostheses," *J Cardiac Surg* 3 (1988), 501–5.

26 J. Butany, C.M. Feindel, and T.E. David, "The Toronto SPV Bioprosthesis: Review of Morphological Findings in Eight Valves," *Semin Thorac Cardiovasc Surg* 11 (4 suppl. 1) (1999), 157–62.

27 Tirone E. David, Christopher M. Feindel, Joanne Bos, Joan Ivanov, and Susan Armstrong, "Aortic Valve Replacement with Toronto SPV Bioprosthesis: Optimal Patient Survival But Suboptimal Valve Durability," *J Thorac Cardiovasc Surg* 135(1). (Jan 2008), 19–24.

28 David, interview, 23 Aug. 2018. See also David et al., "Aortic Valve Replacement with Stentless Porcine Aortic Bioprosthesis."

14. Training

1 Meeting with Bernard Goldman and Hugh Scully, 4 Apr. 2018.
2 Todd K. Rosengart, Erle H. Austin, Harvey J. Pass, and Richard W. Weisel, "Introduction: Great Institutions in Cardiothoracic Surgery, Second Edition," *Seminars in Thoracic and Cardiovascular Surgery* 28 (2016), 609–10.
3 Bigelow to R.M. James, 23 Sept. 1955, Bigelow Papers.
4 In a letter to F.G. Dolan (Halifax), Bigelow says, "Bill Mustard and I have arranged a course in Cardiovascular Surgery that is available here now." (Bigelow to Dolan, 2 Jan.1958, Bigelow Papers.
5 Reznick's comments in this chapter are drawn from Richard Reznick, interview, 3 Dec. 2018.
6 Memo, "Cardiovascular Surgery Postgraduate Training," attached to a cover letter, Bigelow to D.L.C. Bingham (Queen's), 6 Jan.1958, Bigelow Papers.
7 T.J. Giles, RCPS, to H.S. Doyle, asst superintendent TGH, 13 June 1962, UTARMS, A1981–0047/007.
8 Goldman, *Cardiac Surgery in Canada*, 476.
9 Baird, "Development," 11.
10 Goldman note to Shorter, 15 Apr. 2019.
11 *Department of Surgery, Annual Report, 1987/88*, 6.
12 Goldman, "Personal TGH Staff History," 2018.
13 Neil A. Watters to Bigelow, 27 Jan. 1966, Bigelow Papers.
14 Terrence Yau, interview, 21 Jan. 2019.
15 W.G. Bigelow to W. Drucker, 14 Oct. 1966, attachment "Cardiovascular Division Toronto General Hospital," UTA A1989/0030/002.9.
16 Bigelow to McLean at Royal Vic, 22 Oct. 1962. The same letter went out to a number of other services in Canada.
17 Bigelow to Wilson, 17 July 1963, Bigelow Papers.
18 Bigelow to Wolf Sapirstein, 7 Nov. 1959, Bigelow Papers.
19 Key members of the division, such as Ray Heimbecker, Ron Baird, and Wolf Sapirstein – who would shortly go to St. Michael's Hospital – were not salaried by the General but were considered "full-time workers in research." Ron Tasker was supported by a Markle Scholarship. F.G. Kergin to William Oille, 24 Aug. 1961, UTARMS, A1981–0047, box 003.
20 James Yao, "Division of Cardiovascular Surgery, Toronto General Hospital, A Guide for Assistant Residents and Junior Interns," 1964, Bigelow Papers.
21 UTARMS, Donald R. Wilson interview, Hannah Oral History, no. 46, 15.

22 Yao, "Guide for Assistant Residents and Junior Interns."
23 Bigelow to J.A. Key, 21 Oct. 1968; Bigelow Fonds, TGH Archives, 0094–13–26.
24 Bernie Goldman, interview, 4 Feb. 2009, from research for Shorter, *Partnership for Excellence.*
25 Tirone David, interview, 23 Aug. 2018.
26 Minutes of the Surgeons-in-Chief and the Inter-Hospital Coordinating Committee, 23 Sept. 1971, Bigelow Fonds, TGH, 0094–13–0-5.
27 Scully, in David interview, 23 Aug. 2018.
28 Baird interview, *Downtown Toronto Hospital News*, Aug. 1987, 1.
29 Bigelow to W.A. Oille, 1 Feb. 1963, Bigelow Papers.
30 Interview with Scully and Goldman, 4 Apr. 2018.
31 Goldman, in Harry Rakowski interview, 12 Dec. 2018.
32 Barry Rubin, interview, 10 Oct. 2018, 12.
33 Rubin, interview, 12.
34 Rubin, interview, 13.

15. Research

1 Unless otherwise noted, the material in this chapter attributed to Richard Weisel comes from an interview with Richard Weisel on 8 Nov. 2018.
2 Richard D. Weisel, "Cardiac Surgical Scientists at the Institute of Medical Science U of T." (Private document kindly conveyed to the authors.)
3 *The Toronto Hospital, Annual Report, 1987/88*, 192.
4 Hugh Scully, in Vivek Rao interview, 27 Aug. 2018.
5 Goldman comment, in Rao interview, 27 Aug. 2018.
6 "Stephen Fremes Wins Lister Prize," [Department of Surgery], *Surgical Spotlight*, Winter 2005–6, 11.
7 Shorter, *Partnership for Excellence*, 137–8.
8 *Ontario Medical Review*, November/December 2019.
9 Note in *Surgical Spotlight* [Department of Surgery, University of Toronto], Fall 2004, 6.
10 Goldman comment, in Weisel interview, 8 Nov. 2018.
11 For an overview see R.D. Weisel, "Myocardial Preservation: Then and Now," *American Academy of Cardiovascular Perfusion* 25 (2004), 68–72.
12 Scully, in John Wedge interview, 28 Nov. 2018.
13 See J. Li ... R.D. Weisel, and R-K Li, "Young Bone Marrow Sca-1 Cells Rejuvenate the Aged Heart by Promoting Epithelial-to-Mesenchymal Transition," *Theranostics* 8 (2018), 1766–81.
14 Nicolas Noiseux et al., "The IMPACT-CABG Trial: A Multicenter, Randomized Clinical Trial of CD133+ Stem Cell Therapy During Coronary

Artery Bypass Grafting for Ischemic Cardiomyopathy," *J Thoracic Cardiovasc Surg* 152 (2016), 1582–8.

15 University of Toronto, Department of Surgery, *Annual Report,* 2006–07, 10.

16. Cardiologists

1 Sallie Teasdale to Hugh Scully, 1 Nov. 2018.

2 Bigelow, "Some Recommendations Regarding Basic Policy," 7 Feb. 1962, Bigelow Papers.

3 H.E. Aldridge to W.F. Greenwood, 19 Feb. 1971, Bigelow Fonds, TGH, 0094–13–0–29.

4 Unless otherwise indicated, material in this chapter came from an interview with Heather Ross, 20 Nov. 2018.

5 Goldman comment, in Barry Rubin interview, 10 Oct. 2018.

6 Comments by Rakowski in this chapter are drawn from Harry Rakowski, interview, 12 Dec. 2018.

7 H. Rakowski et al., "Echocardiographic and Doppler Assessment of the Fetal Heart," in *Two-dimensional Echocardiography and Cardiac Doppler* (Baltimore: Williams and Wilkins, 1988).

8 Goldman, comment, in Rakowski interview, 12 Dec. 2018.

9 E.D. Wigle to Bernard Goldman, 1 Aug. 1973, Bigelow Papers; as late as June, however, the cardiologists were rejecting the notion of a second balloon pump and said they would acquire one only if cardiac surgery didn't. Wigle to Bigelow, 5 June 1973, Bigelow Papers.

10 These details from Goldman, in Scully interview, 10 Dec. 2018.

11 David S. Jones, *Broken Hearts: The Tangled History of Cardiac Care* (Baltimore: Johns Hopkins University Press), 189–90.

12 This paragraph relies on information in "25 Years for CVIU," [TGH] *Monitor,* Aug. 1981, 2.

13 Otto P. Rahkonen et al., "The First Ten of Everything: A Review of Past and Current Practice in Pediatric Cardiac Percutaneous Interventions," *Congen Heart Dis* 10(4) (July–Aug. 2015), 292–301.

14 This perspective is provided in an overview: Timothy S. Hornung, Lee N. Benson, and Peter R. McLaughlin, "Catheter Interventions in Adult Patients with Congenital Heart Disease," *Current Cardiol Reports* 4(1) (Jan. 2002), 54–62.

15 Lloyd L. Black and Bernard S. Goldman, "Surgical Treatment of the Patent Ductus Arteriosus in the Adult," *Ann Surg* 175(2) (Feb. 1972), 290–3. The findings were first presented at a conference in 1971.

16 John D. Dyck, Lee N. Benson, Jeffrey Smallhorn, Peter McLaughlin, and Richard Rowe, "Catheter Occlusion of the Persistently Patent Ductus Arteriosus," *Am J Cardiol,* 62 (1988), 1089–92.

17 David Harrison, Lee Benson, Charles Lazzam, Janice Walter, and Peter McLaughlin, "Percutaneous Catheter Closure of the Persistently Patent Ductus Arteriosus in the Adult," *Am J Cardiol* 77(2) (May1996), 1094–7; D.A. Harrison, P.R. McLaughlin, "Interventional Cardiology for the Adult Patient with Congenital Heart Disease: The Toronto Hospital Experience," *Can J Cardiol* 12(10) (Oct. 1996), 965–71.

18 C.A.C. Pedra ... L. Benson, "Transcatheter Closure of Atrial Septal Defects Using the Cardio-SEAL Implant," *Heart (British Cardiac Society)* 84(3) (Sept. 2000), 320–6.

19 D.A. Harrison, P.R. McLaughlin, C. Lazzam, M. Connelly, and L.N. Benson, "Endovascular Stents in the Management of Coarctation of the Aorta in the Adolescent and Adult: One Year Follow Up," *Heart (British Cardiac Society)* 85(5) (May 2001), 561–6; see also T.S. Hornung, Lee N. Benson, and Peter R. McLaughlin, "Interventions for Aortic Coarctation," *Cardiology in Review* 10(3) (May–June 2002), 139–48.

20 Michael J. Mullen, Bryan F. Dias. Fiona Walker, Samuel C. Siu, Lee N. Benson, and Peter R. McLaughlin, "Intracardiac Echocardiography Guided Device Closure of Atrial Septal Defects," *Journal of the American College of Cardiology* 41(2) (15 Jan. 2003), 285–92.

21 Barry Rubin, interview, 10 Oct. 2018.

22 Massimiliano Meineri, interview, 6 Nov. 2018.

23 Among Ross's contributions, which number more than three hundred, see, for example, H. Ross, K. Tinckam, V. Rao, and L.J. West, "In Praise of Ventricular Assist Devices: Mechanical Bridge to Virtual Crossmatch for the Sensitized Patient," *J Heart Lung Transplant* 29(7) (July 2010), 728–30.

24 See, for example, Yasbanoo Moayedi ... Heather J. Ross, "A Primer on Quality Improvement for Heart Failure Clinicians," *Circulation Heart Failure* 10(5) (May 2017). DOI: 10.1161/CIRCHEARTFAILURE.116.003722.

25 "Journey to the Bottom of the Earth," *PMCC Clinical and Research Report* 8 (2) (Winter 2013), 11.

26 "Interview With Dr. Mitesh Badiwala," *U of T Med J* 94 (Mar. 2017), 15–18.

27 Vivek Rao, interview, 27 Aug. 2018.

28 Bernard S. Goldman, "The Life and Hard Times of a Coronary Surgeon," *Can J Cardiology* 23(3) (March 2007), 183–8.

17. Nurses

1 Murray, *Medicine in the Making*, 217.

2 Murray, *Quest in Medicine*, 134.

3 Heimbecker to Dr. Charles, Connaught Medical Research Laboratories, 12 Jan. 1960, Bigelow Papers.

4 Murray, *Medicine in the Making*, 217.

5 Bigelow, *Cold Hearts*, 124.

6 See, on this, Hannah Institute for the History of Medicine, Oral History Interviews (Dr. E. Bruce Tovee), vol. 42, 80. UTARMS.

7 Bigelow, "Requirements for Cardiovascular Surgery," 12 Sept. 1957, attached to Medical Advisory Board Minutes, 21 Nov. 1957, TGH Fonds, TH 7.2.5.

8 Bigelow to W.F. Greenwood, 24 July 1964, Bigelow Papers.

9 Bigelow to Jean Dodds, superintendent of nurses, TGH, 9 Jan. 1962.

10 Bigelow to Jean Dodds, 15 Nov. 1961, Bigelow Papers.

11 Bigelow to Jean Dodds, 1 Nov. 1965, Bigelow Papers.

12 Goldman to Shorter, personal note, 15 Apr. 2019.

13 Bigelow to architect G.M. Barstow, 28 May 1958, Bigelow Papers.

14 Scully, in interview with nursing supervisors, 14 Nov. 2018.

15 OR nurses, interview, 31 Oct. 2018. Comments from Heidi Duringer and Leda Parente in this chapter are from this interview.

16 Bigelow, *Cold Hearts*, 201.

17 Goldman personal note to Shorter, 15 Apr. 2019.

18 Scully, in interview with OR nurses, 31 Oct. 2018.

19 Nursing supervisors, interview, 14 Nov. 2018.

20 Martin O'Malley, *Hospital: Life and Death in a Major Medical Centre* (Toronto: Macmillan, 1986), 105.

21 Danna Blakley to Bigelow, 29 July 1966.

22 Source requested anonymity.

23 Joan Hollobon, "Iraqi Woman, 31, Has Brand New Future after Insertion of Plastic Heart Valves," *Globe and Mail*, 2 June 1973, 5.

24 Nursing supervisors, interview, 14 Nov. 2018.

25 Wayne Johnston, interview, 12 Dec. 2018.

26 Nursing supervisors, interview, 14 Nov. 2018.

27 Richard Reznick, interview, 3 Dec. 2018.

28 Linda Jussaume, in nursing supervisors interview, 14 Nov. 2018.

18. Perfusionists

1 Richard Weisel, interview, 8 Nov. 2018.

2 On these events, see Goldman, *Heart Surgery in Canada*, 529.

3 H. Barrie Fairley, "Recollections of the Toronto General Hospital," in Robert J. Byrick, ed., *A Commemorative History of the Department of Anaesthesia* (Toronto: Department of Anaesthesia, 2004), 121.

4 Trimble to J.C. Fortin (manager of operating rooms), 2 Sept. 1969, Bigelow Papers.

5 The material in this chapter from perfusionists Jennifer McDonough and Nancy Pretty came from an interview that included Hugh Scully, 31 Oct. 2018.

6 Scully, in McDonough and Pretty interview, 31 Oct. 2018.
7 See the website of the Institute, https://michener.ca/discover-michener/michener/history-2/.
8 It had been gospel in the division that hypothermia of some degree was necessary for cardiac surgery. But in 1991 research reported from St. Michael's Hospital, traditionally a rival of the General, challenged this. Led by Tomas Salerno and Samuel Lichtenstein, the St. Michael's group compiled statistics on 113 consecutive patients, operated on with "continuous warm blood cardioplegia." Ninety-six per cent of the patients had "spontaneous return of rhythm."

19. Anesthetists

1 Gerald O'Leary to Hugh Scully, 6 Nov. 2018.
2 Stephen J. Evelyn and Iain MacKay, "Anesthetic for Cardiac Surgery," *Current Researches in Anesthesia and Analgesia* 33 (1954), 186–94, presented on 26 Oct. 1953, at an international anesthesia meeting in Quebec City.
3 H. Barrie Fairley, "Recollections of the Toronto General Hospital," in Robert J. Byrick, ed., *A Commemorative History of the Department of Anaesthesia* (Toronto: Department of Anaesthesia, 2004), 119.
4 H. Barrie Fairley, "Hypothermia for Adult Cardiovascular Surgery: A Technique of Anaesthesia," *Can Anaes Soc J* 4(2) (April 1957), 96–103.
5 Fairley, "Hypothermia," 121.
6 Vivek Rao, interview, 27 Aug. 2018, Scully sitting in.
7 Fairley, "Hypothermia," 96–103.
8 H.B. Fairley to Bigelow, 15 June 1962, Bigelow Papers.
9 This section is based on an interview with Gerald O'Leary, 6 Nov. 2018.
10 François Béïque et al., "Canadian Guidelines for Training in Adult Perioperative Transesophageal Echocardiography," *Can J Cardiol* 22 (2006), 1015–27.
11 Massimiliano Meineri, in O'Leary interview, 6 Nov. 2018.
12 Goldman personal note to Shorter, 15 Apr. 2019.
13 Goldman comments in Richard Weisel interview, 8 Nov. 2018.
14 Sallie Teasdale to Hugh Scully, 1 Nov. 2018.
15 Linda Harris, in interview with nursing supervisors, 14 Nov. 2018.

20. Tirone David

1 Terrence Yau, interview, 21 Jan. 2010.
2 Michael Posner, "Magic Hands: If You Ever Need Heart Surgery, This Is Your Man," *Toronto Life* 35 (20) (Dec. 2001), 74.
3 "King of Hearts: Dr. Tirone David,"http:///www.everythingzoomer.com/king-of-hearts-dr-tirone-david/.

4 Much of the material at the start of this chapter is drawn from a 2012 interview with Tirone David in a Brazilian-Canadian magazine, "From the Bottom of the Heart, http://wavemagazine.ca/2012/08/03/from -the-bottom-of-the-hearrt.

5 Martin McKneally, "Tirone David: Passion and Creative Genius in the Pursuit of Technical Perfection," [Department of Surgery], *Surgical Spotlight*, Fall, 2004, 4–5.

6 Tirone David, interview, 23 Aug. 2018.

7 Material in the above paragraphs is, unless noted, is largely from [Tirone David interview] "From the Bottom of the Heart." http://wavemagazine .ca/2012/08/03/from-the-bottom-of-the-heart/.

8 "Celebrating Dr. Susan Lenkei," *PMCC Clinical and Research Report* 7(2) (Dec. 2011), 6.

9 David, interview, 23 Aug. 2018.

10 Baird, "Development," 12. As per David's CV, 1977 seems to be the correct date for his arrival at Toronto Western Hospital.

11 Harry Rakowski, interview, 12 Dec. 2018.

12 These paragraphs on David's move to the Western are based on Baird, "Development," 11–12; and David to Scully, 5 Nov. 2017, in Scully Papers.

13 Goldman to Shorter, personal note, 15 Apr. 2019.

14 Stephanie Brister, interview, 29 Nov. 2018.

15 Harry Rakowski, interview, 12 Dec. 2018.

16 David, interview, 23 Aug. 2018.

17 Henry Hess, "New System Speeds Recovery for Heart-Surgery Patients," *Globe and Mail*, 3 June 1993, A4.

18 David, interview, 23 Aug. 2018.

19 T.E. David and C.M. Feindel, "An Aortic Valve-sparing Operation for Patients with Aortic Incompetence and Aneurysm of the Ascending Aorta," *J Thorac Cardiovasc Surg* 103 (1992), 617–21.

20 Chris Feindel, while readily acknowledging David as the designer of the operation, nonetheless collaborated in the early days. Feindel, interview, 11 Dec. 2018.

21 David, interview, 23 Aug. 2018.

22 "An Interview with Tirone David," [U of T] *Surgical Spotlight*, Summer 2017, 15.

23 Myunghyun Lee et al., "History of Cardiovascular Surgery at Toronto General Hospital," *Seminars in Thoracic and Cardiovascular Surgery* 28(3) (autumn 2016), 700–4, 701.

24 Tirone David et al., "The Importance of the Mitral Apparatus in Left Ventricular Function Following Repair of Mitral Regurgitation," *Ann Thorac Surg* 36 (1983), 1176–82.

25 Goldman, *Heart Surgery in Canada*, 459.

26 Tirone E. David, Glorianne C. Ropchan, and Jagdish W. Butany, "Aortic Valve Replacement with Stentless Porcine Aortic Bioprostheses," *J Cardiac Surg* 3 (1988), 501–5. This was introduced clinically in 1991.

27 Tirone David, "Replacement of Chordae Tendineae with Expanded Polytetrafluorethylene Sutures," *Journal of Cardiac Surgery* 4(4) (Dec. 1989), 286–90.

28 T.E. David et al., "Heart Valve Surgery in Patients with Active Infective Endocarditis," *Ann Thorac Surg* 49(5) (May 1990), 701–5; David, "Left Ventricular Rupture after Mitral Valve Replacement," *J Thorac Cardiovasc Surg* 93(6) (June 1987), 935–6; David, "Techniques and Results of Mitral Valve Repair for Ischemic Mitral Regurgitation," *J Card Surg* 9(2)Suppl (March 1994), 274–7; David et al., "Surgery for Acute Type A Aortic Dissection," *Ann Thoracic Surgery* 67(2) (Aug. 1999), 1999–2001.

29 Tirone E. David, "Surgical Repair of Postinfarction Ventricular Septal Defect," *Circulation*, 82 (suppl IV) (1990), IV-243–IV-247; David, "Surgical Treatment of Postinfarction Ventricular Septal Rupture," *Austral As J Cardiac Thorac Surg* 1 (1992), 7–10.

30 For the 1990 date, see Tirone E. David et al., "Geometric Mismatch of the Aortic and Pulmonary Roots Causes Aortic Insufficiency after the Ross Procedure," *J Thorac Cardiovasc Surg* 112(5) (Nov. 1996), 1231–9.

31 Tirone E. David et al., "The Ross Procedure: Outcomes at 20 Years," *J Thorac Cardiovasc Surg* 147(1) (Jan. 2014), 85–94.

32 Tirone E. David, "Ross Procedure at the Crossroads," *Circulation* 119(2) (20 Jan. 2009), 207–8.

33 "Creativity in Medicine," [Department of Surgery], *Surgical Spotlight*, Spring–Summer 2008, unpaginated.

34 John Wedge, interview, 28 Nov. 2018.

35 Bryce Taylor, interview, 15 Nov. 2018.

36 Scully, interview, 23 Feb. 2018.

37 Lillian Newberry, "Heart Doctor's Colleagues Say He's Not Only Good – He's Fast," *Toronto Star*, 8 Mar. 1985, A4.

38 "King of Hearts: Dr. Tirone David," http://www.everythingzoomer.com/king-of-hearts-dr-tirone-david/.

39 Scully, in David interview, 23 Aug. 2018.

40 Scully, in David interview, 23 Aug. 2018.

41 David, interview, 23 Aug. 2018.

42 "Group to Battle Hospital Overlap," *Globe and Mail*, 15 Mar. 1965, 4.

43 Baird, "Development," 14

44 "An Interview with Tirone David," [U of T] *Surgical Spotlight*, Summer 2017, 14.

45 Bernard Langer and Bernard Goldman, interview, 30 July 2018.

46 Langer and Goldman, interview, 30 July 2018.

47 These details on the merger are from the interview with perfusionists Nancy Pretty and Jennifer McDonough, 31 Oct. 2018.

48 Undated note from Tirone David to Hugh Scully [2017]. In Scully Papers.

49 Baird, "Development," 34.

50 David, interview, 23 Aug. 2018.

51 "An Interview with Tirone David," [U of T] *Surgical Spotlight,* summer 2017, 14.

52 Newberry, "Heart Doctor's Colleagues," A4.

53 "An Interview with Tirone David," [U of T] *Surgical Spotlight,* Summer 2017, 15.

54 "Dr. Tirone David: Looking Back on a Long Successful Career," http:// uhn.ca/corporate/News/Pages/dr_Tirone_David_Looking_long _successful_career.aspx.

55 Michael Posner, "Magic Hands."

56 "A Heart Impossible to Fix?" https://uhnfoundation.ca/stories/heart-impossible-fix-knowledge-can/ .

57 Posner, "Magic Hands."

58 Vivek Rao and Carolyn M. David, "Historical Perspectives of the American Association for Thoracic Surgery: Tirone E. David," *J Thorac Cardiovasc Surg* 153(4) (April j2017), 741–3.

59 Gerald O'Leary interview, 6 Nov. 2018.

60 *Toronto Star,* 8 July 1995, A1.

61 See the study of outcomes in CABG in octogenarians, 1990–2005: The conclusion: "CABG is increasingly common in octogenarians, with steadily improving outcomes over time." Manjula Maganti, Vivek Rao, Stephanie Brister, and Joan Ivanov, "Decreasing mortality for CAB surgery in octogenarians," *Can J Cardiol* 25 (2009), e32–e35.

62 These paragraphs are based on Lisa Priest, "Heart Surgery Backlog Hits All-time High," *Toronto Star,* 14 Oct. 1995, A1, A4.

63 Goldman, *Heart Surgery in Canada,* 455–6.

64 Bernard Goldman, letter, *Globe and Mail,* 5 Mar. 1997, A14.

65 Paul Taylor, "Live TV Show Lets Doctors Get to Heart of the Matter," *Globe and Mail,* 22 June 1991, A7.

66 Department of Surgery, *Annual Report, 1995–96,* 14.

67 Goldman, e-mail to Shorter, 23 Jan. 2019.

68 Posner, "Magic Hands."

69 Posner, "Magic Hands."

70 Gerald O'Leary, interview, 6 Nov. 2018.

71 Posner, "Magic Hands.

72 "'Toronto Fest' at the Annual Meeting of the American Association for Thoracic Surgery," [Department of Surgery] *Surgical Spotlight,* Summer 2005, 11.

73 "'Toronto Fest,'" [Department of Surgery].
74 Vivek Rao, interview, 27 Aug. 2018.
75 Lynda Mickleborough, interview, 21 Nov. 2018.
76 Stephanie Brister, interview, 29 Nov. 2018.

21. Vivek Rao

1 "Interview with Dr. Barry Rubin," *U of T Med J* 94 (June 2017), 30–2.
2 Renee Sylvestre-Williams, "From Science Fiction to 'Almost Routine,'" *PMAC Clinical and Research Report*, Winter 2016, 41–2.
3 Rao's comments in this chapter are drawn from Vivek Rao interview, 27 Aug. 2018.
4 Vivek Rao et al., "Results of Combined Pulmonary Resection and Cardiac Operation," *Ann Thorac Surg* 62 (1996), 342–7.
5 Wallace Imen, "New Technique Keeps Donor Hearts Fit," *Globe and Mail*, 18 June 1997, A10.
6 Rao quoting Tirone David, Rao interview, 27 Aug. 2018.
7 Shelley McKellar, *Artificial Hearts: The Allure and Ambivalence of a Controversial Medical Technology* (Baltimore: Johns Hopkins University Press, 2018), passim.
8 Chris Feindel, interview, 11 Dec. 2018.
9 Prithi Yelaja, "Heart Pumps Beat Drugs, Study Finds," *Toronto Star*, 17 Nov. 2001, A29.
10 André Picard, "Woman Survives Heart Pump Removal," *Globe and Mail*, 28 Mar. 2002, A9.
11 Information about the introduction of these devices, unless otherwise noted, comes from Vivek Rao, "Mechanical Circulatory Support Program, 2019," PMCC PowerPoint lecture. I am grateful to Dr. Rao for sharing a copy of this with me.
12 "Pocket Controller Makes Life Easier for Patients," *PMAC Clinical and Research Report* 9(1) (Summer 2013), 4–5.
13 Sylvestre-Williams, "From Science Fiction to 'Almost Routine.'"
14 "A New Lease on Life," *PMCC Clinical and Research Report* 10(2) (Winter 2015), 6.
15 See H. Kawabir ... H. Ross, and V. Rao. "Outcomes of 100 Continuous Flow Left Ventricle Assist Devices: The Toronto General Hospital Experience," *Canadian Journal of Cardiology* 31 (2015), S195–S196.
16 "Vivek Rao Named One of Canada's 'Top Under 40,'" [Department of Surgery], *Surgical Spotlight*, Summer 2007, 10.
17 E.A. Rose et al., "Long-term Use of a Left Ventricular Assist Device for End-Stage Heart Failure," *NEJM* 345 (15 Nov. 2001), 1435–43.

18 "Celebrating Heart Month at UHN With the Next Generation in Cardiac Care"; http://www.uhn.ca/corporate/News/Pages/celebrating_heart _month_at_uhn_with_the_next_generation.aspx.

19 Jon Wells, "Life and Death on the Transplant List," *Hamilton Spectator*, 24 Feb. 2011.

20 Jonathan Forani, "Heartfelt Commitment Spans a Generation," *Toronto Star*, 31 Jan. 2015, M12.

21 Jasmine Miller, "Mechanical Heart Helps Battle Rare Disorder," *Toronto Star*, 31 Jan. 2015, MT1.

22 André Picard, "With Every Heartbeat, He Beats the Odds," *Globe and Mail*, 10 Sept. 2007, A3.

23 W.E. Stansfield et al., "Multicenter Canadian Experience with the Heartware HVAD – 5-Year Update," *J Heart Lung Transplant* 35 (2016), S125–126.

24 Vivek Rao, "Surgical Ventricular Remodeling: Should We STICH or Not?" *Curr Opin Cardio* 32 (2017), 744–7.

22. The Peter Munk Cardiac Centre

1 The Hudson quotes in this section are from an interview, 29 Nov. 2018.

2 Tirone David, interview, 23 Aug. 2018.

3 Tom Closson, interview, 10 Dec. 2018.

4 "The Toronto Hospital Cardiac Centre," *Globe and Mail*, 9 Dec. 1993, B4; "Cardiac Care to Undergo Consolidation," *Globe and Mail*, 10 Dec. 1993, A18.

5 "Prestigious American Cardiologist Visits PMCC for Inaugural Lectureship," University Health Network, https://www.uhn.ca /corporate/News/Pages/prestigious_american_cardiologist_PMCC.aspx.

6 Patricia Best, "A New Gold Standard in Heart Care," *Globe and Mail*, 10 May 1997, D5.

7 Leslie Papp, "Metro Cardiac Centre at Leading Edge of Heart Care," *Toronto Star*, 13 May 1997, A16.

8 Tennys Hanson, interview, 6 Feb. 2019.

9 Chris Feindel, interview, 11 Dec. 2018.

10 Barry Rubin, interview, 10 Oct. 2018.

11 Shelley White, "International Fellows Come to Learn the 'PMCC Way,'" *PMCC Clinical and Research Report*, Winter 2018, 11.

12 Rubin, interview, 10 Oct. 2018.

13 Rubin, interview, 10 Oct. 2018.

14 Tanya Talaga, "Gold Tycoon's Heartfelt Gift of $37 Million Sets Record," *Toronto Star*, 31 May 2006, A4.

15 Hayley Mick, "An O.R. on the Cutting Edge," *Globe and Mail*, 5 Nov. 2009, L3.
16 Massimiliano Meineri, in interview with Gerald O'Leary, 6 Nov. 2018.
17 Patrick White, "Peter Munk Donates $18 Million to Heart Research," *Globe and Mail*, 24 Nov. 2011, A16.
18 Posner, "Magic Hands."
19 Richard Blackwell, "Nation Builder 2010," *Globe and Mail*, 31 Dec. 2010, A3.
20 *PMCC Clinical and Research Report* 10(1) (Summer 2014), 4–5.
21 *UHN Annual Report*, 2014/15, 21.
22 "'Toronto Fest' at the Annual Meeting of the American Association for Thoracic Surgery," [Department of Surgery] *Surgical Spotlight*, Summer 2005, 11.
23 Tennys Hanson, briefing note, 28 Jan. 2019.
24 Vivek Rao, interview, 27 Aug. 2018.
25 Rubin, interview, 10 Oct. 2018.
26 Heidi Duringer, interview, 31 Oct. 2018. Leda Parente and Hugh Scully participated.
27 Hanson, interview, 6 Feb. 2019.
28 *UHN Annual Report*, 2014–15, 47.
29 Hanson, interview, 6 Feb. 2019.
30 Scully, in Hanson interview, 6 Feb. 2019.
31 Rubin, interview, 10 Oct. 2018.
32 "Interview with Dr. Barry Rubin," *U of T Med J* 94 (June 2017), 30–2.
33 "Cardiac Rehabilitation: Investing in Heart Health," *PMCC Clinical and Research Report* 8(2) (Winter, 2013), 4.
34 "A Prescription for Exercise," *PMCC Clinical and Research Report* 11(1) (Summer 2015), 3.
35 Rubin, interview, 10 Oct. 2018.
36 Vivek Rao, interview, 27 Aug. 2018.
37 Scully comments in Butany interview, 24 Oct. 2018.
38 Rubin, interview, 10 Oct. 2018.
39 Rubin, interview, 10 Oct. 2018.
40 David S. Jones, *Broken Hearts: The Tangled History of Cardiac Care* (Baltimore: Johns Hopkins University Press, 2013), 15.
41 L. Mauri et al., "4-Year Results of a Randomized Controlled Trial of Percutaneous Repair versus Surgery for Mitral Regurgitation," *J Am Coll Cardiol* 62(4) (23 July 2013), 317–28.
42 Mitesh Badiwala, "Trans-catheter Aortic Valve Implantation," [Department of Surgery], *Surgical Spotlight*, Spring–Summer 2008, unpaginated.
43 Bryan Borzykowski, "Inside the Mind of Munk," *PMCC Clinical and Research Report*, Winter 2016, 21.
44 M.D. Osten et al., "Transcatheter Aortic Valve Implantation for High Risk Patients with Severe Aortic Stenosis," *Catheter Cardiovasc Interv* 75(4) (1 March 2010), 475–85.

45 Marjo Johne, "Heart Valve Innovations," *PMCC Clinical and Research Report*, Winter 2018, 8.

46 Feindel, interview, 11 Dec. 2018.

47 OECD, *Health at a Glance 2011: OECD Indicators* (Paris: OECD Publishing, 2011), 91, tab 4.6.2.

48 Camilla Cornell, "Rapid Assessment Saves Lives for Those with Aortic Valve Disease," *Toronto Star*, 31 Jan. 2015.

49 "Meeting the Challenges of Aortic Disease," *PMCC Clinical and Research Report* 9 (2) (Winter 2014), 4–5.

50 For pig research on this, see R. Ribeiro … V. Rao, and M.V. Badiwala, "Is Cold Storage Possible in DCD Heart Transplantation? A Pre-clinical Study," *J Heart Lung Transplant* 37 (2018), S125–S126.

51 Mitesh Badiwala, interview, 23 Jan. 2019.

52 Cedric Manlhiot et al., "Comparison of Cardiac Surgery Mortality Reports Using Administrative and Clinical Data Sources: A Prospective Cohort Study," *CMAJ Open*, 4 Sept. 2018, E316–E321.

53 André Picard, "Cardiac Death Rates 100% More than Predicted? Sometimes Numbers Aren't Exactly What They Seem," *Globe and Mail*, 4 Sept. 2018, A2.

54 Tirone David, interview, 23 Aug. 2018.

55 Daniel Otis, "A Team Approach to Mending Broken Hearts," *Toronto Star*, 31 Jan. 2005, M8.

56 Daniel Otis, "A Group of Multidisciplinary Medical Doctors Work to Solve Some of the Country's Most Complex Cardiac Cases," *Toronto Star*, 31 Jan. 2005, M8.

57 Quotes from William ("Bill") Williams in this section are from an interview on 27 Nov. 2018, with Scully and Goldman.

58 UHN, *PMCC Clinical and Research Report* 7(1) (July 2011), 4.

59 Adrienne H. Kovacs et al., "The Toronto Congenital Heart Disease Transition Force," *Progress in Pediatric Cardiology* 34 (2012), 21–6.

60 Department of Surgery, *Annual Report*, 1999–2000.

61 Adrienne H. Kovacs et al., "The Toronto Congenital Heart Disease Transition Force."

62 "The Faces of Heart Disease," *PMCC Clinical and Research Report*, Winter 2017, 5.

63 Matthias Greutmann et al., "Increasing Mortality Burden among Adults with Complex Congenital Heart Disease," *Congenit Heart Dis*, 2014; no vol. nr. or page range.

64 William Williams to Shorter, 27 Nov. 2018. The facts in the above two paragraphs are largely taken from Jennifer L. Lapum et al., "Historical Investigation of Medical Treatment for Adult Congenital Heart Disease: A Canadian Perspective," *Congenit Heart Dis*, 14(2) (March 2018), 185–192; DOI: 10.1111/chd.12716.

65 A. Kinsell … V. Rao, "Comparison of Heart Transplantation Outcomes between Adult Congenital Heart Disease and Matched Adult Cardiac Patients in a Single Quaternary Reference Centre," *J Heart and Lung Transplant* 37 (2018), S422.

66 William Feindel and Richard Leblanc, *The Wounded Brain Healed: The Golden Age of the Montreal Neurological Institute, 1934–1984* (Montreal: McGill-Queen's Press, 2016).

67 Comments by Feindel come from Chris Feindel interview, 11 Dec. 2018.

68 May Warren, "Toronto Man's Heart Rebuilt in Worst Case Doctors Had Ever Seen," *Toronto Star*, 16 Dec. 2015; PMCC, "The Faces of Heart Disease," *PMCC Clinical and Research Report*, Winter 2017, 52–3.

69 Rubin, interview, 10 Oct. 2018.

70 "PMCC: 'The Dragon's Den' of Health Care," *Globe and Mail*, 9 Oct. 2013.

71 UHN, *Annual Report*, 2012–13, 42.

72 *PMCC Clinical and Research Report*, Winter 2018, 4.

73 Vivek Rao, interview, 27 Aug. 2018, Scully sitting in.

74 Glorianne Ropchan, section, in Goldman, *Heart Surgery in Canada*, 506.

75 Ropchan, section, in Goldman, *Heart Surgery in Canada*, 507.

76 See *Ontario Medicine*, 30 Sept. 1984.

77 Terry Kieser, in Goldman, ed., *Cardiac Surgery in Canada*, 503.

78 Comments by Brister appear in Stephanie Brister interview, 29 Nov. 2018.

79 Information in the above four paragraphs is largely drawn from Dave McGinn, "Queen of Hearts," *Globe and Mail*, 9 Feb. 2008.

80 Bobby Yanagawa, Khaled D. Algarni, Terrence M. Yau, Vivek Rao, and Stephanie J. Brister, "Improving Results for Coronary Artery Bypass Graft Surgery in the Elderly," *European Journal of Cardio-Thoracic Surgery* 42 (2012), 507–12.

81 Marilyn Dunlop, "Doctors Remove Clot From Lung," *Toronto Star*, 23 Mar. 1991, 1. See also S.J. Brister et al., "Pulmonary Thromboendarterectomy in a Patient with Giant Cell Arteritis," *Ann Thorac Surg* 73 (2002), 1977–9.

82 Brister interview, 29 Nov. 2018.

83 University Health Network, "Cardiac Surgeon Calls It a Career: Dr. Stephanie Brister Retires," https://www.uhn.ca/corporate/News/Pages/Dr_Brister_Retires.aspx.

23. The Next Gen

1 Vivek Rao, interview, 27 Aug. 2018; University Health Network, "Doctors' Day Spotlight: Dr. Maral Ouzounian," www.uhn.ca/corporate/News/Pages/doctor_day_maral_ouzounian.aspx.

2 University Health Network, "Doctors' Day Spotlight."

3 University Health Network, "Doctors' Day Spotlight."

4 Maral Ouzounian, Amine Mazine, and Tirone E. David, "The Ross Procedure is the Best Operation to Treat Aortic Stenosis in Young and Middle-Aged Adults," *J Thorac Cardiovasc Surg* 154(3) (Sept. 2017), 778–82.

5 Mitesh Badiwala, interview, 22 Jan. 2019.

6 Information in this section is taken largely from Mitesh Badiwala, interview, 22 Jan. 2019.

7 "Interview with Dr. Mitesh Badiwala," *U of T Med J* 94 (Mar. 2017), 15–18.

8 Unless otherwise noted, the material in this section and the next is from an interview with Terrence M. Yau, 21 Jan. 2019.

9 For an overview, see A.B. Prowse, N.E. Timmins, T.M. Yau, R.K. Li, R.D. Weisel, G. Keller, and P.W. Zandstra, "Transforming the Promise of Pluripotent Stem Cell-Derived Cardiomyocytes to a Therapy: Challenges and Solutions for Clinical Trials," *Can J Cardiol* 30 (2014), 1335–49.

10 "Terrence M. Yau, Pump Man," *Globe and Mail*, 5 Jan. 2008, M5.

11 "Terrence M. Yau, Pump Man," *Globe and Mail*.

12 Osman O. Al-Radi, Vivek Rao, Ren-ke Li, Terrence Yau, and Richard D. Weisel, "Cardiac Cell Transplantation: Closer to Bedside," *Ann Thorac Surg* 75(2) (Feb. 2003), S674–S677.

13 N. Noiseux, R. Weisel, T.M. Yau, et al., "The IMPACT-CABG Trial: A Multicenter, Randomized Clinical Trial of CD133+ Stem Cell Therapy during Coronary Artery Bypass Grafting for Ischemic Cardiomyopathy," *J Thorac Cardiovasc Surg* 152(6) (Dec. 2016), 1582–8.

14 "Ontario's First Cardiac Stem Cell Transplant Performed at the Peter Munk Cardiac Centre," 26 Jan. 2012. https://www.uhn.ca/corporate/News/Pages/ontario_first_cardiac_stem_cell_transplant_performed_at_pmcc.aspx.

24. Conclusion

1 Noah Miller, "The 10 Best Hospitals in the World," *Newsweek*, 5 Apr. 2019, https://www.newsweek.com/2019/04/05/10-best-hospitals-world-1368512.html; "The World's Best Hospitals, 2020," http://www.newsweek.com/best-hospitals-2020; "The World's Best Hospitals, 2021," http://www.newsweek.com/best-hospitals-2020.

2 Department of Surgery, Faculty of Medicine, "Five Year Review, 2009–2014," 15.

3 "Best Global Universities for Surgery," *U.S. News and World Report*, 25 Oct. 2019, https://www.usnews.com/education/best-global-universities/surgery.

4 Times Higher Education World University Rankings 2020, https://www.timeshighereducation.com/world-university-rankings/university-toronto.

5 Richard Reznick, interview, 3 Dec. 2018

6 Goldman-Scully, interview, 4 Apr. 2018.

7 PMCC, *Clinical and Research Report*, "The Faces of Heart Disease," Winter 2017, 42.

8 Bigelow, "Some Recommendations Regarding Basic Policy," 7 Feb. 1962, Bigelow Papers.

9 Harry Rakowski, interview, 12 Dec. 2018.

10 "The Toronto Hospital's Goal: To Create the Finest Hospital-Based Research Institute in the World," *Globe and Mail*, 25 May 1998, C2.

11 Allan Hudson, interview, 29 Nov. 2018.

12 "Bernie Goldman: Saving Children's Hearts," [U of T] *Surgical Spotlight*, Fall, 2016), 18.

13 See A.J. Cohen, A. Tamir, S. Houri, et al., "Save a Child's Heart: We Can and We Should," *Ann Thorac Surg*,71(2) (Feb. 2001), 462–8.

14 *Jerusalem Post*, 26 Nov. 2005. On SACH, see Lior Sasson et al., "Mending Hearts," *J Pub Health Management Practice* 22 (2016), 89–98; B.S. Goldman et al., *Mending Hearts Building Bridges* (Toronto: SACH, 2014).

15 B.S. Goldman et al., *Mending Hearts, Building Bridges* (Toronto: SACH Canada, 2014).

16 [U of T] *Excelsior: Official Newsletter of the Department of Surgery* 7(6) (Feb. 2018), 1.

17 Alex Ballingall, "U of T Professor's Legacy Warms the Heart," *Toronto Star*, 13 May 2014, GT2. See also *Canadian Jewish News*, 2 Feb. 2018.

18 Barbara Sibbald, "Doctor in a Hurry," *CMAJ*, 161 (10 Aug. 1999), 306.

19 Sibbald, "Doctor in a Hurry."

20 Scully, interview, 10 Dec. 2018.

21 Scully, in Mitesh Badiwala interview, 22 Jan. 2019.

22 Barbara Sibbald, "Declining CABG Rate Means Fewer Jobs for Surgeons," *CMAJ* 173 (Sept. 13, 2005), 583–4.

23 Chris Feindel, interview, 11 Dec. 2018.

24 Bryce Taylor, interview, 15 Nov. 2018.

25 Department of Surgery, Faculty of Medicine, "Five Year Review, 2009–2014," 31–2.

26 Sibbald, "Declining CABG Rate."

27 Christopher M. Feindel et al., "The Canadian Society of Cardiac Surgeons Perspective on the Cardiac Surgery Workforce in Canada," *Canad J Cardiol* 28(5) (Sept.-Oct. 2012), 602–6.

28 Vivek Rao, interview, 27 Aug. 2018.

29 David S. Jones, *Broken Hearts: The Tangled History of Cardiac Care* (Baltimore: Johns Hopkins University Press, 2013), 14.

30 Taylor, interview, 15 Nov. 2018.

31 Rakowski, interview, 12 Dec. 2018.

32 John Wedge, interview, 28 Nov. 2018.

33 Scully, in Wedge interview, 28 Nov. 2018.

34 Wedge, interview, 28 Nov. 2018.

Index

Photographs are indicated by **bold** and plate number (**pl**).